The Clinical Psychiatry of Adolescence

Clinical Work from a Social and Developmental Perspective

Derek Steinberg
M.B., B.S., M.Phil., D.P.M., F.R.C. Psych.
*Consultant Psychiatrist, Adolescent Unit, Bethlem Royal
Hospital and the Maudsley Hospital, London*

JOHN WILEY & SONS

Chichester · New York · Brisbane · Toronto · Singapore

Library of Congress Cataloging in Publication Data:

Steinberg, Derek
  The clinical psychiatry of adolescence.
  (Wiley series on studies in child psychiatry)
  Includes bibliographical references and index.
  1. Adolescent psychiatry. I. Title. II. Series.
RJ503.S75 1983   616.89′022   82-13476

ISBN 0 471 10314 4

British Library Cataloguing in Publication Data:

Steinberg, Derek
  The clinical psychiatry of adolescence.—
  (Wiley series on studies in child psychiatry)
  I. Adolescent psychiatry
  I. Title
  616.89′022   RJ503

ISBN 0 471 10314 4

Photosetting by Thomson Press (India) Limited, New Delhi and
Printed in Great Britain by Page Bros. (Norwich) Ltd.

Series Preface

During recent years there has been a tremendous growth of research in both child development and child psychiatry. Research findings are beginning to modify clinical practice but to a considerable extent the fields of child development and of child psychiatry have remained surprisingly separate, with regrettably little cross-fertilization. Much developmental research has not concerned itself with clinical issues, and studies of clinical syndromes have all too often been made within the narrow confines of a pathological condition approach with scant regard to developmental matters. The situation is rapidly changing but the results of clinical-developmental studies are often reported only by means of scattered papers in scientific journals. This series aims to bridge the gap between child development and clinical psychiatry by presenting reports of new findings, new ideas, and new approaches in a book form which may be available to a wider readership.

The series includes reviews of specific topics, multi-authored volumes on a common theme, and accounts of specific pieces of research. However, in all cases the aim is to provide a clear, readable, and interesting account of scientific findings in a way which makes explicit their relevance to clinical practice or social policy. It is hoped that the series will be of interest to both clinicians and researchers in the fields of child psychiatry, child psychology, psychiatric social work, social paediatrics, and education—in short all concerned with the growing child and his problems.

Preface: Guide to the Book

For a sub-speciality of a sub-speciality adolescent psychiatry is remarkably wide ranging. It is not possible to go far in clinical work with disturbed adolescents without wider issues of education and family life, ethics and the law, sociology, politics, and administration presenting themselves as matters of major practical importance. Correspondingly the psychiatrist working with disturbed adolescents and their families works also with other medical specialists, teachers, social workers, psychologists, and administrators, among members of many other professions.

The majority of disturbed adolescents need the help of other people rather than the skills of clinical psychiatrists; indeed, recent developments in our understanding of the nature of emotional problems, and the part social, education, and family factors play in the origins of problems and their resolution, have to some extent drawn attention away from the concept of individual psychiatric disorder in adolescence. Nevertheless there is a large minority of boys and girls with major individual difficulties most appropriately and sometimes most effectively helped by specifically psychiatric approaches. Clinical psychiatry, moreover, has much to teach professionals in other fields of work with disturbed young people as well as much to learn.

It is for such reasons that this book has a dual theme. On the one hand it is intended to be a clinically orientated textbook; to this extent its core approach is that of the medical model, by which I mean the diagnosis and treatment of individual disorder. This definition of the clinical psychiatrist's primary task is not intended to be a rigid boundary, but rather an acknowledgement of psychiatry's limits, and the many ways in which the clinical psychiatrist and the adolescent patient need the help of other people, and of other styles of work. Hence the second theme: the problems and opportunities of working with and through other people in the interests of adolescents.

The book is written from, and for, the particular viewpoint of the clinical psychiatrist, from a conviction that clarity about one professional approach helps rather than hinders collaboration between people who work in different ways. Collaboration requires special, non-clinical skills, and it is important for the clinical psychiatrist to appreciate that the more specialized any professional worker is in a broad field, the more he or she must be able to work, learn, train, and teach with others. Effective collaboration is important in adolescent psychiatry. In no field of work is stability and consistency more important and in no field is it harder to attain. We are dealing with growing, developing young people in rapidly changing cultural circumstances where concepts of right and wrong, normality and abnormality, which are at the foundations of psychiatric practice, are controversial.

Part One describes the ways in which adolescents present to psychiatrists, how the situation as well as the boy or girl is assessed, and how problems develop.

Part Two gives an account of the range of problems and disorders seen, and outlines approaches to their management.

Part Three discusses management in more detail, including both clinical care and aspects of collaborative and consultative work.

The Index includes references to some problems used to illustrate the text. These are not case histories, but short extracts from them used to illustrate problems and ways of managing them. Care has been taken to ensure that the people and organizations involved cannot be identified by the details given, and the examples are drawn from a number of quite different settings in which I have trained, worked or been associated over some 16 years.

In these various settings I have been fortunate in working with people who have seen the problems of childhood and adolescence from a number of quite different perspectives. It is impossible to acknowledge all by name, and the bibliography can only be a guide to that much of other people's wisdom that gets into print. I am particularly appreciative of the Tavistock Clinic's teaching on consultation, and attachment theory, and especially the study group led by Dorothy Heard and John Bowlby and their colleagues; of the stimulating experience of working with David Taylor and Christopher Ounsted at the Park Hospital, Oxford; of several years teaching with the Sociology Department of the University of Surrey (whatever the merits of various sociological points of view, they raise most important questions for psychiatrists), and of the Association for the Psychiatric Study of Adolescence, an organization with a happy aptitude for bringing people from very diverse backgrounds together in formal and informal learning. These different viewpoints have helped put into a useful perspective the rigorously won data and carefully developed approaches of the Maudsley, for whose range, depth and stimulus I am grateful. But I am most indebted to my friends and colleagues at the Adolescent Unit at Bethlem, from who I have learned much and continue to learn. Finally, I am grateful for the hard work of Jean Winship, Celia Gunn and Kathleen Phillips for their typing and collating of the manuscript, and to my wife Gill for preparing the index.

Derek Steinberg

Adolescent Unit,
Bethlem Royal Hospital,
1983

Contents

Part I
Diagnosis

Chapter 1

Concepts of Disorder and the Presentation of Problems

INTRODUCTION

The process by which adolescents become psychiatric patients has as much to do with the feelings and behaviour of other people, and with social customs and routines, as with anything happening inside their heads. The same is true of the reverse process by which a boy or girl is helped back towards the normal development from which he or she has deviated.

The implication of this is that the clinical psychiatrist, in making an assessment, must be as concerned with the adolescent's circumstances and relationships as with his or her individual psychology and physiology. These include the young person's family, friends, school, neighbourhood and cultural setting, and a complex matrix of attitudes, beliefs, feelings, and behaviour. These many factors determine three broad categories of phenomena:

1. How the adolescent and his or her family have developed over the years.
2. How things are today.
3. What has led to his or her referral to a psychiatrist.

Correspondingly, in planning management the psychiatrist must consider the adolescent's care, upbringing, education, and social and occupational future as well as considering whether *treatment* is needed.

In assessment, the psychiatrist should be as prepared to say when there is no evidence of psychiatric disorder as to diagnose disorder when it is present. The vagaries of the referral process are such that there is no reason to assume that most children and adolescents referred have something wrong with them; disturbed behaviour and mood are often clearly sustained by the adolescent's situation, and this should make us circumspect in diagnosing individual disorder.

3

Nevertheless, psychiatrists tend to be reluctant to make no clinical diagnosis.

From the point of view of management, the psychiatrist should similarly be willing to affirm when no psychiatric treatment is required, but instead some modification of the boy's or girl's care, education, training or control. The fact that the adolescent has been referred indicates that there is some sort of problem requiring a helpful response, even if there is no disorder requiring treatment, and the source of help will then be the boy's or girl's family, teachers or other professional workers. The clinical psychiatrist, as well as being competent in his primary task of diagnosing individual disorder and carrying out psychiatric treatment, must be able to collaborate with others who are involved with young people, and to work with the families of the boys and girls he sees. With some adolescents who are referred the best way of proceeding may be consultation without the psychiatrist seeing the boy or girl at all.

This 'job description' raises many issues. What is normal behaviour in an adolescent, what is psychiatric disorder, and how does it differ from problematic feelings or behaviour apparently sustained by social or family influences? How can the psychiatrist intervene at these various individual and emotional levels, to gain information and to plan a helpful response? By what means, with what skills, with whose assistance and with what authority? What technical, ethical, legal, and interpersonal issues arise when important components of a psychiatrist's work deal not only with the adolescent, but also with the boy's or girl's family, teacher, other professional workers and indeed other authorities and organizations, such as the police, the courts, the school, the education department, the social service department? When these other groups do not see the problem in quite the same way as the psychiatrist this may become a problem in itself, and not simply a mild difference of opinion. A social worker and family may insist that an adolescent is ill and should be in hospital and not have to face the difficulties of going to school, say, or appearing in court; the psychiatrist may believe the reverse would be in the best interests of the boy or girl concerned. A psychiatrist may believe an adolescent with, for example, emotional problems and epilepsy could manage in a school rather than a hospital if only the staff were less anxious about his disorder; but they *are* very anxious, and the head teacher feels unable or unwilling to help generate the necessary advice and support that would make a return to school a success. Perhaps he knows the education department would not support him if things went wrong. In child and adolescent psychiatry there is an infinite variety of such permutations of clinical disorder, non-clinical problems, and ways in which they are perceived, reacted to, and maintained by immediate or more distant relationships and social attitudes. In adolescent psychiatry in particular the issues are often sharpened by the capacity for action (and indeed its legal sanction) of the adolescent himself or herself. Younger children tend to be less influential, or at least their wishes are not so readily articulated and given legal and social support.

So to the traditional problems of assessment and treatment in psychiatry, the adolescent psychiatrist must add as his proper concern the issues which involve other people in the care and education the young person needs, and negotiation about the attitudes and feelings of parents, professional workers, and others. The importance of collaborative work across professional disciplines is rather taken for granted, disposed of again and again under the magic formula 'the multidisciplinary approach'. Multidisciplinary work is in fact extremely demanding; professional workers who do not think so are characteristically at the top or bottom of professional hierarchies, and misleading themselves or being misled; more effective collaboration between those responsible for adolescent care would help resolve some intractable problems, but there are many difficulties in the way.

Chapters 2, 3, 4, and 5 develop the theme of the breadth of factors which must be considered, provide a historical perspective for the place of clinical psychiatry in work with adolescents, and explain the reasons for the diagnostic approach taken in this book and summarized in Chapters 6 and 7. However, before embarking on this somewhat lengthy discussion some of its conclusions will be presented in outline, to help explain the usage of some terms in this book.

THE IMPORTANCE OF ATTEMPTING DEFINITION

Everyone knows that it is impossible to reach satisfactory, generally agreed definitions of such crucial concepts for psychiatry as normality and abnormality, right and wrong, good and bad, psychiatric disorder, 'disturbance', their relationship to mental illness, and even the scope of psychiatry itself. Excessive concern with definitions may even seem a somewhat unhealthy preoccupation to those anxious to get on with the job of treating patients. Nevertheless, even though foolproof definitions of such terms is beyond the capacity of this book, there are in adolescent psychiatry a number of reasons why it is important to make an attempt to demarcate certain areas of need and response.

First, problems present to adolescent psychiatrists in a most haphazard way; this is a recurring theme in this book, and will be taken up again from several different aspects. Psychiatric disorder exists among adolescents who are never referred to psychiatrists, while many adolescents without psychiatric disorder are referred for treatment.

Second, and following from this, many adolescent problems that present to psychiatrists neither have their origin in the boy's or girl's individual psychological functioning, nor are primarily mediated through it. Instead, problems manifest in terms of family, marital, educational, social or legal difficulties, which means the involvement of siblings, parents, teachers, education welfare, and social workers, probation officers, the police and the courts, all with their quite different ways of seeing things, different aims, different jargon, and indeed different and sometimes conflicting expectations of psychiatrists. In diagnostic assessment the clinician needs some alternative

Table 1   Reasons for attempting 'definition' of psychiatric disorder in adolescent psychiatry

---

1. To clarify the role of psychiatrists and identify their proper areas of concern
2. To clarify the roles of others in the care of young people and affirm the place of non-psychiatric help
3. Because it affects practical issues of responsibility
4. Because it affects practical issues of authority
5. Because of the importance for child development and psychotherapy of clarity about authority and responsibility
6. Because it is ethically desirable

---

conceptual frameworks in addition to those of individual psychiatric disorder, and this requires some definition of the latter; a corollary of this is that the notion of individual psychiatric disorder is a useful concept despite some tenacious sociological and political views that it is not. Clarification of what is *psychiatric*, in both diagnosis and treatment, helps the process of clarifying what is best understood in non-psychiatric terms (see Table 1). It is most important to be clear about what is, for example, a social, educational, or legal problem, or for that matter a social, educational, or legal solution.

Third, *responsibility* is a most important issue in psychiatry and in the care of children generally. Children or adolescents may be regarded as less than fully responsible for themselves because of: (a) their chronological age and legal status; (b) their personality and maturity; (c) the particular matter in question (for example coming to the clinic alone, agreeing to treatment, leaving home); (d) mental handicap; (e) psychiatric illness. To the extent that an individual boy or girl is not fully responsible, adults must be so: that is to say, they must accept responsibility for the sort of issues listed above. But which adults are responsible? Mother and father together, ideally, but very often in child and adolescent psychiatry parents disagree in an unhelpful way: indeed, there may be serious marital discord, serious parental incompetence, or parental psychiatric disorder. In such circumstances, the social services department may share or take over parental responsibility, informally or by application of the Children's and Young Persons Act. If a psychiatrist is involved he is responsible for his own work like any other professional worker, but of course will be fully *clinically* responsible for his patients while not having full *parental* responsibility, which he must share with his colleagues and the child's parents or social worker. Within this complex net of relationships, the issue of psychiatric disorder or its absence therefore significantly affects the adolescent's responsibilities, parents' responsibilities, the responsibilities of other professional workers, and the clinical responsibility of the psychiatrist.

Fourth, *authority* is of crucial importance in work with adolescents. Much of the above paragraph applies to questions of authority too, for as responsibility retreats (or is pushed back) someone else's authority tends to replace it. But the terms are not neatly antonymous because where problems, methods, and roles are not clearly defined in a particular child's case, adults may find themselves with authority but no responsibility, or responsibility without authority. Authority, like responsibility, may derive from recognized expertise in a relevant field (for example clinical skill, if clinical skills are relevant to the case); from social including hierarchical status; from legal status; or by personality, which may or may not be a good thing depending on the circumstances. Authority is not only a matter of authority to act; it affects also authority to complain, and many adolescents present because of other people's complaints. It can be important to decide who is in a position to complain, for example when different members of a broken and separated family have different and perhaps conflicting complaints about a boy or girl.

Fifth, both authority and responsibility have a separate significance for both upbringing and psychotherapy with adolescents. One of the tasks of adolescence is to get the balance right between self-assertion on the one hand and compliance with adult authority on the other. This is a difficult transition to make and a difficult balance to achieve, which is why adolescent disturbance is frequently manifested as aggressive misbehaviour or shyness and overcompliance. In questions of care and education and in therapy, the responsibility a boy or girl is encouraged to take, and the authority he or she is expected to accept, will again hinge on, among other things, questions of psychiatric disorder on the one hand and the appropriateness of the particular adult authority, medical or otherwise, on the other.

Finally, it is dubious ethically as well as administratively muddling unless it is made clear to all concerned whether a boy or girl is a patient, a pupil, or a client in one or other setting or professional relationship. At its crudest, most psychiatrists will have experienced the problem of the parent (and occasional professional worker) who has not 'told the boy or girl yet what sort of doctor you are'. Correspondingly, it seems to me important that an adolescent attending a day centre of some sort should know whether he is attending as a patient for treatment, as a pupil to learn something, as a trainee to acquire an occupational skill, or for punishment. (If the centre has more than one of these functions, this too can be said.)

There are relatively subtle ways in which professionals can be misleading about whether or not a boy or girl is a psychiatric patient, and in many cases the effect will be to contribute to the muddle, misunderstanding or dishonesty to which psychiatric disorder and psychiatric treatment are vulnerable. But there are many ways in which the false attribution of psychiatric disorder, or the failure to recognize it, can result in serious injustice too, whether as official policy in the USSR for example, or by neglect and gaze-aversion in the provision of resources for the mentally ill and mentally retarded in many Western countries. Do we also provide treatment services where we should provide good housing, good schooling, and proper employment? Probably we do, and perhaps social and welfare agencies for young people and their families blur the boundary between the proper responses to disadvantage and disorder to the detriment of both.

Disease, disorder, disturbance, and other problems

The first step in diagnosis is to map out the presenting problems in terms of their *location* and their *nature*. The location and nature of *psychiatric* problems are complex and will be discussed later; at this stage we are concerned with a broad categorization which must be made first before the diagnosis is refined. There is no point, for example, in proceeding at once to a prolonged, intricate examination of a boy's or girl's neuropsychiatric functioning and mental state if it is quite clear that the way the adolescent is being handled by his parents is making him unhappy.

Before beginning this process we need to examine briefly some terms which are troublesome because they defy watertight definition, and are used in different ways by different people.

Problems

The fact that a boy or girl has been referred to a psychiatrist is immediately and sufficiently a *problem*. It would be a problem even if it were all an administrative misunderstanding, which is not unknown. The concept of the problem is a convenient way in which to start, because it assumes no particular type of problem (for example poor upbringing, mental illness, naughty behaviour), and depends on no special concept of social or individual dysfunction.

Problem orientation as a style of clinical thinking and keeping medical records (POMR) has been recommended for general medicine by Weed (1968a, 1968b, 1969) and McIntyre *et al.* (1972) among others, and applied to psychiatric practice by Fowler and Longabaugh (1975) and Liston (1976), as a means of identifying and dealing systematically with a range of problems requiring specific action (for example disorientation, dehydration, ketosis, hyperglycaemia, infection, gastritis, poor self-management of diabetes, housing and marital problems) rather than simple diagnosis of a disease state (for example diabetic ketosis). Of course the principle of diagnosis remains important, but the traditional emphasis of clinical medicine has been to focus on the hypothetical nature of the underlying disorder and giving it a name (the disease) with the symptoms and signs being merely indicators of it. Problem definition is a supplement not an alternative to this, and a way of bringing systematic management more clearly into focus for practical clinical purposes and for teaching (McIntyre *et al.*, 1972).

Whatever the pros and cons for general medical practice, the principle, if not the detailed practice is most relevant to adolescent psychiatry, where some problems are psychiatric in nature and require a psychiatric response, while

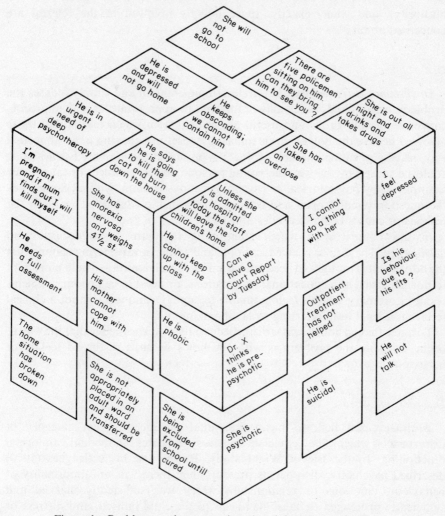

Figure 1   Problems and presentations in adolescent psychiatry

others (in the same referral) are social or educational in nature and require a quite different response. The task of diagnostic assessment is to identify these different types of problems and needs, in addition to making a precise clinical diagnosis in the traditional sense (see Figures 1 and 2).

The *problem*, then, exists as soon as the referral is made. Problems can present with as many variations as a Rubic cube and the psychiatrist's first task is to decide who is involved (he must compile a list of the dramatis personae), how they are involved (for example formal and informal relationships, legal authority), and what, exactly, those directly involved in the referral are concerned about.

Disturbance

Disturbance is frequently used in describing children and simply focuses the problems on the child, which may or may not be appropriate. It is an imprecise, conveniently ambiguous and useful provisional term which means that those involved believe the boy or girl is unusually upset or behaving in an abnormal way, leaving open the question of how the presumed abnormality has arisen. It could be caused by the way the young person is being handled, or taught, for example, or by physiological or psychological dysfunction 'within'. Sometimes the question remains open and a child is regarded as 'disturbed' without the reasons or causes being clearly established.

In this context it is worth mentioning the terms *maladjustment* and *delinquency*. The former is an educational and administrative term meaning that the adolescent is thought to need education in a special setting to help him adapt to normal social and educational expectations, or because behaviour problems result in ordinary schools feeling unable to cope. Delinquency is not a clinical term but a legal term referring to law-breaking.

To agree that an adolescent is disturbed is only to acknowledge that the way to begin assessing the problem is with the boy's or girl's disturbed feeling or behaviour as a focus.

Disorder and disease

Disorder (used here to mean individual disorder) is that category of disturbance which the clinician believes indicates individual abnormal functioning. In the Isle of Wight study, Rutter and his colleagues (1970) described psychiatric disorder as present when there was an abnormality of behaviour, emotions or relationships which was sufficiently marked and sufficiently prolonged to cause handicap to the child himself, and distress or disturbance in the family or community. This definition, which of course is descriptive, not aetiological, does allow statistically abnormal behaviour or feelings (such as constant sadness) to be regarded as individual disorder when it is in fact a normal reaction to, say, constant neglect by the parents. As already stated, it is impossible to make an entirely watertight definition, but for the purposes of this book I would add to the above definition the notion of the individual boy or girl being liable to function abnormally within other settings and relationships too and contributing at some level and in an abnormal way to the disturbed relationships.

Psychiatric disorders, to adapt Slater's and Roth's (1969) definition of psychiatry, are disorders where psychological phenomena and approaches are important as causes, as signs or symptoms or as curative agents. (Drug overdoses, neurodegenerative disorder and anorexia nervosa are three representative examples.) Disorder has traditionally been categorized in terms of the disordered system (for example cardiovascular disease) or the treatment (for example 'surgical conditions'). The state of child and adolescent psychiatry makes it necessary for psychiatrists to be Janus-faced on this issue, to regard some disorders as *psychiatric* in the sense that the adolescent's psychic functioning is disordered at some level (for example neurophysiologically, psychoanalytically, or in terms of his or her repertoire of social behaviour) or in the sense that a psychiatric approach to assessment and perhaps treatment seems the most appropriate one. In this respect it is worth affirming that (as pointed out, for example, by Rutter *et al.*, 1970) *psychiatric disorder* does not necessarily indicate a need for *psychiatric treatment*.

Disorder, then, is used in the following pages to mean individual abnormal functioning. If the abnormal functioning is apparently due to an abnormality in the development and maturation of a particular capacity (for example, delay in the development of speech or reading ability) the problem is categorized as *developmental disorder*. If it is believed that some psychological or psychophysiological process of disorganization has become superimposed on development (normal or abnormal), this is closer to the concept of *disease*.

The disease concept in psychiatry has been extensively and helpfully discussed elsewhere (see Clare, 1976, 1979a; D.C. Taylor, 1979) and will not be taken further here except to confirm its use as representing a handicapping and/or distressing internal process which has become self-perpetuating to a significant degree, that is it is not (or at least, no longer) substantially maintained by external circumstances. The word 'disease' has tended to become associated with severity so that someone with, say, hay fever or a cold does not normally regard himself as having a disease in the sense that arthritis, pneumonia or cancer is a disease. This common usage conveys real meaning, even though it is perhaps not theoretically defensible, and accordingly I have tended to use *psychiatric disorder* for those syndromes which are relatively minor (like some forms of anxiety or depression), or relatively circumscribed in their effects (like many obsessional and phobic conditions), and reserved the term *disease* for those seriously and widely disruptive conditions like manic-depression and the schizophrenias.

An aspect of individual functioning that may be part of normal variation, developmental progress or lack of it, or due to disease, is *intellectual functioning*. A boy's or girl's intellectual level may contribute to the problem or be part of it (for example undiagnosed neurodegenerative disorder; or a child of normal intelligence who for some reason is in a school for educationally retarded children) but is an observation, not a disorder in itself.

Physical ill-health or disability, minor or major, can be a direct or indirect cause of problems. Occasionally a physical disorder will be found to contribute directly to the child's problems in the case of an unrecognized major disease or indirectly when a chronic (or past) illness has left a legacy of handicap or family anxiety.

The distinction between disease processes and disorders of development is in some respects an unsatisfactory one, although for some conditions the distinction is a valid one indicating broadly the sort of problem being dealt with and the sort of help needed. Thus a manic-depressive adolescent may be regarded as having inherited a genetic tendency to a disease, a neurochemical imbalance which can be treated effectively by lithium; while a child with specific reading retardation may be regarded as having a specific maturational problem in one capacity, corrected by special teaching. For our purposes at the stage of problem-sorting it is useful to distinguish these two sorts of disorders and needs, but it is important to recognize, first, that some disorders seem to have the components of both (for example autism, some forms of schizophrenia, and major abnormalities of personality development; see Chapters 13 and 14) and that the developmental process and its variations can also be regarded as a unifying concept in phychiatry and many disorders understood in developmental terms rather than in terms of disease processes (see Chapter 4; and also Ounsted, 1972; Eisenberg, 1977; Chess, 1980, Rutter, 1980a).

Illness is a tentative but important term referring to the attribution of illness by others or by the person concerned (he must be ill; I feel ill). Whether what is observed or experienced reflects an underlying individual disorder is another matter; it may not. D.C. Taylor (1979) describes illness in the following terms: it is about experiences and roles; it represents disease, but is valid as an experience and a role in the absence of discernible disease; illness varies in the way it represents disease; and the diagnosis of illness is description in the language of medicine. Illness consists therefore of symptoms or signs perceived or illness attributed, whether or not there is evidence of disease. In one way or another, it is a social judgement based on the medical model, and this model may be 'capable of being validated (as disease) or not worth validating, or not yet technically possible to validate. Or it may be purely conceptual and have the function of standing for disease' (D.C. Taylor, 1979).

Figure 2 is a summary of this broad taxonomy of the components of problems as variously perceived by the adolescent, his or her family, and the professional workers involved up to the time of the referral. The categories, of course, are not mutually exclusive; on the contrary, putting together a helpful diagnostic formulation requires the clinician to take account of their relative significance, and how they interact. It will be noticed that the classification consists, untidily, of potentially verifiable facts, and opinions which may be incorrect but are significant none the less. Thus a teacher may insist that a boy is mentally ill when he is not. The teacher's view remains a fact, and indeed a highly significant fact, even if it is incorrect.

This elaborate set of several different individuals' perceived and felt difficulties

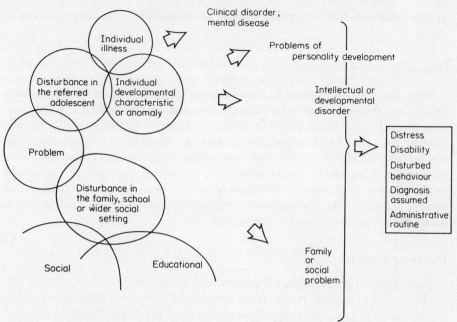

Figure 2   The components of problems and how they present

can be presented to the psychiatrist in only a limited number of ways, as shown below.

HOW PROBLEMS PRESENT

The final common path of the problem complex on the way to the psychiatrist consist of distress, disability, disturbing behaviour, presumed diagnosis, or administrative routine.

Distress

Distress, which may be the child's or an adult's, refers to uncomfortable feelings of, for example, anxiety or sadness, but whether they are appropriate or exaggerated, normal or pathological, does not matter at this stage, because for the present we are concerned with sorting out who is presenting what to the psychiatrist, rather than what it means.

Disability

This refers simply to the notion that the boy or girl cannot do something it is felt that he or she should be able to do, for example, to see, hear, read, play, make friends. (Parents may complain of *their own* disability: 'I can't get him to school'.)

Disturbing or disturbed behaviour

Disturbing behaviour refers to the concern or complaint about the adolescent's behaviour; the boy or girl may claim to be quite unconcerned, or at least not choosing to present it as a problem for the psychiatrist. The only component to a referral may be adult complaints about an adolescent's behaviour. The adolescent, truculently or evasively, may state quite explicitly that it is not a problem for him, and he wants no involvement with a psychiatrist. Disturbing behaviour is not necessarily misbehaviour; a boy or girl may seem unhappy or bizarre to adults, who are concerned on the adolescent's behalf, and seek help which the adolescent insists is not wanted.

Presumed diagnosis

This refers to the assumption that parents, teachers, and others may make that the disturbed behaviour results from illness. A teacher may describe a child as psychiatrically ill; a general practitioner or a child psychiatrist seeking a second opinion may say the same. The 'receiving' psychiatrist may or may not agree. Thus a child causing anxiety at school may be sent to a psychiatric clinic because the teachers believe the boy or girl may be psychiatrically disordered, this being their interpretation of behaviour they are unused to. Occasionally parents and child may present at the clinic with no complaint of distress, disability or disturbing behaviour at all, having been 'sent along' by someone in authority. Whose, then, is the problem?

Administrative routine

This happens too. The rules of an organization may require that in certain circumstances a psychiatrist be asked to see the boy or girl, for example adolescents taken to a children's reception centre or being routinely assessed for court appearance at a remand centre. It may or may not be appropriate, in the individual case or as a system. The point is that adolescent and psychiatrist can meet on this basis without anyone having any particular complaint or concern about anything; such anxiety as exists has then become institutionalized rather than related to the individual, only to reappear if the rules are not followed, for example if the psychiatrist declined to see the boy or girl concerned.

The attempts at demarcation of the last few pages are only of importance if they have implications for management, which they often do. To return again to the recurring theme of the complexity and arbitrary nature of adolescent referrals, it matters whether, for example, a diagnosis of enuresis or schizophrenia is made by a psychiatrist, another physician, a teacher, a parent or someone else, and how far the psychiatrist accepts this opinion. In practice it can be problematic when, for example, an experienced and respected psychiatrist makes a firm diagnosis of depressive illness in an adolescent and refers him for individual treatment to another psychiatrist whose opinion is that the boy or girl is reacting unhappily to family circumstances.

Correspondingly, disturbance identified in an adolescent by the staff of a chaotic children's home is not the same problem as disturbance identified by the staff of a children's home which is highly competent; concern about educational failure and lack of academic interest in a boy or girl is a judgement that will depend very much on the academic aspirations of a family, which may be low, high or even an obsessive preoccupation; anxiety about a child's development may depend on what information the parents have about normal development; and complaints that a parent cannot get an adolescent to do things (for example go to school) may depend on how much cooperation and support that parent has from the other parent or from the school. All this may be fairly obvious, but coping with such aspects of the problem is not always a straightforward matter.

IMPLICATIONS FOR CLINICAL WORK: A CONSULTATIVE–DIAGNOSTIC APPROACH

The usual emphasis of clinical work is individual disorder: the clinician assesses the individual's symptoms and signs, makes a diagnosis, and institutes individual treatment. The greater proportion of diagnostic and therapeutic work, particularly in adult psychiatry, for example, can be on a one-to-one basis.

It will be clear from what has been said so far that this is the exception rather than the rule in adolescent psychiatry. Individual diagnosis and often individual treatment remain the focus of clinical work, but other people are always involved too. Individual disorder, when it exists, presents amid a complex matrix of other people's problems: the adolescent may be depressed, but in addition his father is uncomprehending and irritated; his mother anxious; the parental relationship is strained, his elder brother contemptuous and his younger sister alarmed and confused; his teachers variously sympathetic, annoyed, and not sure how to help or what to expect; the general practitioner puzzled; and an education welfare officer who has become involved is not sure what to do. What they are helped to understand and do can be crucial in the boy's or girl's management.

The clinical psychiatrist will need information about the adolescent's difficulties from the other people involved, and while he is about it, will form opinions about their personalities and attitudes and be alert to the possibility of clinical disorder too. But these are *diagnostic* functions, and in addition the clinician should in parallel take a consultative approach too.

Consultation as a technique is discussed in Chapter 20. It is a term used in many different ways, but is used in this book in the special sense developed by

Caplan (1964, 1970) among others, to refer to the process by which the consultant (who need not be a psychiatrist, or even a clinician) helps the person who is consulting him (the consultee) to clarify for himself the difficulties he is presenting and explore possible solutions without the consultant taking over responsibility for the problem or its resolution. The consultee is left in an autonomous position, and can take or leave whatever emerges from consultation. It is a 'peer–peer' relationship, to use the jargon of the field, which a diagnostic doctor–patient relationship is not.

It is important to make the difference clear, and two brief examples should help.

Example 1
The director of a children's home is concerned about one of the residents, a boy of 14, believing him to by psychiatrically disturbed, and asks the visiting psychiatrist for help. The psychiatrist takes a history and examines the child, finds no evidence of clinical disorder, and reassures the director (or, finds a disorder and arranges treatment). This is a traditional piece of clinical work.

Example 2
The director of a children's home is concerned about one of his residents, a boy of 14, believing him to be psychiatrically disturbed, and asks the visiting psychiatrist for help. The visiting psychiatrist explores what the director means by psychiatric disturbance; what is the boy saying or doing that is causing concern? Are other members of staff worried? Are any members of staff not worried? What about the other children? How are the different staff and children coping with the boy among them who, for whatever reason, has generated anxiety and drawn attention to himself? What have they tried that helps? What has not helped? What do they fear may happen? The psychiatrist helps the director see how he can help the boy using his own skills and those of his staff. This is a consultative approach.

An important advantage of the latter approach is that *to the extent that the boy does not have an individual disorder that requires specialist diagnosis and treatment,* the fact that the problem is resolved means that something useful has happened among the staff members, for example more skilled and understanding perception of the children's behaviour and feelings and ways of helping them, more useful conversations and exchange of information between staff, perhaps more confidence in dealing not only with the boy concerned but also with similar matters in future. In short, the staff have learned something that they might not have learned if the psychiatrist had taken the adolescent on for a few private sessions of mysterious 'therapy' at his clinic.

But suppose the boy did have an individual disorder needing specialist treatment? Or even that he needed to confide in someone not connected with the children's home? If the clinician is able to adopt a dual consultative–diagnostic approach he will be alert to the possibility of individual problems in the boy that the staff cannot handle *and* conscious of the importance of leaving the staff in as competent and effective a position as possible both in general and in relation to the adolescent concerned.

In 'pure' consultation the psychiatrist would make a point of not seeing the boy, which could occasionally leave the staff coping with more than they could reasonably be expected to handle, to the boy's disadvantage. In routine clinical work, the staff would grow used to the expert who always seems to manage children better than they can, and the number of children referred to him would gradually grow. A consultative–diagnostic approach provides a useful compromise in that the psychiatrist offers consultation always, and direct clinical work sometimes; and when clinical work is undertaken, the consultative approach helps to make the most of what others can contribute. It has the following advantages:

1. Many adolescent problems referred to psychiatrists are helped satisfactorily by this approach, with staff and children benefiting more than would have been the case had the adolescent been booked into a clinic.
2. This approach does not prevent individual problems that the 'first-line' staff cannot handle from coming forward; on the contrary, it clarifies most quickly which children should see the psychiatrist. (A good general practitioner, for example, knows when a parent can cope with a child's problems and when he should see the child himself, and the parents learn too.)
3. When an individual problem has been identified, the other adults involved are in a position to help, and have not been undermined. Few adolescents need psychiatrists; all adolescents need parents (or their substitutes) and teachers, and they continue to need them even if a psychiatrist is seeing them once or twice a week.

Assessment, then, consists of both consultation and clinical diagnosis in adolescent psychiatry, because the dual approach meets the realities of the problems that are actually presented in day-to-day work. The diagnostic component, the deduction of disorder by the specialized appraisal of symptoms and signs, identifies what the clinical psychiatrist can contribute to the adolescent's care. The consultative component clarifies what other people can contribute, and this is always important.

Chapter 2

Adolescent Psychiatry in Perspective

INTRODUCTION

This chapter and Chapters 3, 4, and 5 are diversions from the question of diagnostic assessment, which is taken up again in Chapters 6 and 7.

As we have seen the practice of adolescent psychiatry is complicated by the shifting sands on which it is practised. In clinical work with this age group the symptoms and signs of disorder must be assessed against the background of the very considerable changes taking place between the ages of 10 and 20. Much has been made of the emotional turbulence and change of adolescence – perhaps too much. At least as significant are the quite dramatic changes in physical build and physiology, intellectual ability and verbal and social skills, the changes in the family and the changes in what the community expects of (and permits) boys and girls as they move through this period of life. The latter cultural changes vary not only from adolescent to adolescent or neighbourhood to neighbourhood, but from time to time, so that during the time it takes a child to become an adult many changes in social fashion, belief and attitude and even the law will take place.

Central to adolescence is the boy's or girl's move from childhood dependence to taking a place in the adult world. This transition may take place smoothly or otherwise. Those things which may interrupt this passage may include major or minor psychiatric disorder, but other things too, and it is part of the adolescent psychiatrist's task to sort out who needs the help of clinical psychiatry, and who needs something else that may be more to do with education or upbringing than treatment.

This may not be clear, or if clear (at least to the clinician) the other people involved with the boy or girl, parents and teachers for example, may not agree. It is no great relief to parents or teachers to be told by a psychiatrist that the adolescent in question is psychiatrically normal, indeed well, if the adults cannot

18

cope with the young person's behaviour and consider it bizarre and alarming. Must the adolescent still change in some way, and if he or she does not have a psychiatric problem, what sort of professional worker is in a position to help the boy or girl change? But he or she may not wish to change; what then? Again, perhaps the parents or teacher should change *their* expectations or behaviour? How is this going to be put to them, and if they are prepared to consider change, who is to help them do it? The involved adults may have to change as much as the adolescent.

The law's provisions too are crucial to the handling of children and adolescents at every level – psychiatric, educational, and social – and the psychiatrist will find some more helpful or clear than others; moreover what the law and the community require and expect is undergoing constant transformation, not steadily and in one particular direction, but jerkily, inconsistently and erratically, with frequent changes of general direction, whether we are considering experiments in educational approach, the vagaries of government policies, or dramatically changing patterns in fashion, in social opportunities and the lack of them, or in child care and child psychiatric practice. In many ways the adult world is itself undergoing a cultural adolescence of sorts, with all the exploration, failed experiments, excitement, anger, disappointment, and ambivalence involved, yet developing boys and girls need adults to be confident, secure, and mutually trusting.

To take up the theme of the first chapter, the problems found among newly referred adolescents will be found to fall broadly into the following categories:
1. Problems of the adolescent's individual functioning most helpfully conceptualized in the terms of clinical psychiatry.
2. Problems of individual functioning best conceptualized in other terms, for example in terms of problems in some aspects of physical or social development.
3. Problems best conceptualized in terms of the patterns of relationships within the adolescent's family.
4. Problems best conceptualized in terms of relationships and attitudes in the wider social network, for example at school, with peers, in terms of the law, or the nature of the adolescent's involvement, or need for involvement, with other professional workers.

These categories are not mutually exclusive. Diagnosis means to know thoroughly, and to understand why a boy or girl has been referred to a psychiatrist requires consideration of all these areas, as does making practical management plans.

Sometimes (how often depends on how the psychiatrist selects his or her clientele) it is possible for psychiatrist and adolescent to do all the work they need to in neatly circumscribed sessions, week by week, meeting in the psychiatrist's consulting rooms; individual psychotherapy with older adolescents can be conducted on such lines. My own view is that this is an exceptional way to work with younger adolescents and applies largely to those in their late teens leading relatively independent lives and managing well enough socially, educationally or in their work. But for most adolescents, certainly those living with families or substitute families and under the age of 18, the wider issues referred to apply most insistently, and must be faced.

My conception of the clinical adolescent psychiatrist is very much as a psychiatric 'general practitioner' rather than a specialist psychotherapist, who works with young people between about 10 and 20, and who should be as comfortable with neurological, pharmacological, and developmental concepts as with individual psychodynamics, family dynamics, and social, educational, legal, and ethical matters. Not that he needs to be skilled in all these areas, or could be, but it must be possible to converse and work constructively with those who are. He or she needs to be a practical clinical practitioner who is prepared to help negotiate the best course through psychiatric and other professional assistance for the boys and girls who come his or her way. If this means that the adolescent psychiatrist is a generalist of sorts, someone who will work with the best of what is available (and many competing alternatives are available), rather than a 'committed', high-powered therapist operating in one particular direction, then while this has its disadvantages it is also one of clinical psychiatry's strengths.

THE ADOLESCENT AND THE PSYCHIATRIST

Most specialist clinicians can take their clientele more or less for granted. Their skills are more or less known, particularly to the general practitioner who makes the referral, and who has the same general professional background and speaks the same language. To some extent this is shared by the general public; we all know, within reasonable limits, who should take on for treatment the boy or girl with a fracture, with meningitis, with renal failure; the referral pathway from home and school to family doctor and then to specialist team is clear.

In adolescent psychiatry the picture could not be more different. On the one hand there is an extremely large number of young people about whom adults are, for one or other reason, concerned. How many depends of course on the sort of problems included, the particular age group considered and the locality; but taking together the studies referred to later, and including all the boys and girls with family, social, emotional, and educational problems for whom it could be said that some sort of special psychological–social help is needed, the number can reach the order of 20–25% of the adolescent population.

On the other hand there is an extraordinary diversity of services available. For example, there is the psychiatrist as individual psychotherapist, as counsellor, as group therapist, and as family therapist; as clinician in charge of psychiatric units, and as 'facilitator' or 'coordinator' of child guidance teams; as leader of a therapeutic community, consultant to a children's home or special school, as psychodramatist, crisis-intervention therapist, and director of units for the mentally retarded. Psychiatrists have pioneered and developed all these areas of work, and antipsychiatry too for that matter. Conversely, almost all of the areas of work listed can be and are undertaken by other professional workers too; social workers, psychologists, specialist teachers, psychotherapists, counsellors, education welfare officers, probation officers, and others.

Given the range of social, family, emotional, behavioural, and educational problems on the one hand in an adolescent population, and the varieties of professional help available on the other, and given also the near-impossibility of delineating psychiatric disorder, it is not surprising that the process of referral of adolescent to psychiatrist is in general an arbitrary business, and correspondingly the adolescent psychiatrist is much more in the position of a general practitioner than a specialist in the sense that the people in his waiting room may be there for a score of possible reasons in addition to the possibility of there being something wrong with them.

Of course, this is true of other professions and specialities too, although in general to a lesser extent; certainly this factor strongly characterizes adolescent psychiatric practice, and strongly influences the approach the clinical psychiatrist should take.

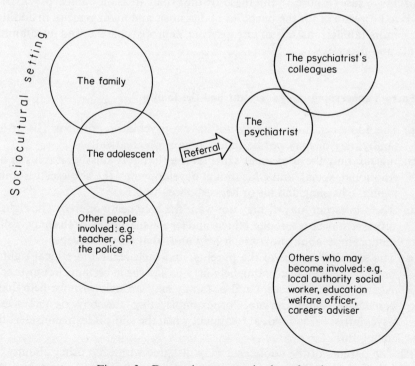

Figure 3   Dramatis personae in the referral

A number of other factors are influential, and account for the complexity and difficulties of adolescent psychiatry far more than any particularly anarchic or chaotic characteristics of individual adolescents, which in any case are more myth than reality. An aim of this book is to provide a strategy for assessment and management of the problems of adolescents which takes account of all the difficulties and dilemmas that arise in practice, not as a blueprint but as a general way of proceeding. At the outset it is worth outlining the range of factors the clinical psychiatrist must be aware of when a boy or girl is referred in order to place the clinical aspect – the diagnosis and treatment of individual disorder – in perspective.

These factors may be broadly categorized as those to do with the adolescent and his immediate family; those to do with other people and professional workers already involved with the adolescent, and perhaps with his or her referral; factors both abstract (for example 'normal' and 'abnormal') and concrete (for example the neighbourhood) to do with the wider socio-cultural setting; those to do with psychiatry, and therefore the psychiatrist and his or her immediate colleagues, for example in the clinical team; and those to do with professional workers on whose help the psychiatrist may call in the adolescent's interest. The dramatis personae and setting of course vary in detail and emphasis from case to case (Figure 3). But these are the broad areas the clinical psychiatrist needs to be aware of for the purposes of diagnosis and management, in addition to the more familiar matters of intrapsychic, neuropsychiatric, and intrafamilial events and processes.

1. Factors concerning the adolescent and the family

(a) The adolescent may or may not have a psychiatric problem. His or her family may or may not be functioning problematically.

(b) It is not only the adolescent's mental health that is at issue; it is his or her emotional, social, and educational development—the adolescent's upbringing, schooling and his or her response to both.

(c) The adolescent may or may not want the help being offered. The right to refuse it may be a complex ethical and legal issue. Or, he or she may wish to compromise about how much help and what sort to accept.

(d) The same (c) is true of the parents, and their legal and ethical right to prevaricate about accepting help may be at issue in certain circumstances.

(e) Alternatively, adolescent and/or family may strongly wish for help that is considered inappropriate, for example, that the boy or girl sees a psychiatrist for individual treatment when the clinical team considers this unhelpful.

(f) The parents of the adolescent may disagree with each other about what help to insist upon, encourage or support; the marital circumstances (for example impending divorce) or issues of parental personality and mental health may make parental authority unclear.

2. Factors to do with other people involved by the time of referral

(a) It is as often as not a matter of controversy whether or not the adolescent's mood and behaviour constitute a disorder, and, if so, whether psychiatric treatment (itself a most variable commodity) is what is needed.

(b) Correspondingly, there may be considerable pressure for the psychiatrist to take over responsibility, regardless of the psychiatrist's feeling that he or she is able to help.

(c) Social, legal, and educational authorities may not agree with the adolescent and his parents about which help should be accepted.

(d) Those already involved with the adolescent (family, teachers, local authority social worker) may vary in their willingness and ability to continue contact with the adolescent in collaboration with the clinical team, for example, a helpful involved social worker may be about to leave, or a boy's or girl's school place may be in jeopardy.

(e) As with the adolescent and family, there may be a wish to negotiate with the psychiatric team about how much to go along with the help offered.

3. Factors to do with the wider socio-cultural setting

(a) As with 2(a) above, the ways in which a boy's or girl's problems may be conceptualized vary enormously, not only in psychiatric terms (for example as individual or family disorder) but as right or wrong, good or bad.

(b) The services available vary widely from locality to locality as does their use. Neighbourhood, family doctor, and court attitudes to particular groups of adolescents and to psychiatric and other services are variable and arbitrary. The routes to different services vary too; there may be lengthy waiting lists or complex administrative procedures for entry to certain resources (for example therapeutic communities, physically secure units, schools).

4. Factors to do with psychiatry, the psychiatrist and the clinical team

(a) Whom the psychiatric team should see, how the assessment should proceed, what form of treatment to adopt, and the effectiveness and outcome of treatment in adolescent psychiatry (and in other fields of work with adolescents) are for the most part open questions.

(b) Good research is time-consuming and difficult, and new approaches are hard to evaluate. Helpful findings are slow to be implemented.

(c) Clinical teams have work to do to maintain effective collaboration and their success in this varies from time to time and place to place: this is particularly significant for work with adolescents and their families.

(d) Teaching, training, and supervision in adolescent psychiatry is time-consuming, and often receives low priority compared with 'service needs'. Colleagues' skills and experience vary widely among psychiatrists as among other professionals.

5. Factors to do with other professional workers whose help may be needed

(a) As with 4(c) there is variation in the working relationships at both personal and organizational levels between clinical team and agencies and professionals with whom they might hope to collaborate in an adolescent's interests.

(b) Professionals who need to collaborate may, in addition, disagree with each other about the adolescent's needs.

(c) As with 3(b) resources and facilities vary in availability from locality to locality and from time to time, with changes of personnel as well as in economic fortunes. A children's home may change its working philosophy with a change of leadership, or close down altogether. New resources may open up but not be widely known. Personal knowledge of a very large number of alternative resources for referral or collaboration is necessary; official lists are soon out of date.

To list these points is not merely a masochistic exercise; it is impossible to practise clinical psychiatry with adolescents without actively working with other people and other agencies, whether the immediate task is assessment, treatment, or making follow-up arrangements.

The sort of boy or girl the adolescent has become by the time the referral is made will depend on the interaction between his or her biological and psychological characteristics and a wide range of disparate social factors, including those listed above. Some will have helped shape the adolescent's personality development so far; some will have had more to do with the particular circumstances – recent events and the adolescent's response to them – which have led to the psychiatric referral (see Figure 4). And, of course, these factors will continue anyway, whatever the psychiatrist does or does not do, because the boy or girl will continue to develop and have some sort of upbringing, education, and pattern of relationships.

Therefore, in his assessment of what has helped make the adolescent what he or she has become at the point of referral, the psychiatrist has to consider, among other things, what parents, teachers, and others have done or not done so far; and in making plans for the present and the future, the possible contribution of parents, teachers, and others must be considered. The specifically psychiatric contribution should be seen in this context.

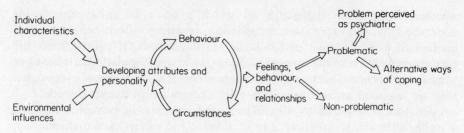

Figure 4   The referral process in a developmental perspective

This wide range of factors to be considered may appear complicated, as indeed they are, for the possible permutations of cultural and social attitudes at different times and at different places, the feelings, attitudes and behaviour of parents, teachers and others, and the responses of psychiatrists and other professionals are immense. Elsewhere I have suggested a way of simplifying this by broadly categorizing what happens to developing children and adolescents, and what may happen to them as a result of professional intervention in terms of *treatment, training or education, care* and *control* (see Figure 5; also Steinberg, 1981c, 1982a).

Treatment, which characterizes the medical–clinical model (see page 50) refers to special techniques of correcting disorder. If there is no disorder there is no indication for treatment, and the use of the term 'treatment' loosely to refer, for example, to special forms of education or correction is, I believe, unhelpful and misleading. Relatively few children and adolescents need treatment.

Training (*and education*), however, is needed by all children. It is the means,

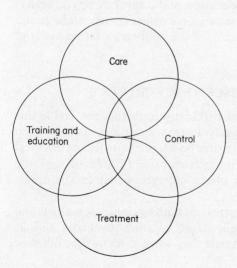

Figure 5   The broad categories of adult responses to children and adolescents

whether informal or systematic, by which a boy's or girl's capacity for understanding, self-expression, imagination, creativity, social behaviour, and intellectual and academic performance are developed. Of course, there are treatments which take the form of training (for example social skills training or some forms of behaviour therapy) and hence there is some degree of overlap, but they are regarded as treatment if they are undertaken to correct disorder.

Care, too, is required by all children, and includes the provision of food, warmth, affection, stimulation, a sense of value and security and predictability, and the dawning experience of the relationships that underwrite and provide these things. Again, education in its widest sense, whether in social behaviour, creativity or academic skills is a characteristic of proper care, and overlaps with it but the distinction is worth making; the two are fundamentally different.

Control, the setting of limits, is an essential part of care, education, and treatment, but in essence distinct from them. A child may be controlled without particular regard to his or her care, education, or treatment. Control is exercised in suitable ways, as part of the careful and loving balance exercised between parents and child, where limits are explored constructively but the child not allowed to go too far. At the other extreme, a wildly misbehaving adolescent may need physical control as a priority.

In extreme situations, care, control, and treatment become co-extensive, for example a severely and acutely psychotic child who must, for the moment be put to bed, sedated, and closely observed, or a physically deteriorating anorexic patient whose most basic physical needs must be attended to. Sometimes control is a precondition of treatment, for example when an aggressive, absconding adolescent thought to need psychotherapy must first be contained in one place with some order in his or her life in order to receive treatment.

When the adolescent is referred to the psychiatrist, it is helpful to think of the history in terms of what pattern of care, education, and control the boy or girl has experienced so far and how this makes sense of his or her current feelings and behaviour, and what implications there are for the adolscent's future needs in these terms too.

THE SCOPE OF ADOLESCENT PSYCHIATRY

Much of what is said about adolescent psychiatry in this section and in this book applies to child psychiatry too. The distinction sometimes made between the two fields is largely artificial; it is defensible on a limited number of practical grounds, but for most purposes the continuity from earliest childhood to young adulthood is more important than any of the differences that can be drawn between them.

Nevertheless, adolescent psychiatry is practised both by child psychiatrists and by those whose training and experience is largely in adult psychiatry and, as already pointed out, psychiatrists in this field may work in many very different ways and settings. Thus a report of the Royal College of Psychiatrists (1978) found that child and adolescent psychiatrists were working in any of the following settings:

1. Hospital departments of child and adolescent psychiatry: out-patient; day-patient; in-patient.
2. Hospital child psychiatrists without a department providing a consultative service to paediatricians, surgeons, and physicians admitting suicidal adolescents.
3. Child guidance clinics administered by the National Health Service.
4. Paediatric assessment centres.
5. Private practice and private clinics.
6. Child guidance clinics administered by local authority education departments.
7. Schools and units for children categorized as maladjusted – day and residential.
8. Colleges of further education, and universities.
9. Social service assessment and observation centres, community schools, and children's homes.
10. Remand homes and classifying centres, probation hostels and borstals.
11. Voluntary agencies such as the National Society for the Prevention of Cruelty to Children, private and charitable children's homes, the Marriage Guidance Council, the Samaritans, organizations such as CRUSE (for widows) and Release (for adolescents in difficulties with the law), the Richmond Fellowship (for after-care hostels), and the Spastics Society.

To these might be added various therapeutic communities such as Peper Harow in Surrey and the Cotswold Community in Wiltshire; units with physically secure provision such as the St Charles Youth Treatment Centre in Brentwood, Essex, and Southwood (for girls) and Orchard Lodge (for boys) in South London, and the special hospitals (such as Broadmoor and Moss Side); and finally the schools for special disabilities such as blindness and deafness.

The same report noted that child and adolescent psychiatrists worked with psychiatric and medical social workers, local authority social workers and those from voluntary agencies, residential child care staff, educational psychologists, clinical psychologists, remedial teachers, child and adult psychotherapists (medical and non-medical), medical specialists in mental handicap, child health, obstetrics, neurology and other specialities, as well as adult psychiatrists and general practitioners; nurses, teachers, home and bedside tutors, play leaders, and occupational therapists.

These are the agencies and professional groups with whom adolescent psychiatrists, and therefore adolescents and their families, work. Together they constitute an elaborate network of skills and resources, departments and units, within which boys and girls are looked after, educated, and treated, from which they are referred to psychiatrists, and to which psychiatrists refer them.

The range of methods and schools of thought in adolescent psychiatry are variegated too. The subject matter of many conferences in adolescent psychiatry in the United Kingdom and in the United States and the content of journals, books, and proceedings from both sides of the Atlantic, testifies to the predominance of psychodynamic and social approaches to psychiatric work with adolescents (see, for example. *Proceedings of the Association for the Psychiatric Study of Adolescence (APSA), 1970–1976; Centre for the Study of Adolescence: Monographs 1968–1974; Annals of the American Society for Adolescent Psychiatry, 1972 et seq.; Journal of Adolescence 1978* and subsequent volumes). At the risk of oversimplification, a tendency towards a polarity within the adolescent psychiatric field may be demonstrated; on the one hand, the 'mainstream' adolescent psychiatry which has burgeoned in the past 15 years has emphasized psychodynamic and social conceptual models and therapies for young people with for the most part emotional and conduct problems and delinquency; and on the other hand, epidemiological studies and work on the major mental disorders, habit disorders and handicaps have tended to be the focus of work where longer established child psychiatric departments, particularly academic centres, have turned their attention to adolescent problems.

The variety of aims, methods, practitioners, and institutions in the field can be disconcerting but is understandable because of (a) the nature of the problems with which workers in the field are trying to deal, and (b) the historical development of the different professions and services, which grew out of quite different ways of perceiving (and dealing with) the problems of children and adolescents.

Chapter 3

Clinical Psychiatry in Relation to the Problems of Adolescence

INTRODUCTION

What documentary evidence and word of mouth tell us about the care and upbringing of children by large sections of the human race throughout much of the world for much of the time does not make happy reading. In Europe and the West, childhood appears to be a relatively recent concept, emerging in the 18th century and becoming consolidated in the 19th century when it became increasingly important (and required more thought, effort, and resources) to prepare children for taking part in an increasingly industrialized civilization (Aries, 1962; Rosen, 1970).

It is not clear how deviant or deficient children and adolescents were dealt with in earlier times, but in general the authority of Church, state, and home tended towards the absolute (if transient) over their particular domains, and those who would not or could not cope or fit in were often punished very harshly or neglected. It may come as a surprise to learn just how brutish our ancestors of only 100 or 200 years ago could be, not in terms of exceptionally appalling behaviour, which continues today, but in terms of acceptable norms. Standards of behaviour and intellectual expectations were not generally high (we are misled by the well documented writing and thinking of the gifted and prominent) and a growing child would have been nagged, cuffed, beaten, prodded, and cajoled into following the occupation of his or her parents or, perhaps, going off to the sea or military service. Teachers and churchmen were the earliest child specialists to take a special interest in those developing into adults, followed by the Masters of Guilds when trades and professions began to organize themselves. As the community became more complex, demanding, and heterogeneous, adults found

29

it increasingly important and increasingly difficult to get the young into line and ready for adulthood. As a result older children became more noticed, in some senses more wanted and more important, probably fitter, competent and more articulate (and thus most clearly differentiated from those who were not), and more was expected of them. They, or some of them, became more powerful too, in a limited way, and as there were more alternative philosophical and political views available in the rapidly developing adult community, there was more to criticize and contend with too; hence the development, for example of the *Sturm und Drang* (storm and stress) radical movement in Germany in the eighteenth century (Rosen, 1970). This pluralistic process of cultures rapidly evolving towards ever greater complexity, alternatives, opportunities, and demand added complexity to the task faced by children and their families and teachers as boys and girls moved towards autonomy and independence.

More and more outside helpers were called in to help deal with those who presented problems; first clergymen, teachers, craftsmen, guildsmen, and workhouse authorities; the police and their antecedents; then welfare workers, and in the present century social workers, psychologists, physicians, and specialist teachers. The following section traces some of this history in outline, and sets out to propose a place in the care and upbringing of children for one of the more recent arrivals on the scene, the clinical psychiatrist.

THE DEVELOPMENT OF SERVICES FOR ADOLESCENTS

Problems in communication, cooperation, and mutual understanding between professional workers in the adolescent field are often commented upon (Dunham, 1980; Steinberg, 1981c). There is nothing particularly unusual about interprofessional and intraprofessional dissension, controversy, and competition, indeed it is a time-honoured characteristic of academic and clinical institutions, and has its healthy aspects too. However, this has to be set against the needs of troubled or neglected adolescents and their families for a sense of mutual trust, respect, and cooperation among the professionals to whom they are referred for help. Anxiety and argument among professional workers and resulting uncertainty, unpredictability, and poor planning can mirror the experience that adolescents and their families have experienced through several generations; indeed the clumsy and chaotic way in which unhappy and muddled people of all ages may try to provoke professionals into responding to them (usually labelled as manipulative behaviour) often demonstrates the flaws in the relationships between professional workers. Dunham (1980) has accounted for these differences in such terms as problems in sharing information, ignorance of the other profession's aims and procedures, differences in terminology and theoretical positions and the tendency for each professional group to regard its own point of view as the best available. To this I would add the interpersonal strain which is provoked when adults with their different personalities and backgrounds try to cope with the powerful feelings generated by adolescents in difficulties, and the quite different origins, history, and development of various professional groups.

Early legal measures

The king said now again at Witlanburgh to his witan and bade tell to the archbishop by Theodrede biscop, that to him seemed pitiful that men should slay men so young, or for so little, as he heard that everywhere was done. Said that to him seemed and to those with whom he took counsel, that men should slay none younger than a fifteen winters' man, unless he could defend himself or flee, and would not yield, then let men force him, the greater or the less, whoever it were. And if he will yield, let him be set in goal, and so let him be redeemed.

If his kindred will not take him, nor be surety for him, then swear he as the bishop shall teach him, that he will shun all evil, and let him be in bondage for his price. And if after that he steal, let men slay him or hang him as they did to his elders. (Cadbury, 1938)

This ruling for boys of 14 and under by King Athelstan of England, Alfred's grandson, who reigned from AD 924–939, had something about it of the probation order and court order. It was well ahead of its time, since torture, imprisonment, and death were meted out to all including children for such offences as 'stealing, felling a tree, associating with gipsies and pickpocketing' (Cadbury, 1938) for the next 800 years.

Children have been treated thoughtlessly and badly throughout history (see Aries, 1962; De Mause, 1974). In Western cultures in the Middle Ages children who survived were expected to follow in their parents' footsteps, for example as farm labourers or servants, and in so far as they came to the attention of the authorities were regarded as having no special rights and needs until the age of seven or eight, when they were treated as young adults. The idea of a mid-childhood and adolescent period during which a young person was prepared for adult life came later, partly for altruistic reasons and partly from expediency. Thus the medieval guilds saw the need for both reasons to train children for employment and regulate the hours that they worked. Laws enacted in the time of Henry VIII required very large numbers of vagrant children between 5 and 14 to be bound to masters as apprentices, and in 1601 a comparatively enlightened statute enabled the children of parents unable to support them to be apprenticed too. There has always been a surplus of unwanted, neglected or rootless children, dealt with in different ways. Some primitive communities killed them or let them die; now we have institutions for them. As recently as the nineteenth century, as described graphically by Millham and his colleagues (1978a), thousands of boys were required each year to replace those drowned at sea in the Mercantile Marine.

Over recent centuries, the trend has been towards a gradual increase of humanitarian attitudes towards children as individuals and as people, with a recognition that the increasingly complex and technical world needed from each new generation, fit, competent, reasonably trained young people to operate industry and the professions at various levels just as for a time in Britain they were needed to man the Empire. Adolescence, in some cultures a fairly brief and ritualized transition from childhood to adulthood, in the advanced technical cultures became a prolonged period of partial responsibility and further training extending into the early twenties and in some respects beyond. With this gradual shift from children perceived as play things, soldiers, labourers or future leaders to young people who were needed as educated and trained young adults, increasingly elaborate educational expectations and systems were added to natural parenting, apprenticeships, and official discipline (see, for example, Payne, 1916; Cadbury, 1938; Craig, 1946; Hibbert, 1963; Aries, 1962; De Mause, 1974; Millham *et al.*, 1978a; Millham, 1981). Educational developments are taken further on page 36.

The dissolution of the monasteries in the sixteenth century removed by far the most important source of charity for the poor and this deficiency was exacerbated by the disbanding of the vast armies after the Wars of the Roses and the enclosure of land which threw many farm labourers out of work. A succession of Acts required towns and parishes to look after their poor and to raise first voluntary and then compulsory contributions for this purpose, culminating in the first Poor Law of 1601. Subsequent history of the Poor Laws and the amendments to them is elaborate, but among the effects of the Poor Laws was the establishment of poorhouses and workhouses which were ultimately separated into hospitals for the sick, homes for children, and institutions for the aged and the unemployed. In addition, special establishments were set up for two groups: the blind or deaf, and the dumb or insane.

More recent legislation, and the development of social services

The Beveridge Report of 1942 recommended the abolition of the Poor Law which was replaced by the wide-ranging provisions of the National Assistance Act 1948 which sought to establish legislation based on the novel concept of general social welfare, and out of which the legislation and many provisions of the social service departments of local authorities and the National Health Service have developed. The most significant developments as far as children and adolescents are concerned have been the successive Children's and Young Persons Acts, of which there have been many from 1933 to the present. The 1969 and 1975 Acts have been particularly important and their main effect, at least as far as child psychiatric and related services are concerned, has been to shift the emphasis of the law away from conviction for crime and towards the provision of adequate care and control for children and adolescents, not only in terms of institutional provision, but in trying to ensure that children are properly supervised, cared for and controlled by their parents, or by others if their parents cannot or will not cope—which is not so far in principle from King Athelstan.

The details of various legislative Acts and their implications will be mentioned later; at this stage it is sufficient to say that the reasons for using a court order to transfer parental authority and responsibility to the local authority are, in the words of the Act, when the child's proper health or development is being avoidably impeded or neglected; because he or she is not receiving suitable education; or because he or she is guilty of an offence, excluding homicide. The effect of such legislation, particularly at a time when the limitations of psychiatry are becoming clearer, and when traditional controls and punishments are becoming unfashionable or unacceptable, has placed an astonishing, increasing, and some would say inappropriate burden on social service departments and social workers. Certainly it has led to considerable controversy (see Brewer and Lait, 1980).

The roots of the social work profession are hard to describe with any certainty. Social work began, where in some fields it still continues, in independent charitable and welfare organizations, sometimes on a local and almost individual basis, sometimes as small organizations that become national institutions, such as the National Society for the Prevention of Cruelty to Children which began in Liverpool in 1883, drawing from the experience of an equivalent society in New York (Allen and Morton, 1961). The beginnings of social work as a profession, with training programmes and qualifications, began in Britain and in the United States in the 1920s and 1930s (see, for example, Flexner, 1915; Lubove, 1971). The hospital social worker's role developed out of the function of the 'lady almoner' whose original task was the assessment of the patient's financial means. In psychiatric work he or she became the psychiatric social worker, whose equivalent 'in the field' was the mental welfare officer. These various categories of social worker disappeared under the recommendations of the Seebohm Committee of 1967 and the Social Services Act of 1970 so that the social work specialists, for example in child care, mental health and subnormality became 'generic' social workers within a single profession and hierarchy. As widely predicted, now that the professional hierarchy and career ladder is firmly established, with social work in at least this sense on a par with other professional groups, the possibilities and advantages of specialization are again being explored.

There is little in life that the concept of social work cannot be stretched to encompass. In practical terms, social workers in adolescent psychiatric work can and do arrange transport, help pay bills, get adolescents into psychiatric care and out of it, prepare court and other reports, take family and personal histories, undertake liason, consultation, counselling, marital work, individual casework and family therapy and every aspect of academic work; and private practice too. Some social workers have begun to consider what their profession is for, and where it is leading. In rudimentary political terms, it has been asked whether social workers provide a particularly insidious form of social control (the 'soft police') or are radical activists undermining the established social fabric:

questions that can easily be applied to practically anyone doing anything that impinges in some way on people's behaviour and freedom of action. At a more philosophical level Ragg (1977) has pointed out that the social worker can operate in two quite distinct ways: as a *diagnostician*, perceiving *needs* in terms of theoretical systems which he or she but not the client understands; or as an *advocate*, helping to clarify and describe the client's *wants*. Clearly the former comes close to the medical model, and the latter to the legal–political model in which the professional's task is to help his client speak. 'Treating the client as a person demands that he be treated as wanting, and the description of wants does not allow the caseworker to act as the expert diagnostician' (Ragg, 1977).

Should the social worker, then, be social advocate or therapist? If he or she can be either, who decides which in the individual case? For if the social worker decides, he or she is acting as diagnostician. If the argument is accepted that it matters whether care, control or treatment is being offered by the professional worker, then this rather difficult question deserves thought.

Residential care is a separate aspect of social service department provision; some of the types of facility are listed on page 49. Residential care poses many problems for children and staff (see, for example, Wolkind and Rutter, 1973; Tizard, 1974; Rutter, 1979a; Wolkind and Renton, 1979;) About 100,000 children are officially in the care of local authorities in England and Wales at any given times (DHSS, 1977) and the evidence is that they are a group at considerable psychiatric risk, with conduct disorders common, particularly among the boys, a tendency to long-term institutionalization and long-term problems, and the experience of having many different care staff looking after them. Wolkind (1977) has shown that prolonged contact with the same care staff member is associated with lower rates of severe disorder, but such stability of personal relationships in such settings is unfortunately exceptional, and care staff tend to receive less than adequate training, supervision, support and status, factors which together encourage a high staff turnover, add to the children's problems and may account for an unknown but probably substantial number of referrals for admission to psychiatric units (Steinberg, 1981c; Steinberg *et al.*, 1981). Alternatives to residential care have been explored, for example in the recent Family Placement Project in Kent, where selected families are paid to foster boys and girls with delinquency and behaviour problems (Hazel, 1978, 1981), an experiment which has had some good results and deserves fuller evaluation.

When children are taken into care they are taken to social service reception and assessment centres, sometimes as emergencies, unless a home is already allotted to them. In these centres they receive social, psychological, educational, and psychiatric assessments and plans are made for their future, many children going on to community homes with educational facilities, the successors to the old approved schools which, in principle, went out with the 1969 Act.

Forensic developments

Prisons are a relatively recent development in historical terms, progressive in their time, since fines, the pillory, the stocks, both corporal punishment and execution used to suffice for both children and adults well into the 19th century. By then two sorts of places of confinement had been established: prison, where the inmates paid for their own maintenance (they were private establishments) and which had their origin in providing custody while the Crown extracted its fines; and the Bridewells, paid for by the Poor Law, to contain and provide work for the unemployed and those who would not work. The original Bridewell (an ancestor of Bethlem) was granted to the City of London in 1552 by Edward VI as a house of correction for vagrants and became one of the five royal hospitals. O'Donoughue describes vividly the sittings of its court.

The minutes of the last meetings have been read, a procession of vagrants and petty criminals, marshalled by the porter and beadles, begins to filter in by way of the back staircase. They have been begging in the streets, they have no visible means of subsistence, or they have been pilfering from the haberdasher's shop in Newgate Market. Most of them, no doubt, are 'old customers', 'old guests' and 'notorious varlets'. Against the names of such in the court books monotonously occurs the laconic formula 'punished and set to work'. Punishment of course, meant the lash...
...But this morning it happens that tenders have been received from contractors, who offer to ship vagrants and petty misdemeanants, if healthy and strong, to Virginia, and the court empowers the treasurer to spend a certain sum of money per head on their transportation. Possibly a few of these Bridewell boys and girls, if they escape massacre and the plague, were the ancestors of some of the first families in Virginia. (O'Donoghue, 1929)

O'Donoghue's book carries a photograph of the monument at Jamestown, Virginia, marking the spot where indentured servants, formerly prisoners at Bridewell and including many in their teens, landed in the reign of James I.

The prisons have always had an uneasy and ambiguous task; the containment of nuisances, the protection of the public from dangerous people, the custody of people unable to organize themselves or their lives, punishment, reform, and treatment. The history of prisons, particularly up to the 19th century reform, is a horrifying one and throughout it children and adolescents from the age of eight have been prominent victims (see Hibbert, 1963).

The age of criminal responsibility has been progressively raised and is now 10. Even if a child under 10 has committed a criminal offence, he or she can be dealt with only in care proceedings. The minimum age to be sentenced to prison is 17, although young people can be held in prison below this age if awaiting trial and no children's home or centre can contain them. Young people of 15 or over can be sent to a borstal institution, although in fact this is unusual below the age of 17, and they may also be sent to detention centres. Both detention centres and borstals are run by the Home Office via the prison service, and the latter institutions take their name from the first attempt at Borstal Prison, near Rochester, Kent, in 1902, to provide a special training approach to young offenders. Different borstals vary in the type of adolescents they accept and the degree of security provided; some are open, some closed, and some provide special security. Two are for girls. Their working philosophy is based on social and occupational training.

Younger children, whether convicted of offences or in need of care and control may be sent to community homes (the descendants of the approved schools) and those who are considered to need greater security may be sent to special secure units such as the Royal Philanthropic School at Redhill, the Kingswood Schools in Bristol, the St Charles Youth Treatment Centre in Brentwood, and Orchard Lodge or Southwood (for girls) in South London. They are essentially social service establishments, run on residential care lines, with considerable psychiatric and psychological collaboration.

Millham *et al.* (1978a), Cawson (1979), and Millham (1981) have studied the children referred to these special closed units and concluded that the population in them did not differ significantly from that of the general approved school (community school) population in terms of family background, psychiatric disturbance or personality, and although the young people referred had some special characteristics, two-thirds being persistent absconders, they also tended to be a young group (mostly 12–14 years), not markedly delinquent, and not particularly physically aggressive. Such violence as there was had been towards the staff or residents of institutions from which they were referred. The authors also concluded that older (over 15) more delinquent young people were probably being sent to borstals rather than being committed to care.

Residential care and management is discussed in Chapter 18. For the purposes of this chapter it may be noted that this wide range of settings exists, and, as with so many facilities for young people, the referral process tends to be arbitrary, the goals and methods of the various regimes variable and ambiguous and the results difficult to evaluate and at best uncertain.

By no means all forensic developments were residential. Courts in the 19th century tried 'binding over to be of good behaviour' as a strategy (as Athelstan had tried 1,000 years earlier) and the assistance and supervision which accompanied this, initially on a voluntary basis, became the Probation Service from 1907 onwards.

Developments in education

It is interesting that we must turn again to the monasteries to see the beginnings of education in Europe. "Literacy was virtually co-terminous with the clergy; far into the Middle Ages, even kings were normally illiterate. The clergy controlled virtually all access to such writing as there was' (Roberts, 1976). Not that education is only about writing – 'like most other living things', said Gilbert

Murray, instancing poetry, "it cannot be defined' (Micklem, 1948). The Egyptians, Greeks, and later the Romans had schools, and with the rise of Christianity monastic schools were set up to instruct children in the faith (Stuart, 1926), with serious education for girls trailing behind (Stuart, 1933). For centuries education, such as it was, was left to parents, special tutors for the rich, the churches, and the small number of grammar schools (later to become the 'public schools') founded from the 14th century onwards. As urban life and the trade guilds developed more people wanted to learn the rudiments of reading, writing, and arithmetic and the elementary schools, usually taken by the parish priest and the local helpers, grew in the 16th and 17th centuries. State intervention in schooling in England and Wales was relatively late. The Education Act of 1870 created school boards and subsequent Acts (1902, 1918, 1944) successively introduced compulsory secondary education and raised the school leaving age to 14 and then to 16. It now seems as proper to expect children to cease full-time education and go to work at 16 as it once seemed natural at 14, 13, and 10. Perhaps the time will come when full-time education will be seen as a necessity for all well into later adolescence.

All this is not remote from the clinical psychiatry of adolescence; what young people become, for good or ill, depends on their constitution, their parenting, various internal and environmental events, and their education. The development, behaviour, and achievements of children are powerfully affected by the schooling they receive, and conduct and emotional problems, delinquency and educational attainment are closely associated (Rutter, 1974; Rutter and Madge, 1977; Rutter et al., 1979), while many problems manifest as problems at school, or are helped by educational means.

Special schooling for children handicapped in various ways existed before the 1944 Education Act, but since this Act there have been considerable advances in the provision made, on both day and residential bases, for children with physical handicaps, including 'delicate' schools for children considered physically vulnerable and schools for deaf and blind young people and various degrees of mental retardation (including the educationally sub-normal, or ESN) and those categorized as maladjusted.

There are two other professions with whom adolescents and adolescent psychiatrists have contact. School counsellors are teachers who have had further training in counselling and operate in some schools, usually counselling individual children and sometimes operating special units for children who need extra help to adapt socially. Counselling has developed in university and college campuses too, as a profession in its own right. The *Dandy* and *Beano* comics in the 1940s and 1950s used to feature, in pursuit of Keyhole Kate, Hungry Horace or some other character, the 'truant catcher', armed necessarily with a giant butterfly net. The school attendance officer, to give him his correct term, has evolved into the education welfare officer, whose office operates very much as a school's social service and welfare department.

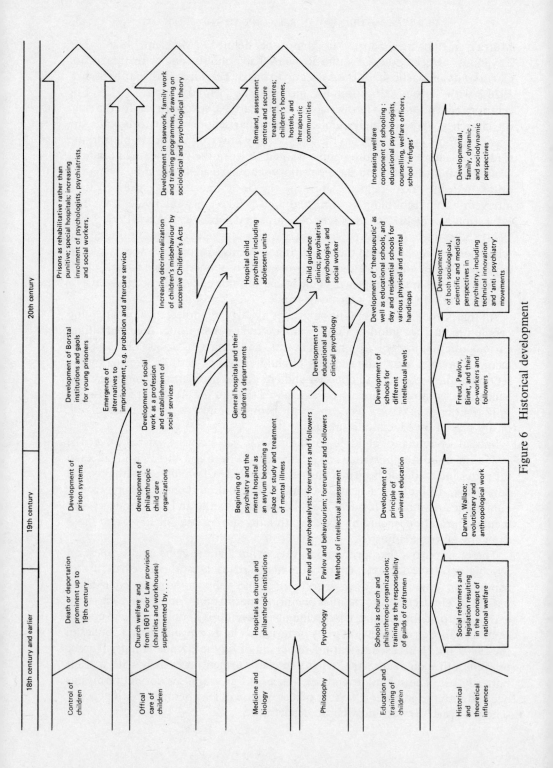

Figure 6 Historical development

Education, like social work, overlaps with concepts of therapy too. Maria Montessori (1870–1952), a physician in Rome, concluded from her interests in child anthropology that educational help was more important than medical treatment for mentally retarded children, and developed what came to be known as the Montessori method, based on early use of non-directed stimulating play, particularly with physical activities, and this was extended to educational methods for ordinary children too.

Education through self-directed activity and play was also the basis of the method devised by Friedrich Froebel (1782–1852) and the use of activity, creativity, and art in a child's development and education was developed too by Rudolf Steiner (1861–1925), again for children of all levels of intelligence. Schools and communities based on such principles, and particularly those of Rudolf Steiner are to be found in many parts of Britain and Europe. While they stress individuality as establishments and for their pupils, they have in common an emphasis on community life and responsibility, arts, crafts, music, and rural activities which seem to help some intellectually and emotionally handicapped adolescents function at their best. Their emphasis on the positive, normal aspects of their pupils, rather than on their disorders and disabilities, and the range of medium-term, long-term, and even life-long facilities, makes them an immensely useful resource. Like all self-supporting communities with special philosophies, Rudolf Steiner schools and communities take time to get to know and liaison between them and psychiatric clinics and hospitals can take some considerable effort on both sides, but it is very frequently worth while, and their achievements with some young people can be considerable.

Therapeutic communities

Somewhere between the triangle of care, education, and psychotherapy come the therapeutic communities. The principles of the therapeutic community are frequently discussed and hard to describe with precision; they form something of a mythology within child and adult psychiatry. Well known examples in Britain include Finchden Manor (Burn, 1964), the Henderson Hospital (Whiteley, 1970; Whiteley and Zlatic, 1972; Whiteley 1975), Peper Harow (Rose, 1977), Shotton Hall (Lennhoff and Lampen, 1968, 1975; Lampen, 1978), and the Cotswold Community in Wiltshire and Red House School in Kent. Accounts of these and other therapeutic communities and how they work (Jones, 1946, 1968; Main, 1946; Bettelheim, 1950, 1960; Bettelheim and Sylvester, 1952; Martin, 1962; Docker-Drysdale, 1968; Clark and Yeomans, 1969; Clark, 1977) and the more systematic attempt at description by Rapoport (1960), taken together, convey a sense of the prominence if not the importance of charismatic leadership; permissiveness (in the sense of the individual 'being himself') but with the discipline, imposed by confrontation, of the whole community as a group; democracy, that is the community's rules are those made by the group;

willingness on everyone's part to express and expect strong feelings, for example of anger, anxiety, and sadness as well as excitement and affection; public participation by all, in all matters of any significance; a tendency to the community developing a powerful ethos, mythology, and its own private language and rituals; and, at a theoretical as well as practical level, consciousness of the importance of clarity about roles, rules, and authority. Despite the non-hierarchical, democratic ideal of many therapeutic communities, there is often considerable dependence on the leadership, and the community is vulnerable to change and even collapse when the leadership changes.

This ideal of a democratic, self-helping community is often profoundly modified for work with children and adolescents, where responsibilities are earned by young people who behave responsibly, but ultimate authority rests firmly with the staff. Problems of authority in such settings have been most helpfully discussed by Lampen (1978).

The results of therapeutic communities are hard to evaluate. One important difference to, say, hospitals and which partially accounts for this is their difference in goal. A clinical setting should aim for specific symptomatic improvement among other things; a therapeutic community, despite its adherence to the concept of treatment (therapy) could be said to be more concerned with the concept of personal development rather than the conception of disorder. Of course a hard line cannot be drawn between the two, but the emphases are different.

In comparison with children's homes, therapeutic communities tend towards the application of a particular therapeutic–developmental system and the requirement of the staff to understand it and implement it consistently, and examine their motives and difficulties in doing so. They tend to have better trained staff and better supervision of work, and to give high priority to personal commitment and reasonably long tenure of appointment for staff who fit in. It is difficult for staff who do not learn to fit in to stay very long because of the constant and open emphasis on the community's ethos and requirements. The same can be true of the community's clientele, although different therapeutic communities may be expected to vary, and indeed vary from time to time, in their tolerance.

Interestingly from the point of view of the development of institutions, Manning (1975, 1976), who describes the therapeutic community as a social movement rather than a medical innovation, believes the therapeutic community as a principle is in decline – a natural third stage following the first two stages of turbulent development and enthusiastic mobilization.

Now it has more limited but more realistic aims: providing therapeutic resources for certain problems; gaining experience in organisation development, in close association with a tolerance for self-criticism and research. The therapeutic community is coming in from the cold and will continue to play a modest role in the field of residential institutions through its special experience of individual and social processes.

Developments in psychology

It is almost impossible to differentiate developments in the profession of psychology from developments in education, care, psychotherapy, and psychiatry.

As with psychiatry, psychology's roots were in philosophy, science, and quasi-science; before the 19th century it consisted largely of philosophy and relatively primitive ideas about physiology. Experimental psychology began in the 19th century, becoming established with the opening of psychology laboratories by Wilhelm Wund in Leipzig in 1879 and G. Stanley Hall in Johns Hopkins University in the United States in 1883, developments which laid the foundations for work by teams rather than isolated individuals (see, for example, Flugel, 1933; Miller, 1964; Hilgard and Atkinson, 1967).

Of particular relevance to the foundations of subsequent clinical practice was the work, in the early 1900s, of Ivan Pavlov (1849–1936) on physiological conditioning, the founding of behaviourism by John Watson (1878–1958), and the development of the psychological theories of psychoanalysis by the psychiatrists Sigmund Freud (1856–1939) and Carl Jung (1875–1961). Conditioning and behaviourism showed how the mind and body could acquire habits, accidentally or by systematic training. Psychoanalysis held that feelings and fantasies of which people are not conscious were nevertheless profoundly influential in their lives and behaviour. Despite it being common to criticize the limited and mechanistic viewpoint of behaviourism, and the speculative and static dogmatism of psychoanalytic theory, in fact a wide range of other theoretical positions and treatment approaches have developed from both these roots, and continue to do so. Certainly the many forms of behaviour therapy, and the psychodynamic therapies used with individuals, families, and groups, can be traced to these origins.

A different sort of psychology was more orientated to measurement and description rather than intuition and experiment. Also at the turn of the century, Binet and Simon devised the first intelligence test (1905), followed by many modifications of methods of intellectual assessment such as the Stanford–Binet test developed by Louis Terman at Stanford University in 1916, and the Wechsler Intelligence Scale for Children developed in the 1940s. These developments in the intellectual assessment of children were encouraged by developments in universal education which in turn contributed to them; indeed, they were part of the increasingly responsible official approach to children seen in the 19th century and already noted as a relatively recent phenomenon in human history.

In parallel with these developments, the anthropological and biological studies of mental life pioneered by Charles Darwin and Francis Galton led to centres and laboratories where children were measured and studied, culminating in the foundation by William Sully of the British Child Study Association in 1893, whose main object was 'to encourage teachers to study the individual child and seek advice [there] on their more difficult problems' (Warren, 1975).

Moving to psychology today, the clinical psychiatrist will find psychologists' skills as wide-ranging as those of psychiatrists and social workers, and again with considerable overlap with the work done by both professions. In the United Kingdom there are broadly two sorts of psychologist: educational psychologists, trained in teaching as well as psychology and employed by the education department in the School Psychological Service; and clinical psychologists, again with training in psychology but their in-service training and practice in hospital settings. Both may work in academic centres and undertake teaching and research. Different psychologists, educational and clinical, have their professional preferences, but the special psychological skills of particular value to the clinical team are the psychologist's competence in making reasonably objective, standardized observations, for example of intellectual capacity or more specific cognitive skills; of assessing behaviour patterns and situations upon which certain patterns of behaviour are contingent; and of undertaking the planning, supervising or teaching of techniques in the behaviour therapies. But in addition, and like every other professional in the child care field, psychologists are able and often willing to carry out one or other of the psychotherapies too. Like psychiatrists and social workers, psychologists are to be found working as individual, marital, sexual, family or group counsellors or psychotherapists; as behaviour therapists, educational or vocational consultants; and leading special child treatment centres and therapeutic communities. In these capacities they may be employed by central or local government or independent bodies or work in private practice.

Developments in general psychiatry

Child and adolescent psychiatry has developed in parallel with considerable advances in general psychiatry, paediatrics, and general medicine too. The increasing sophistication in the use of medication since the 1950s, improvements in diagnosing and treating disorders such as asthma, diabetes and epilepsy, the diagnosis and prevention of the causes of mental retardation are a handful of improvements among many. One development of particular significance for adolescent psychiatry, however, was the increased understanding of social and group dynamics which received a special impetus during the two world wars when military psychiatrists were operating among more sophisticated, better educated officers and men than in previous mass conflicts, so that psychological understanding of the effects of near-intolerable stress on individuals and groups, informed by psychodynamic and behaviour concepts, could be put into practice (see, for example, Miller, 1940; Sargant, 1957, 1967). These military experiences were influential early in the development at the Tavistock Clinic in London of work on neuroses in civilian life and on aspects of the social psychology of groups, hierarchies, and organizations (Dicks, 1970). Such developments in our understanding of group processes and social dynamics have been of considerable importance to adolescent psychiatry, not so much for the treatment of individual adolescents, but in understanding the natural groups in which they grow, the therapeutic groups and communities in which they are treated, and the children's homes and schools in which they are placed.

Such sociological and sociopsychological thinking provided a receptive climate of thought for work from another perspective, that of the family, which for a time was considered by some another sort of battlefield and as much a malign influence on humanity (see, for example, Laing and Esterson, 1964; Cooper, 1967; Esterson 1970), a position from which many of the earlier protagonists have somewhat backtracked. Certainly the concept of the schizophrenogenic family and the psychotogenicity of the 'double-bind' (Bateson *et al.*, 1956) are no longer widely accepted, but the work of Bateson and his colleagues Jackson, Haley, and Weakland in the 1950s at Pao Alto Mental Research Institute laid the foundations for the developments of 30 years during which we have begun to see what family processes can do for good or ill, for children and their parents.

The development of child and adolescent psychiatry

The psychiatric disorders of children do not feature particularly prominently in the history of psychiatry, perhaps because it was taken for granted over the centuries that there was no discrimination between children and adults whenever the Church, the law or other authorities did something on behalf of the deranged, troublesome or incompetent young or old.

It is difficult to distinguish early accounts of odd behaviour, mental illness, and mental defect from each other. An early reference to what might now be described as mass hysteria was the children's pilgrimage of Vendôme, in France, when it was said that 30,000 children flocked to follow a shepherd boy who claimed to have seen a vision of God.

These thousands of delirious children set out for Marseilles, notwithstanding the opposition of their parents and the King, and resolutely facing all the terrors and hardships of the journey, they eventually arrived at the sea, but only to be the victims of the merchants, who sent them off in ships to the East, where the little fanatics were sold as slaves. (Hyslop, 1925)

Robert Burton (1577–1640) in the *Anatomy of Melancholy* referred to the influence of parents on children by inheritance (Burton, 1927 edition):

That other inbred cause of Melancholy is our temparature, in whole or in part, which we receive from our parents and also by being excessively strict or by too much remissness, they give them no bringing up, no calling to busy themselves about, or to live in, teach them no trade or set them in any good course... many fond mothers especially, dote so much upon their children, like Aesop's ape, till in the end they crush them to death...

Robert Burton is worth reading for his comments on children and parents. Hunter and Macalpine (1963) give several accounts of disturbed children including the 'egregious cunning of the boy of Bilson' (1622) who mixed ink in his urine to feign possession, clearly a dangerous practice but fortunately diagnosed. They quote the conclusions of Bingham (1798–1849) that children rarely become insane, but when they do 'strong mental excitement and injudicious development of the moral faculties' are the causes.

As in so much of the history of child care, expediency as much as interest focused attention on abnormal children; thus Payne describes how eighteenth-century industrialists trafficking in child labour might be persuaded to accept, for example, one idiot with every 20 other children sold for labour; in most cases the mentally ill or retarded child – in retrospect the boy or girl might have been either – 'mysteriously disappeared' (Payne, 1916).

In the nineteenth century, however, serious medical interest began to be shown in the emotional and intellectual problems of children, for example by Henry Maudsley (1867) and Charles West (1848). Maudsley described monomania, choreic delirium, cataleptoid insanity, epileptic insanity, mania, melancholia, and moral insanity in children and took a developmental perspective, pointing out that as the child's mind developed its more elaborate organization permitted more elaborate phenomena such as hallucinations and delusions to occur; 'the insanity met with in children must of necessity be of the simplest kind; where no mental faculty has been organized no disorder of mind can well be manifest'. West took a similar view, and expressed the view that most doctors under-estimated the prevalence of mental disorder, mistaking it for the more familiar idea of idiocy.

Special hospitals for idiocy were already being established, perhaps stimulated by the publication in Itard's study of his attempts to educate the Wild Boy of Aveyron found in the woods and his assertion that innate defect, while not curable, could be minimized by special training (Humphrey, 1932; Bowden, 1979). Asylums for idiots were established in London and elsewhere from 1847 onwards, for example at Darenth and Earlswood and the Idiots Act (1886) required conditions for admission, care, and inspection to match those already in existence for lunatics. Further Acts followed, including the Elementary Education (Defective and Epileptic Children) Act of 1914 which required local authorities to provide special education for the mentally retarded.

As already pointed out, this was a period when more attention was being paid to children, the authorities were becoming interested in their education and welfare, and dramatic propositions were being made about the nature of man and the mind by Darwin, Galton, and Freud. Another important step was the establishment of the British Child Study Association by J. Sully who with A.

Baine and Galton categorized the children at Darenth and Earlswood into grades of imbecility (including, incidentally, assessment of digit span, one of the most useful and enduring of tests) and apparently influenced Binet when he developed his intelligence scale some 20 years later (Forrest, 1974). Of course it had long been appreciated that a minority of children showed gross mental deficiency, but the new measuring devices and the attention focused on children's educability by the introduction, in England, of universal education, made finer differences in intellectual ability both appreciable and significant, and led in due course (1913) to the appointment of the London County Council's first psychologist, Cyril Burt (Warren, 1975).

Developments in the United States, and as a result in England too, were strongly influenced by the teaching of Adolf Meyer (1866–1950), whose particular approach is best appreciated by comparing it with the Kraepelinian school. Emil Kraepelin's approach was descriptive and nosological; taking for granted the natural existence of mental disorder, he proceeded to describe and classify the forms it took, based on careful clinical description and follow-up of patients over many years. Clearly this fits best when the process being considered has the features of an internal disease state, and correspondingly his clarification of the forms manic-depressive illness, the organic psychoses and dementia praecox (schizophrenia) took, and the differences between them, were landmarks in the development of psychiatry.

Meyer, however, was more concerned with the uniqueness of each individual rather than with what he or she had in common with others, and saw each illness as a psychobiological reaction, involving physical, psychological and environmental influences, all of which were relevant to the patient's history. Meyer's approach had more to contribute to the understanding of personality problems, and in particular enabled a multi-factorial, clinical and social developmental perspective to be taken which is why it looked as if it would help illuminate the problems of children. Meyer's influence and that of his followers in psychiatry and outside led to the formation of the National Committee of Mental Hygiene in the United States in 1909, the Chicago Juvenile Psychopathic Clinic in the same year, the Judge Baker Guidance Centre in Boston in 1917, and the Boston Habit Clinic in 1921, bringing together the work of psychiatrists, psychologists, and social workers.

These developments were closely followed in England, and in the 1920s similar clinics were set up, the first being the East London Child Guidance Clinic, directed by Emmanuel Miller (Renton, 1978), while the first patient ever seen at the newly established Tavistock Clinic in 1920, was a child (Dicks, 1970). The Maudsley Hospital, which opened in 1923, had registered 44 child and adolescent patients in the first year of its operation, its children's clinics (and later Department) developing between 1927 and 1935, the new Children's Department being formally opened in 1939, with places for in-patients.

From then the developments spread; by 1939 there were 46 clinics in Great

Britain, some relying on voluntary workers and some on charity, local authorities first maintaining clinics from 1935 (National Association for Mental Health, 1965; Warren, 1971). These developments were full of an idealism and optimism that were to last some 40 years; what miracles might not medicine, science, and sociology achieve together? Fifty years later, Whitmore (1974) wrote in an ultimately optimistic and certainly constructive paper that the proper responsibility for the child guidance service was not clear, hinting courteously at a competition for its control between health, education and social service departments which has since become more overt (Steinberg, 1981c); uncertainty, misunderstandings and disagreement about terminology, aims and clientele; changes in social work, psychology, psychiatry, and paediatrics which have brought about changes in the task and in the demands of interdisciplinary collaboration; and shortages and maldistribution of staff, so that the unmet demand is large. He also urged caution about using too readily epidemiological evidence of the prevalence of children's emotional and behavioural problems to indicate a need for more clinics. As Rutter (1970; Rutter et al., 1977a) has pointed out not all such problems need psychiatric help.

Meanwhile, the clinics which see adolescents may be found linked to general, psychiatric, or paediatric hospitals (with or without in-patient units, which may or may not include beds for adolescents); partially or wholly organized by health, education or social service departments, though usually uneasily shared between them; and with differing emphasis on the type of assessments made and the nature of the work undertaken depending on the relative experience and influence of the members of staff.

Units for child and adolescent in-patients had begun in the 19th century with the facilities for the severely mentally retarded. In the United States, units were set up in the 1920s, primarily for children with the after-effects of encephalitis and by the 1930s several in-patient units for children and adolescents were describing their experiences (Klopp 1932; Potter, 1934; Beskind, 1962; Barker, 1974 b.c.). It is interesting that the early accounts emphasized the need for a systematically planned programme with academic and occupational as well as clinical components, and control over admissions by the staff so that a therapeutic atmosphere could be maintained. Barker (1974 b.c) gives an interesting account of these developments in the United States and in Britain, pointing out their considerable differences in clientele, methods, and leadership; the direction was not always by a psychiatrist, and the residential units quite often regarded more as homes or schools than hospital departments (see, for example, Aichorn, 1935; Bettelheim, 1950; French, 1963). Throughout the literature the central importance of the social and educational milieu in helping adolescents whatever their problems, the importance of psychological understanding and methods, the varying contribution of psychiatrists (who themselves vary considerably in theoretical orientation), the importance of dealing with staff tension and communication, and the importance of clarity about authority and control, have been recurring and important themes (see, for example, Bettelheim and Sylvester, 1952; Redl and Wineman, 1951, 1952; Rioch and Stanton, 1953; Rinsley, 1963).

In the United Kingdom, the first in-patient adolescent units were opened in 1948 (at St Ebbas Hospital, Epsom, later moving to Long Grove Hospital nearby) and 1949 (at Bethlem); it is of interest that both St Ebbas's and the joint Maudsley–Bethlem Hospitals together took largely voluntary patients, an innovation of the 1930s, and for this reason received many adolescent referrals (Warren, 1971). The St Ebbas's unit has been described by Sands (1953) and the early years of the Bethlem by Warren (1952). Beech House, near Canterbury, was opened soon after (Turle, 1960).

Since then some 30–40 adolescent units have been developed in Britain, particularly over the past 15 years, with a total number of around 700 beds (Association for the Psychiatric Study of Adolescents, 1976; Peterson, 1980). The exact numbers vary depending on how adolescence is defined, whether only primarily psychiatric units are included (as opposed, for example, to those intended primarily for young people with mental retardation) and whether small nests of adolescent beds in children's or adult's wards are included; moreover, some adolescent units tend to come and go over the years. They vary considerably in their philosophy and clientele (see Allchin *et al.*, 1967; Berg and Griffiths, 1970; Evans and Acton, 1972; Bruggen *et al.*, 1973; Wardle, 1974; Framrose, 1975; Perinpanayagam, 1978; Wells *et al.*, 1978; Bedford and Tennent, 1981; Steinberg *et al.*, 1981). Many of these units developed in their existing adult mental hospital settings, and continue to be influenced by them, characteristically with recurring conflict with the parent hospital about autonomy and resources; an intriguing parallel with adolescence itself.

An editorial in the first issue of the *Journal of Adolescence* has outlined a number of the developments in adolescent psychiatry which led to the foundation in Britain in 1969 of the Association for the Psychiatric Study of Adolescents, and particularly a conference on adolescent psychiatry organized three years earlier at which the speakers included a nurse, a teacher and psychotherapist, an administrator and a psychiatrist (*Journal of Adolescence,* 1978). Multi-professional clinical work, teaching, research and organization has been a special hallmark of child and adolescent psychiatry's development, and is reflected in the leadership and membership of both the Association for the Psychiatric Study of Adolescents and a rather more academically orientated fellow in the field, the Association for Child Psychology and Psychiatry, founded in 1956 (MacKeith, 1976). These two organizations, and the Child and Adolescent Psychiatry section of the Royal College of Psychiatrists, have together made important contributions to the broad field's development and its representation at all levels at which social policy is formulated.

To this complex network of organizational, legal, social, educational, psychological, and medical developments must be added enormous variation in schools of thought. It would be an elaborate exercise indeed to try to summarize the different conceptual models and methods in use in contemporary psychiatry (see, for example, Clare, 1976; Tyrer and Steinberg, in preparation), and the recent pattern of changing fashions in diagnosis and management. It is intriguing that in the family therapy approach to adolescent problems insistence on the authority and expertise of the professional worker and the firm setting of limits currently appears to be in the ascendant, while these qualities are apparently less fashionable and even actively discouraged in the community at large, at least in the West; and the first academic paper which finds a place for the spanking [*sic*] of young children in certain circumstances has now appeared. (Bean and Roberts, 1981).

Different conceptual models of development, diagnosis, and treatment, and how to integrate some of them in practice are recurring themes in subsequent chapters. As far as actual resources are concerned, how might the range of facilities for adolescents look from the viewpoint of, say, a child psychiatrist who works in a child guidance clinic in England? (see also Figure 7.)

He or she will probably have as immediate colleagues a social worker or two, an educational psychologist and perhaps a part-time child psychotherapist and one or two secretaries; probably more than half the clinic's clientele will be adolescents.

Anywhere between 5 and 50 miles away there will be an in-patient adolescent unit, probably likely to be able to cope with only a segment of the spectrum of young people's cases referred to it. The occasional very ill adolescent or one who has taken an overdose will be seen in the local general hospital, and perhaps, in an emergency, admitted to a paediatric ward. There may be a similar *ad hoc* admission arrangement with the local adult psychiatric hospital. There may be a second adolescent unit, rather inaccessible for administrative or geographic reasons, which takes a different general approach to the nearest one.

Apart from the adolescent unit psychiatrist, there will be contact with the psychiatrist at the clinics in neighbouring towns, and occasional teaching or administrative meetings.

The social service department (by whom his social worker colleagues are employed) will have access to children's homes, reception centres and hostels and, usually with some difficulty, to more physically secure homes on the one hand and long-term homes and hostels run on broadly psychotherapeutic lines on the other. The difficulties are because of distance, selectivity, waiting lists and cost, because many such facilities are outside the usual resources of the local authority and separate funds must be found to support an adolescent being placed there; this may amount to a special commitment of many thousands of pounds for each boy or girl. Admission to hospital, of course, does not result in a direct charge on the local authority.

Exactly the same applies to the education department, which will have its own day and residential schools for children with special needs, but which will not

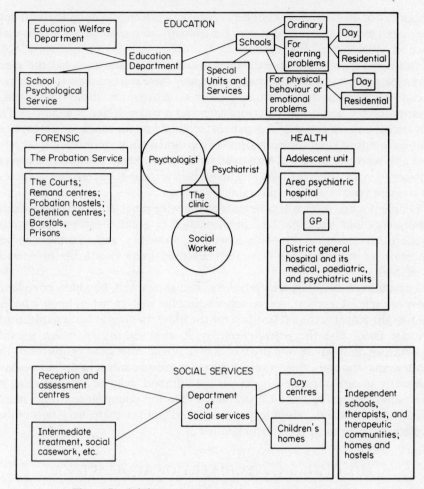

Figure 7   Adolescent services – the view from the clinic

meet the requirements of all. Independent residential schools, perhaps over-lapping in style and quality with therapeutic communities, may be approached on a psychiatric recommendation, and again, paid for separately out of a limited budget. The School Psychological Service, where the clinic's educational psychologist operates independently of the clinic, will run its own assessment, liaison, consultation, and treatment service. How and whether this integrates with the work of the clinic is up to the psychiatrist and psychologist concerned.

Adolescents will be referred from time to time by and to the social service department, sometimes from the courts. Recommendations to a court may include providing any of the resources mentioned above, but sometimes, with or without the psychiatrist's support, an adolescent may go off to a detention centre or borstal, or an older adolescent may be sent to a prison for young adults (if only for assessment on remand) and, very occasionally, to one of the special hospitals such as Moss Side or Broadmoor.

Out-patient and day-patient arrangements will depend on what the clinic arranges, and what is available nearby. Usually there will be access to one or two social service department training centres, usually for those with mental retardation but occasionally a centre caters for a wider degree of handicap. The adolescent unit may provide day-patient facilities, and the education department may have tutorial units or equivalent centres, and a home tutor service, for boys and girls who cannot or will not attend their school. There will also be a careers advisory service which can offer invaluable help for school leavers, and has access to training centres and special training schemes.

Different social service departments offer a wide range of schemes for helping adolescents and their families, supplemented in some areas by the Family Welfare Association and other independent, voluntary, and charitable bodies. There is no substitute for constantly updated local knowledge of what is available.

For adolescents with special problems such as deafness, blindness or epilepsy there are special teachers, special schools and the well-known voluntary bodies such as the Royal National Institute for the Blind, the Royal National Institute for the Deaf, and the British Epilepsy Association, all of which provide information and advice and are well aware of the emotional problems of the adolescents who come their way. Facilities for the mentally retarded adolescent, especially in late adolescence and early adulthood, may be disappointing or profoundly worrying for all concerned, while for young people with major personality problems, chronic psychoses and autism there may be nothing available at all except for a fortunate few.

THE CLINICAL PSYCHIATRY OF ADOLESCENCE

As already pointed out, psychiatrists may work in any number of quite different ways. The point of attempting to define the special function of clinical psychiatry is not to propose a professional straitjacket for the psychiatrist, or any other worker, but rather to define one particular job among many that are needed in the broad field of adolescent care.

Clinical refers to the bedside (Greek—*klinikos*) and points to the essentially medical orientation of clinical work. The medical model is a much maligned term, and much debated (Macklin, 1973; Kety, 1974; Ullman and Krasner, 1975; Clare, 1976, 1979a; Tyrer and Steinberg, in preparation). A recently fashionable school of thought has seen the medical model as either a gross misunderstanding of the true nature of psychiatric problems or as a professional conspiracy by which the 'establishment', usually referring primarily to authorities in the Western world and the northern hemisphere, keeps the people in their allotted places (Laing, 1960, 1967; Szasz, 1961, 1971, 1973; Illich, 1977; Kennedy, 1981). It is certainly a mistake to regard the medical model as primarily concerned with disease processes, if only because the way in which medical practice has always been conducted has recognized that internal physical disease processes are only one aspect of medicine, which is not to say that most medical practitioners have tended to handle the non-organic aspects well.

The essence of medical practice, and therefore the medical model, is primarily concerned with the diagnosis, treatment or prevention of *individual disorder*. Macklin (1973), for example, has summarized the medical model in relation to psychiatry by pointing out that psychological, like physical, ailments present themselves with symptoms (which the patient complains of) and signs (which the clinician sees, feels or hears for himself) and that there is assumed to be an underlying disordered state which produced them. This, in my view, applies as much to the concept of (for example) an Oedipal conflict or abnormal physiological conditioning presumed to be going on 'within' the patient, as to notions of organic disorder. The psychoanalyst, the individual psychotherapist, and the behaviour therapist tend to work on this basis and to this extent employ the medical model. In such work it is believed that the problem is at some level or in some sense within the individual, and that it represents deviation from normal functioning.

This is important in the practice of adolescent psychiatry for two main reasons. First, many adolescents referred to psychiatrists are not individually disordered in this sense. Second, much professional work with these adolescents is not primarily concerned with individual disorder. The task of the teacher is to help develop skills to the full, not to treat disorder; the task of the lawyer is to represent the client's views and position, not to correct what may or may not be wrong with him; most counsellors and some psychotherapists see their role as helping the individual develop his or her full potential and deal with the normal difficulties in living and not with treating disorder. As already pointed out, Ragg (1977) has reminded social workers of the alternative approaches possible within their profession: as representatives and clarifiers of the cases of their clientele; or as diagnosticians and therapists. (It seems to me that family therapists have not entirely clarified this: on the one hand their theory and practice emphasizes the problem (or 'sickness' according to some usage) in the family as a whole, not the individual; yet in their work the symptomatic progress of the referred individual tends to remain the key criterion of referral and discharge. To this extent some family therapists seem to use a dual medical and social dynamic model.)

An important quality of the medical model is the willingness and varying ability of physicians to use biological, social, and psychological (behavioural and psychodynamic) concepts in their attempts to make sense of the individual's current state, and in mobilizing ways of helping so that the interaction between all aspects of the environment and all aspects of individual functioning can be considered in diagnosis and treatment (Ferris, 1936; Eisenberg, 1973, 1977;

Chess, 1979; Rutter, 1980); and of particular importance in the case of children and adolescents is the concept of developmental change. Thus the *medical model* acknowledges the importance of interaction at several levels of functioning (whether, for example, in the maintenance of blood pressure, blood sugar level or schizophrenic beliefs) as the result of interacting physiological, psychological, and social systems; while the *developmental model* adds the dimension of growth and change over time. The developmental model is complex and important and is discussed in Chapter 4. In so far as the subject is health and disorder, the developmental model may be used as a particularly complex version of the medical model and particularly applicable to child and adolescent psychiatry.

Medical practice, then, is concerned with the cause, prevention, and cure of individual disorder understood in biological, psychological, and social terms and clinical practice represents its application to individual problems. The clinical model, therefore, represents a medical theoretical framework and a particular professional–client transaction, in which A, the clinician, professes to understand the ways in which there may be something wrong with B (see Figure 8).

In the broad field of work in which troubled adolescents present:

(a) the clinical approach is quite often inappropriate, which is widely recognized; but

(b) it is often appropriate too, a fact which is *not* so well recognized, particularly by professional workers who tend not to see those boys and girls for whom the clinical model is helpful;

(c) it has a number of important advantages and disadvantages in work with young people.

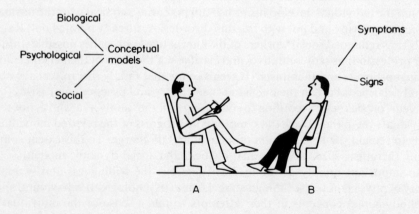

A diagnoses B's disorder

Figure 8   The clinical model of diagnosis and treatment

Table 2   Some advantages and disadvantages of the medical model and the clinical approach

---

Advantages
1. Eclectic: versatile in diagnosis and treatment methods
2. Innovative
3. Authoritative: high status
4. Professional independence and autonomy
5. Capacity for taking on difficult and unrewarding problems

Disadvantages
1. Complex, specialized, expensive
2. Tendency to technical, formal professionalism
3. Apparent strengths may undermine normal coping mechanisms
4. Authority can be used inappropriately; can be practised idiosyncratically with little effective challenge. More economic and efficient ways of helping may be discouraged.
5. Clientele may be chosen arbitrarily: can raise false hopes and professional service may be patchy

---

Some advantages and disadvantages of the clinical approach (see Table 2)

Advantages

1. It is well suited by its eclecticism for exploring complex and difficult problems where more straightforward measures have not succeeded.
2. Similarly, its conceptual range *and* the resources granted by the community to clinical practice can result in considerable innovation in the medical field and outside.
3. The relative authority accorded to doctors can be helpful for patients and the community as well as for doctors themselves, for example in seeing difficult problems and solutions through in the face of legal and ethical uncertainty.
4. Doctors' relative autonomy is in contrast to that of many other professional workers who are answerable to complex hierarchical and bureaucratic organizations. This can be advantageous, particularly in work with adolescents where personal authority is important.
5. For all the above reasons and the sanction for risk-taking socially permitted, doctors are able to take on problems which may be particularly difficult and unrewarding, for example in the fields of chronic illness and handicap.

Disadvantages

1. Clinical practice is inclined to be elaborate, complex, specialized, expensive, or all of these things.
2. It tends towards a technical, formal professionalism that is not the most appropriate way of responding to many of the problems of children and their families.

3. Its implications (of individual disorder) can work against the adolescent, the family and the community taking the responsibilities that they should.
4. Its status, authority, and autonomy can produce excessive compliance and a misplaced faith in magical solutions which can discourage more economic and appropriate ways of helping, and professional idiosyncracies may be very difficult to challenge.
5. Just as the range and status of medical practice allows difficult and challenging problems to be taken on, they may just as arbitrarily be neglected.

Other conceptual models and approaches

There is good reason to regard the *psychoanalytic model* as akin to the medical model in its attribution of individual disorder to the interplay of psychobiological forces which the diagnostician/therapist is trained to understand (see, for example, Eisenberg, 1970; Clare, 1979a).

It has been argued that the *behavioural model* is fundamentally different from the medical model in that it denies the existence of a disease process underlying symptoms, and instead treats the symptoms themselves; nevertheless, the process of individual assessment of abnormal behaviour and the prescription of a programme of treatment (Eysenck, 1960, 1975) with diagnosis and treatment based on a particular theoretical model comes so close to the medical model that to contrast it to the medical approach as Eysenck has done (1975) seems pedantic *except* where the behaviour to be modified is not considered abnormal. This is an important distinction; if a man or woman wished to change a particular preference (for example sexual) by a behavioural programme, this is equivalent to learning a new skill rather than having treatment for a disorder.

Social models are most clearly antithetical to medical concepts of individual disorder and its derivatives. Social factors have long been recognized as crucially important in the origin of psychiatric disorder and in the problems of its definition (Lewis, 1955; Rosen, 1968; Foucault, 1967, 1970) but as already pointed out there is a large body of opinion holding that psychiatry is at worst one of several methods of social oppression (Szasz, 1961, 1971, 1973) or at best a gross misunderstanding of the pain and confusion of many people (Laing, 1960, 1967). The following are the main ways in which social concepts are relevant to adolescent psychiatry:

1. *Social factors as sufficient causes of disorder*

For example, the views of Bateson *et al.* (1956), Lidz (1968), and Laing (1967) that particular patterns of parent–child interaction and communication are so chaotic that the individual who is ultimately designated schizophrenic has been forced to adopt a defensive style that appears 'mad'. This view fades into the antipsychiatry view that this defensive or adaptive position may be wrongly labelled as mad.

2. *Social factors as contributions to disorder*

For example, there is ample evidence that marital breakdown with overt discord accompanied by rejection of a child may well lead to more or less enduring behaviour disturbance (Rutter, 1979c), and that people susceptible to schizophrenic breakdown are vulnerable to certain patterns of family stress (Vaughn and Leff, 1976).

3. *Social factors as phenomena associated with disorder*

For example, conduct disorder is associated with large families, educational backwardness, a deprived and overcrowded home, inconsistent discipline and family discord (Rutter, 1975). These factors, individually, do not cause conduct disorders, and conduct disorder occurs in their absence. But they are environmental factors to be aware of in considering the aetiology and nature of children's problems, preventative policies, and in mobilizing help.

4. *Patterns of social behaviour which may themselves be taken as problems and responded to as such, without invoking concepts of individual disorder*

At this point we move significantly away from the clinical concept of individual disorder. Thus according to the systems theory of a family behaviour, a child with worrying or annoying behaviour would be seen as maintained in that pattern of feeling or behaviour by the way the family operates as a whole (see Bruggen and Davies, 1977). Whether the child is regarded as 'disordered' or not if this perspective is taken seems to depend on the preference of the family therapist. Certainly all emphasize the family, not the individual, as the dysfunctional unit, although as already pointed out the referred adolescent's symptoms seem to be a focus of work for some family therapists for at least some of the time.

Another example is the use of the crisis of, say, a family's or children's home's *inability to cope* with an adolescent's mood or behaviour as the focus of work, rather than the issue of whether or not the adolescent is ill and needs treatment (Bruggen *et al.*, 1973). The problem then selected for work, at least at the point of crisis, is the difficulty the adults have in continuing to carry adult responsibilities.

5. *Social factors as determinants of the use of services*

As will be discussed in Chapter 5, the arbitrary nature of the referral process in child and adolescent psychiatry is well known. We can assume that large numbers of boys and girls are referred to psychiatrists who may well have been referred to quite different professional workers depending on chance factors in people's attitudes, knowledge, and the availability of resources.

6. *Social factors related to wider developmental needs*

Facors 1–5 are related in some way to the concept of disorder and its treatment. But the non-clinical social needs of children, that is upbringing and education in their widest senses, are social aspects of children's lives of which the clinician must be constantly aware since, as already pointed out, they are required by all children whether they also need treatment or not.

7. *Social factors affecting psychiatric authority*

Traditionally medical practice has been characterized or caricatured by two contrasting attitudes: unremitting hard and conscientious clinical and scientific work on the one hand, attempting to match rigorous method with the disarray and muddle of real life; and more or less well-intentioned deception on the other. There are countless anecdotes to illustrate the latter: 'Always say the case is grave', advised a physician whose name fortunately perhaps I cannot trace, and medical writing particularly of the older schools is replete with similar recommendations.* Clinical practice has to balance confident authority, on the one hand, against lack of useful knowledge and the unpredictability of people's lives and progress on the other, and has often achieved an uneasy balance by adopting a paternalistic, protective approach.

Cultural and social attitudes (including the clinician's own) profoundly affect clinical practice (see Table 3). Less subtle considerations affect the authority of psychiatrists too. The attacks of the antipsychiatrists have already been mentioned; and there is of course a politically revolutionary position that anything which contributes to the stability of the social fabric of the community is therefore to be undermined on quasi-moralistic grounds, an approach which has made some psychiatrists oversensitive to constructive criticism from organizations such as MIND (see, for example, Smythe, 1981). Legal and professional developments, too, such as the power of social workers to challenge the psychiatrist's ability to detain patients against their will, cause recurrent disquiet and real problems for psychiatric practice (Timbury, 1981). From a somewhat different angle, reflections about the limitations of psychiatry (Nunn, 1981) are liable to elicit pained rejoinders about ways in which it can be more rewarding (Snaith, 1981).

No specialty rests on more uncertain foundations than psychiatry, and no area of activity is so full of arbitrary assertions, legal and practical inconsistencies, major and minor injustices, instability of status and inconstancy of purpose as the socio-political field. Nevertheless as Eisenberg (1975) has pointed out, it is within this context that far-reaching decisions for the individual and for the

---

*'Keep up the spirits of your patient with the music of the viol and the psaltery,' advised Mondeville, 'or by forging letters telling of the death of his enemies, or (if he be a cleric) by informing him that he has been made a bishop'.

Table 3   Social factors involved in clinical practice

Factors	Example
As *causes* of disorder – or of behaviour labelled as disorder	Bateson *et al.*'s (1956) concepts of the schizophrenogenic family. Or Laing's (1967)
As *contributory factor* in disorder	Vaughn and Leff (1976): vulnerability of some ill patients to certain patterns of family stress
As factors *associated with* disorder	'Clustering' of conduct disorder with such factors as large families, educational backwardness, deprived and overcrowded homes, inconsistent discipline, and family discord. (Rutter, 1975)
Social patterns of behaviour *which may themselves be taken as problems and responded to as such, e.g.* by family work, family therapy or consultation	Using the crisis of inability to cope with an adolescent as the focus of work, rather than the concept of the adolescent's disorder (Bruggen *et al.*, 1973)
Social factors as *determinants of use of services*	The arbitrary nature of the referral process: see Chapter 5
Social factors related to *developmental needs.* Non-clinical	The parenting, educational, recreational, social, legal, and other aspects of children's and adolescents' lives which apply to all children, whether or not they need treatment, and with which the clinician must work
Social factors which affect the clinician's authority to act	Social and cultural attitudes which may result in unhelpful challenges or unhelpful deference to psychiatric authority; legal and ethical issues which complicate clinical decisions

community must be made, and the confident assertion of authority and the making of clear and defensible decisions is particularly important in work with disturbed adolescents.

CONCLUSIONS

1. The clinical psychiatric approach is one among many, and requires reasonable definition and clarity. It is concerned with the diagnosis of individual disorder, and its treatment if necessary, by means which draw upon biological psychological and social conceptual models. It can be overrated and underrated; the problem is that it is overrated for some tasks with adolescents, and underrated for others. The first responsibility of the clinical psychiatrist is to be clear about the nature of his or her special skills, and about what can and cannot be done by psychiatry.

2. The time-consuming nature of properly conducted clinical assessment and treatment, the arbitrary realities of the referral process, and not least the side-effects of being a patient, mean that there will be a number of referred adolescents who need not and indeed should not be seen.

3. Hand-in-hand with giving priority to a competent clinical assessment procedure, the provision of helpful alternatives for those not seen is imperative. The alternatives will include: (a) the availability of comprehensive, accurate, and up-to-date information and advice on alternative services, for many referring agents will not know of most of what is available in adolescent psychiatry and outside; (b) a dual consultative–diagnostic approach (page 15) providing clinical diagnosis and treatment appropriate to the needs of the case, while making time and space for this by developing an efficient consultative service the purpose of which is to clarify what alternative forms of help are needed by whom. This consultative aspect of work provides an essential intermediate function: to 'hold' and help with the considerable anxiety that may be mounting in adolescent, family, and indeed in the referring professional worker while the nature of the problem is clarified. Thus it may be that a boy or girl is ultimately taken on (or admitted to an in-patient setting) for a planned piece of clinical work, understood and agreed by all concerned, after perhaps days or weeks of careful consultation, information-gathering, and preparation, instead of being taken on in the overheated flurry of a quasi-emergency.

4. Working in this way makes time for occasions when lengthy crisis-intervention with a family or institution or urgent clinical work with a boy or girl is necessary. There are adolescents who must be seen quickly, but a non-selective policy will result only in a silting up of the appointments system with young people and their families who not only could wait a little longer, but would get a more helpful and effective response as a result of doing so. Some form of differential approach to referrals must be adopted simply because the arithmetic of referrals to most clinics means that for much of the time there is no alternative. Nevertheless there is a need for studies to be carried out to help predict who it is most helpful to see quickly, the type of work that needs to be done in such circumstances (e.g. family crisis-intervention), and what happens to those who receive alternatives to on-demand clinical care.

5. The two fundamental components of the clinical approach (the diagnosis of individual disorder and a multi-dimensional use of conceptual models in diagnosis and treatment) is a way of proceeding, not an end in itself. No psychiatric diagnosis may be made; there may be no abnormality at all, or an individual problem identified in terms of intellectual performance or some other aspect of cognitive function rather than psychiatric abnormality. Correspondingly, establishment of psychiatric disorder in an individual adolescent does not mean that individual psychiatric treatment necessarily follows. An adolescent may have an emotional or behavioural disorder best managed, for example, by work with his or her family or school.

6. Whatever clinical work is done, the education, care, and control needed by all children and adolescents is needed no less by the adolescent patient too; indeed, in most cases more carefully planned education, care, and sometimes control will be required.

7. Since this chapter has dealt with questions of role and definition it is worth acknowledging that the distinction between treatment for identified individual disorder (i.e. clinical treatment) and work described as 'therapy' is not clear. Certainly many forms of educational and social training, art therapy, psychotherapy, and family therapy have more in common with education and counselling, fostering personal development, than with treatment aimed at correcting disorder.

8. This emphasis on a selective approach to those boys and girls who are referred, does not mean that the practice of clinical psychiatry with adolescents should be a remote operation. In fact the reverse is the case. To be in a position to select adolescents appropriately for clinical work, to help meet their wider educational, family, and social needs in a comprehensive way, and to be able to respond helpfully and effectively on behalf of adolescents not taken on as patients, the clinical team must be more accessible, not less; it should be able and willing to offer information, advice, and consultation, so that its specialized clinical work is balanced by close involvement and familiarity with the community served. The more highly developed a team's clinical skills become, the greater is its responsibility to develop accessible advisory, consultative, and educational functions to complement them, and in these activities are the seeds of preventative work.

Chapter 4

The Emergence of Problems: I. Development

INTRODUCTION

The interaction between individual characteristics and environmental influences determines how the individual adolescent is at any given time; and
should the boy or girl present problems for someone, they may be perceived as
psychiatric in nature and the young person referred to a psychiatric clinic. The
process of becoming a psychiatric patient is therefore a two-stage process: the
first largely determined by biological, psychological, and social factors; and the
second by those responses to the adolescent which taken together constitute the
referral process (see figure 9). This chapter is concerned with the processes of the
first stage, and Chapter 5 with the referral process.

DEVELOPMENT

The processes involved in development are:
1. *Multiple*, i.e. not representable by a single sort of observation, measurement
   or conceptual model.
2. *Developing and changing*, not static.
3. *The multiple and changing factors interact with each other*; they do not operate
   in isolation.
4. *The interaction is dynamic* in the sense that changes in one part of the
   interacting system bring about changes elsewhere.
This is a complex but necessary way of looking at the problems of children and
adolescents and is discussed further on page 64 *et seq.*

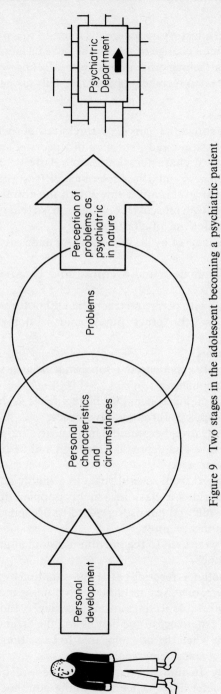

Figure 9   Two stages in the adolescent becoming a psychiatric patient

Example 3

A boy of 15 with a history of epilepsy is referred to a psychiatric clinic because soon after a change of schools he became increasingly moody and aggressive, attacking other pupils physically and verbally and now beginning to threaten members of staff. He tells his parents he would rather be dead.

1. *Multiple factors*

(a) Clinically he shows the signs of a depressive state with high levels of anxiety, low self-esteem and loss of confidence and suicidal ideas.

(b) His personality characteristics seem relatively immature, with marked impulsiveness and a low tolerance of frustration.

(c) His intellectual level is at the low end of the normal range, and he had special difficulty in muscular coordination, so that he shines neither in theoretical classes nor practical work.

(d) His father is angered by his misbehaviour and is distancing himself from him.

(e) His mother is anxious and overprotective because of his sadness and his fits.

(f) Relationships with peers and teachers at school are very poor: he is unpopular, alarms the other pupils and is doing badly at his schoolwork.

2. *Changing factors*

(a) He has recently experienced a somewhat belated spurt in growth and sexual development.

(b) The pattern of his epilepsy is changing as is his response to medication as he passes through adolescence.

(c) Despite his relative personality immaturity, he is more able to articulate aggressive and depressive ideation and be able to act on it, than he was a year ago.

(d) He has changed from several years in a highly structured school where he was the oldest in class, reasonably popular, doing reasonably well and where staff and pupils were used to his epilepsy, to a school where all the opposites apply.

(e) His parents were used to the previous school but are apprehensive about the new one.

(f) The boy's mother is reacting to the new situation by becoming more anxious and overprotective; his father by becoming more irritable and distant. Uncomfortable feelings of anxiety, guilt, and mutual blame dating from the experience of the first fit and the diagnosis of epilepsy, almost forgotten when the boy appeared to be settling successfully at his first school, are surfacing again.

(g) He is nearly 16 and his parents fear he will not manage the expectations of later adolescence and young adulthood as well as he coped with those of earlier childhood. They cannot imagine him leaving home, becoming self-supporting or marrying. They are not sure what sort of institution or organization will be able to help them and him if he has to leave school; he may not manage to get into a training course and finding work seems remote.

(h) His fits are getting worse and more frequent, his doctors are trying different drugs in different doses and beginning to say that the problem is 'psychiatric'.

3. *Interaction*

(a) His new medication is giving him still more difficulty in containing his moods and in concentrating at his work without improving his epilepsy.

(b) His recent physical development is affecting his own moods and other people's expectations of him.

(c) The change of school is also changing other people's expectations of him.

(d) His greater difficulties at school are making his mother more anxious and his father more angry.

(e) His parents' stronger and different feelings are causing discord between them and increasing the boy's anxiety.

(f) His worsening behaviour and performance are making his present teachers and doctors less confident about taking responsibility for him.

(g) This, in turn (f) is adding to his parents' troubled feelings.

4. *Dynamic interaction*

(a) Recent changes in development and schooling have affected his precarious self-esteem and made him more anxious.

(b) He has coped with his anxiety in immature ways, resulting in worse behaviour and more anxiety and developmental and mood changes have exacerbated his epilepsy.

(c) His parents' old anxieties (and differences) about his epilepsy have resurfaced, adding to the tension and insecurity at home.

(d) The doctors have tried to correct this destabilizing process (as shown by his worsened mood and epilepsy) by the use of medication, but this has made him more anxious and irritable and less able to concentrate on his schoolwork; while his teachers' lack of confidence in handling him has made his behaviour more erratic.

(e) The teachers' and doctors' lack of success has added to the parents' anxiety about their son's future and this in turn is making him more anxious. His behaviour and fits worsen.

Development and aetiology

The number of processes outlined in the example above may be daunting, but it is possible to think of aetiology in child psychiatry in oversimplistic terms: an individual, an adolescent for example, is the way he or she is today 'because' of a biochemical abnormality or because of circumstances in early life which led to the formation of a particular intrapsychic conflict. For some disorders in some people relatively straightforward 'X results in Y' models of causation may in due course be confirmed; but the evidence does not make it very likely that such one-to-one aetiological relationships will have wide application, and in the present state of knowledge it is not easy to separate significant from redundant data in a reasonably scientific way.

This does not mean that the aetiology of psychiatric disorder must necessarily be complex, but that more complex models of human functioning, especially those which cross disciplinary boundaries, require exploration before simple aetiological models will work reliably. It could emerge, for example, that children whose intellectual development takes the pattern X, whose emotional development is delayed within normal limits according to pattern Y, and who temperamentally readily become highly aroused, withdrawn and anxious, are likely to become clinically obsessional if in middle childhood their parents behave in pattern Z. This, it must be emphasized, is psychiatric science fiction, but it illustrates the style in which we may have to think and the sort of observations we may have to make to explain longitudinally, interactionally, and multi-dimensionally, how a boy or girl develops normally or abnormally. Such constructions are no more complex than many biochemical, neural or psychodynamic notions, but represent a different, developmental approach to understanding normality and disorder.

CONCEPTUAL MODELS OF DEVELOPMENT

Multiplicity of factors

People function at many levels. The processes involved in family relationships, for example, are influences of a different order to social and cultural factors such as family income, neighbourhood facilities, and moral attitudes (see figure 10). Similarly the pattern of behaviour of an adolescent may be best understood in terms of the way he is handled by his parents, his psychological functioning or his body biochemistry. All these levels require consideration and although all will not be needed in the diagnosis, all need to be understood to make sense of a child's development. This stratification of function, much simplified for the purposes of an overall scheme for development presented here is consistent with the concept of stratification of successive hierarchies of function formulated by Hughlings Jackson (1884) and Sherrington (1906) and integrated with psychodynamic and developmental theory by, for example, Ey (Evans, 1972), Smythies (1966), and Meyersburg and Post (1979).

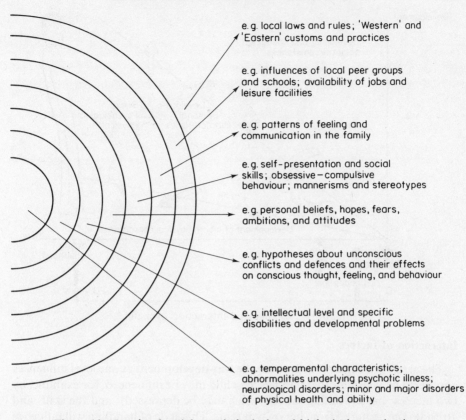

e.g. local laws and rules; 'Western' and 'Eastern' customs and practices

e.g. influences of local peer groups and schools; availability of jobs and leisure facilities

e.g. patterns of feeling and communication in the family

e.g. self-presentation and social skills; obsessive – compulsive behaviour; mannerisms and stereotypes

e.g. personal beliefs, hopes, fears, ambitions, and attitudes

e.g. hypotheses about unconscious conflicts and defences and their effects on conscious thought, feeling, and behaviour

e.g. intellectual level and specific disabilities and developmental problems

e.g. temperamental characteristics; abnormalities underlying psychotic illness; neurological disorders; minor and major disorders of physical health and ability

Figure 10   Levels of social, psychological, and biological organization

Development and change in these factors

Figure 11, simplified to include only broad categories, illustrates change over time, which in fact occurs in all the levels of Figure 10, at different rates and at different times. Ideas of acceptable, normal behaviour change over time just as the adolescent changes over time. Sexual behaviour, for example, often an issue in deciding on an adolescent's maturity, normality or delinquency, is dependent on the current views and mores of the culture and the family, including what they expect and teach and what they tolerate at different ages; the social setting and circumstances; the individual's personal and legal relationship with anyone else involved; what the law allows the individual to do; social skills and habits; actual behaviour; attitudes, ideas, and mood; physical development, emotional maturity, and biochemical state, including, for example, sex hormone function and adrenal functioning. All these factors change, and at different rates and times.

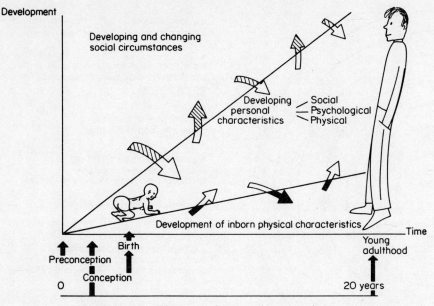

Figure 11   Change and interaction over time

Interaction of factors

The arrows in Figure 11 illustrate the way development at one level influences another. The way a mother handles her child may be influenced, for example, by two factors: her prevailing mood (which may be depressed); and the skills and attitudes she acquired from her own parents. This style of handling will influence the baby's response. But the baby's response may not be determined only by this, it may be strongly influenced by developmental attributes of the child who may be, say, temperamentally less able to elicit warm stimulating responses from the parent and less adaptable to different patterns of handling. This inherent characteristic of the child will add to the difficulties of the depressed, relatively unskilled mother, who will feel less competent, less confident, more anxious and unhappy and perhaps handle the child still less helpfully.

Dynamic interaction

The dynamic concept links separate interactions together to describe the operation of a more elaborate system, change in one part bringing about change elsewhere (see figure 12).

Example 4
A woman with painful and disruptive experiences in her earlier family background marries an unstable, immature man who manages to

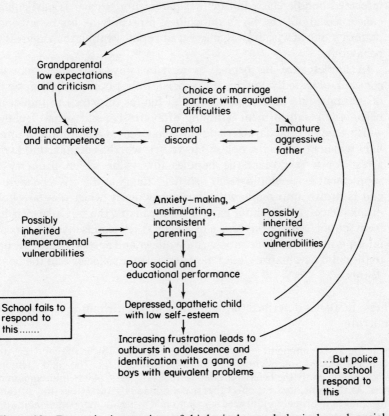

Figure 12 Dynamic interaction of biological, psychological, and social factors

impress her in defiance of her parents' wishes. Bad feeling surrounds the marriage and it is assumed by the mother and father that the children as well as the marriage will be difficult: hence the *preconception* part of the developmental diagram; family and social circumstances in which the child is conceived and into which he or she is born (mother smokes heavily, father drinks heavily and is aggressive, and the advice of the antenatal clinic is largely ignored) begin to operate against the child's development, and when he starts school it is one with poor organization, relatively poor teachers and facilities and the other children have low academic and occupational expectations and interests as well as undisciplined behaviour. Like his father, the boy is not very bright, but in addition has particular difficulty in reading. These are largely inherited vulnerabilities, which could be overcome by skilled teachers, particularly if the child's parents were members of the articulate and informed middle class, but neither parent nor teacher is particularly concerned about the boy's difficulties, especially as his behavioural pattern is one of withdrawal, misery, and apathy rather than aggressive behaviour.

In adolescence he begins to develop physically and sexually, somewhat belatedly, and his poor social skills, poor relationships with his parents, and lack of mature adult figures on which to model his behaviour result in inept handling of aggressive and sexual feelings, which leads to uncharacteristic misbehaviour at school and a street fight which involves the police. His father, who has managed to avoid arrest for a few years (he handles low value stolen property to supplement his unemployment benefit) is angry at the boy's behaviour and is drawn into fights with him, particularly when they are both drunk, once at the school gates which leads to the boy's suspension from school 'until he has seen a psychiatrist'. A bemused family doctor is telephoned by an education welfare officer and agrees to refer the boy to the child psychiatric clinic; the referral letter suggests that the boy is depressed.

Chess (1980) has described the temperamental contribution to development in these terms:

We have found that temperament plays a highly significant role in the child–environment interactional process at sequential age stages of development. The child's temperament influences significantly the behaviour and attitudes of peers, older children, parents, and teachers. At the same time, the effect that these individuals' behaviour and attitudes have on any child as markedly influenced by that child's specific temperamental attributes. Furthermore, temperament, motivation, and cognitive attributes enter into a mutually reciprocal interactional process in helping to shape the child's development at each age period. These findings have been abundantly confirmed by a number of other investigations.

This changing, almost kaleidoscopic pattern may seem impossibly complex, but what is important to grasp is the broad conceptual framework of quite different factors changing and interacting over time, rather than each detail. In practice, which detailed factors are important and require detailed assessment is a matter of clinical judgement; in the example given for instance, it might have emerged that the parents have sufficient warmth and strengths and motivation to bring some order into the family's life and assert some control over their son's behaviour, if (a) they were helped to stand up to their in-laws, and (b) their son had special remedial help at school. The focus in history-taking and in management might be largely to do with family relationships and the boy's cognitive functioning and the sort of teaching he needs. For diagnostic purposes more economical observations and hypotheses must be selected from the range of possibilities; answers to questions such as why does this parent or teacher find this behaviour beyond his or her capacity? Why does this girl have difficulties in this subject and not that one? Why is this boy perfectly well now yet has twice been very disturbed in circumstances which seem identical? This theme, the selection of factors for the diagnostic formulation, is taken up again in Chapter 7.

PHYSICAL DEVELOPMENT

Physiological changes

Puberty is an event, meaning the acquisition of the capacity to reproduce, and it marks the onset of *adolescence*, which refers to the whole period of transition from childhood to adulthood. Together, puberty and adolescence involve changes in physiology, physique, and psychological and social functioning, the latter including changes in the individual's social functioning as well as in social role and expectations.

The marked physiological and physical changes of adolescence are not entirely new. Chromosomal and hormonal activity in foetal life lead to sexual differentiation in the sexually neutral embryo so that internal and external sexual organs develop, but from birth until puberty there is no significant difference between the sexes in sex hormone production, small quantities of both androgens and oestrogens being produced by the adrenal glands in boys and girls. Androgen production in both boys and girls increases at about nine years of age, with a further increase in adolescence that is more marked in boys; oestrogen production rises in both sexes from age seven, with a sharper rise in girls (see Tanner, 1962; Rutter, 1971c, 1980b; and figure 13).

A rise in the level of pituitary gonadotrophins causing the development of ovarian follicles in girls and the testicular tubules in boys is the first event of puberty, and leads in turn to the release of sex hormones which include oestrogen in girls and testosterone in males; up to this time there has been little external physical evidence of the hormonal changes of prepuberty except an increase in activity and energy without any particular change in behaviour towards the opposite sex.

Physical changes

By the age of 11 50% of boys and girls show signs of puberty (Brook, 1981) but there is very wide variation, the onset being in the range 11–16 years in boys and 9–13 in girls, with the subsequent period of physical change being about $4\frac{1}{2}$ years in both sexes and tending to be slightly shorter for girls (data summed up in Rutter, 1980b).

The first sign of puberty in boys is the enlargement of testes from the prepubertal size of a small olive (2 ml) to the size of a large acorn (4 ml) (Brook, 1981), with scanty growth of long, slightly pigmented downy hair at the base of

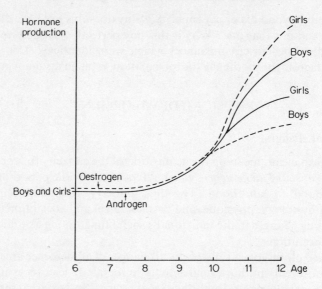

Figure 13   Relative changes between boys and girls in sex
hormone production and puberty (not to scale)

the penis (Tanner, 1962). Subsequent changes are growth and darkening of the
scrotal skin, lengthening and then generally increasing size of the penis, a spurt in
height and laryngeal growth resulting in the changes in voice in adolescent boys.
Axillary and facial hair of the adult pattern appears some two years after the
appearance of pubic hair. Erections of the penis can occur at any age, but are
more frequent now and accompanied by the ability to ejaculate which occurs
early in puberty and is sometimes taken as its first significant sign.

The gain in height at this time is 20 cm (range 10–30 cm) and in weight 20 kg
(range 7–30 kg) with maximum velocity of gain at 14 years (range 12–17). This
general growth is accompanied by other changes, for example in systolic blood
pressure (greater in boys), heart, lung and abdominal size, increased red blood
cell number, a decline in basal metabolism, and increased sebaceous secretion
which, at a time the skin is also changing, produces a tendency to obstruction and
acne. The height increase is due more to increased trunk length than leg length
and contributes to adolescent clumsiness and a need to adapt athletic skills
acquired so far (see, for example, Tanner, 1962; Irwin, 1977; Katchadourian,
1977; Coleman 1980).

Enlargement of the breast buds is the first sign of puberty in girls with elevation
of the breast as a small mound and widening of the areolar diameter (Tanner,
1962), followed by a fine growth of straight downy hair along the labia, later
becoming coarser, darker and more curled, probably earlier in this sequence than
in boys (Eveleth and Tanner, 1977). Menarche, the first menstruation, is usually

taken as the first significant sign of puberty in girls and, like ejaculation in boys, occurs early.

The different sequence in the growth spurt in girls and boys has been reported by Eveleth and Tanner (1977), with boys' height development coming later. This may mean that boys would have more height to gain well after the onset of puberty while for many girls their height spurt would be nearly over once menarche has occurred.

It has often been said that the onset of menstruation has become progressively earlier, with the implication that improved nutrition and possibly other environmental circumstances was leading to earlier puberty at least in girls. Bullough (1981) has re-examined this notion, using classical and medieval documents including those relating to laws about sexual intercourse and marriage and which it may be supposed required accurate information (for example, in Islamic centres it was criminal to have intercourse with a prepubertal girl), and concluded that the age of menarche throughout the world has always been around the age of 12 or 13.

There are later physical changes too, for example in pubic hair which becomes distributed horizontally across the lower abdomen in women and up the linea alba in men, and to the medial surfaces of the thighs in both sexes. The clavicle, the first bone to begin to ossify completes growth and ossification late, around the 18th–25th year, and contributes to the increase in shoulder breadth that may occur in early adulthood.

Most cases of delay in the onset of puberty are constitutional rather than pathological, representing the 3% of normal children who first show signs of puberty after their 14th birthday; how much this runs in families is uncertain. Illnesses such as asthma, pituitary or gonadal disorders, Klinefelter's syndrome (XXY chromosomal abnormality) in boys and Turner's syndrome (XO abnormality) in girls delay or prevent the onset of normal puberty. Possible causes and the most helpful sorts of response are extremely varied; biochemical investigations are not always easy to interpret, and hormonal treatment, when indicated, is fraught with difficulty. Investigation and management require close collaboration between psychiatrist and paediatrician or endocrinologist (see reviews by Money, 1970; Shearin and Jones, 1979; Brook, 1981).

COGNITIVE DEVELOPMENT

Cognition is a large field embodying knowledge and memory, attention and perception, language, reading and mathematical skills, and intelligence – all those mental functions in fact which can be distinguished from emotion, although the relationship between the two is close and complex.

Verbal, mathematical, and visuo-spatial abilities in boys and girls increase throughout adolescence. Such sex differences as there are in the acquisition of verbal ability are unclear. On testing, prepubertal boys and girls perform similarly but with girls slightly more advanced than boys, possibly with language development in girls starting earlier; the advantage girls have in verbal ability is most apparent in adolescence although even then the difference is small, and recent American studies suggest that the difference at least in later adolescence is diminishing. Boys have an advantage over girls in mathematical ability and visual-spatial ability, though studies in the United States are examining the possibilities that the former difference may be strongly influenced environmentally by the type of mathematical education girls receive. Despite the modest differences among normal children and adolescents, disorders of language development are much commoner in boys. (For a review of this field see Maccoby and Jacklin, 1980; Rutter, 1977c; Howlin, 1980).

Intelligence represents 'the broadest and most pervasive cognitive trait' (Butcher, 1970) 'a convenient summary of cognitive ability' (Hindley and Owen, 1978) and more specifically, performance on standardized tests.

It is measured relative to a child's age, because the skills involved increase throughout childhood and adolescence. The intelligence quotient (IQ) is a percentage score comparing a child's performance on standardized tests with the performance of children of comparable age on the same tests. Thus while intellectual ability increases throughout childhood, the IQ could remain the same, and the early psychologists in this field believed that individuals' intellectual potential was indeed more or less fixed from birth (Terman, 1919).

There have been many studies of the stability of performance on intellectual tests over time (see review by Madge and Tizard, 1980) and the overall picture is of no useful predictability being possible for normal children of less than 18 months and then increasing predictive value throughout childhood and adolescence. Madge and Tizard emphasize that while the general impression is that measured intelligence becomes more consistent with age, there is usually considerable variation within the samples of children, with one-third likely to change their tested IQ scores at least 15 points over time, and to do so in a pattern of spurts and plateaux which seem more dependent on individual differences than on general development, although the level the individual starts from seems not to affect subsequent volatility of scores (see Hindley and Owen, 1978); that personal adjustment and environmental factors (particularly likely in child psychiatric clinic attenders) significantly influence intellectual performance and change over the years; and that environmental factors appear to be highly influential in determining the point at which individuals reach an IQ peak beyond which they do not rise. How long through adolescence and into early adulthood intellectual growth in this sense can continue depends on the continuation of intellectual stimulation, according to Vernon (1960) but is thought unlikely to continue beyond about 25–30 years.

Within the normal intellectual range the overall picture is that of the range of cognitive skills developing throughout childhood and adolescence but with intellectual ability as measured by standardized tests (that is comparing children of similar age) tending to be constant so that children's relative positions tend to be broadly similar. On the other hand there is considerable individual variation in which environmental and inherited factors play complex interacting parts. For clinical and educational purposes intellectual testing is a helpful guide to the band within which a boy or girl may be expected to function, but within that band the response to education and stimulation is the best guide to performance, and whether change can be anticipated. In practice this means that the reports of teachers working with a child are as important as the results of psychological tests; each complements the other whether the task is completing a clinical history or monitoring progress.

Children in the mildly mentally retarded range (IQ 50–70) and the moderately to severely retarded (IQ below 50) show greater consistency of IQ scoring over the years, although, as before, testing in infancy shows low predictive value. Environmental changes may account for the improved performance on IQ testing that can take place in the mildly mentally retarded in late adolescence and early adulthood. This improvement is usually slight but may be considerable, and seems not to occur in people with brain damage. It is most marked in those with a history of domestic deprivation who leave home for a better social setting and the improvement which is associated with improved social functioning appears due to the removal from what was an intellectually undermining social environment rather than to any particularly striking quality of the new one (Rutter and Madge, 1977).

The striking advance in mental ability that takes place in puberty and adolescence has been attributed not to any simple spurt in intellectual level but to a qualitative development in thinking and reasoning (Inhelder and Piaget, 1958; Coleman, 1980).

Piaget's work in this area deserves a fuller account than is possible here, for example see Piaget (1955), Bryant (1977), and Piaget and Inhelder (1958). Wood (1980) helpfully places Piaget's theories in their wider conceptual context, in particular emphasizing how the development and perceptual judgement of the outside world requires action and movement within that world, so that the developing of thinking becomes a constructive, creative process, the internal building of conceptual models that work.

The general scheme for Piagetian cognitive development follows this sequence: up to the age of two years (sensorimotor period) the child is stimulation-seeking and object-manipulating, but at first when an object is lost from sight, for example the well-known example of the toy that gets hidden beneath a blanket, as far as the infant is concerned it has gone: out of sight out of mind. During this first period the child begins to create internal notions, models of the outside world which, therefore, for him, begin to endure. 'What happens when we see or hear and *know*, is a complex assimilation to an integrated system of connections between actions and sensations' (Wood, 1980). From two to seven years (preoperational thought period) the child is egocentric and begins to develop elementary ways of classifying what he perceives from the outside world. From 7–11 years (period of concrete operations) the capacity to think in terms of classification and organization becomes more logically developed and the child begins to see relationships between things. The child does not seem aware of the pattern of his own thinking, or that alternative ways of thinking are possible; rather, contradictory information is dealt with by rationalization or altering the data.

In adolescence the period of formal operations begins, and the child is now able to begin to think in more abstract terms, construct hypotheses about what he perceives, and think of imagination and ideas *as* imagination and ideas, which can be manipulated like objects in order to reach hypotheses, propose alternatives and distinguish from each other beliefs, fantasies, probabilities, possibilities.

The capacity to think in this way is clearly intimately related to our notions of intelligence, but intellectual differences between children do not account for the variation from individual to individual in the time at which formal thinking operations begin to develop, which may be early in adolescence or relatively late (Coleman, 1980). In individuals the change occurs slowly, intermittently, and depends on the nature of the issue or problem being worked with. Capacity with formal operational thinking may well wax and wane before becoming an established part of the adolescent's or young adult's intellectual repertoire (Turiel, 1974). These changes have important bearing on clinical phenomenology: in clinical diagnosis we give considerable emphasis to such things as what the adolescent really *believes*, for example, in the assessment of delusional thinking and its differentiation from fears or obsessional thinking; and yet the capacity to hold and express a personal belief with conviction is a maturational task and a developmental skill in which some children and adolescents will be more advanced and established than others.

Is the patient with paranoid schizophrenia a relatively more competent thinker than the patient we describe as hebephrenic? Might a 'schizophrenogenic' lesion, for example, biochemical or family dynamic, express itself differently through different modes of thinking which, at least initially, represent normal developmental variations? As with the earlier example of obsessional disorder, there is no reason to think that this is part of the formulation of some people's schizophrenia, but it illustrates again a way in which psychiatric disorder and its aetiology may be more profitably understood in general. For the particular patient's case, internal or external events at one or other level of organization influence developmental processes – the resultant thinking, feeling and behaviour in turn contributing to events affecting further development and in the process generating that activity or inactivity which is regarded as distress, disability, or symptoms.

Adolescent reasoning and judgement and the development of moral and political thinking

The further development of adolescent thinking from the Piagetian account just outlined represents the wider social circle and broader social issues with which the adolescent becomes concerned, compared with the most immediate and limited areas of interest of younger children. The work of Elkind (1966, 1967) suggests that with adolescence, the individual's egocentrism, inherited from earlier years, becomes aware of and sometimes preoccupied with both real and imagined thinking and attitudes of others (the 'imaginary audience') and in response to which he constructs a 'personal fable', a notion which is comparable with the self-consciousness, sensitivity, and inhibitions associated with adolescence and perhaps a development in emphasis, social conscience, and altruism too.

Studies of altruistic behaviour indicate a rise throughout the later preadolescent period of childhood and possibly into adolescence (Ugurel-Semin, 1952; Kohlberg and Kramer, 1969; Harris, 1970; Graham, 1980) but with adolescents' increased personal resources (social and material) and capacity for abstract thinking compared with that of younger children, and their capacity to take action and influence the world they live in, altruism (tested experimentally by relatively simple giving or sharing exercises) becomes complicated by more sophisticated concepts of what is the right and good policy to support, so that once a threshold of altruistic development is achieved what seems morally right has to be adapted to what seems politically desirable and consistent. The adolescent then can think in terms of freedom versus anarchy, compromise versus radical change, patriotism versus internationalism, and idealism versus expediency, matters which continue to tax the wisdom of his or her elders. Studies of adolescent political attitudes tend to show a move from concrete to abstract thinking and, at about the age of 14 or 15, a move from relatively simple authoritarian solutions to a willingness to allow for there being more than one side to questions, ends being balanced against means and giving more room to humanitarian solutions (see, for example, Adelson and O'Neill, 1966; Conger, 1977; and a useful brief review by Rutter, 1979a and Coleman, 1980).

Awareness of others in a wider abstract sense rather than in the sense of impact and comeback restricted only to immediate relationships, and the concomitant emergence of a sense of self in relation to others is of course also consistent with theories of adolescent development elaborated by, among others, Blos (1962), 1967), Erikson (1964, 1965, 1968), and Winnicott (1971, 1972) and which is discussed in the following section on emotional development.

If an aspect of development were to be singled out as characterizing the most outstanding change from childhood to adolescence, it would be the capacity to take action, if necessary in cooperation with others. This requires adequate cognitive development, but clearly cannot be separated from emotional changes and changes in social skills and social position.

In relation to cruelty to children, Kipling (1937) wrote: 'Children tell little more than animals, for what comes to them they accept as eternally established.'

Adolescents are in the process of acquiring the intellect, mood, physical and verbal capacity, social position, legal right and responsibility to understand the world and make decisions about conservation or change, and where this conflicts with the way adults see, want, and do things the result, as Winnicott (1971), put it 'will not necessarily be nice'.

EMOTIONAL DEVELOPMENT

Introductory note

The study of the emotions and emotional development necessarily straddles art and science. It involves two sorts of interacting phenomena: describable, measurable activity which follows known rules and is reasonably predictable; and ideas, attitudes, and feelings which are crucially important (because they directly affect what people say and do) but which are based on individual, idiosyncratic motivation and processes whose nature can only be the subject of speculation and intuition and which are fundamentally non-rational.

The *measurable material* includes such physiological data as pulse rate, tremor, respiration, electroencephalography, and body chemistry; the reasonably standardized methods of recording verbal reports of subjective moods such as anxiety or sadness; and observations of behaviour such as facial expression, body posture, and movement.

The *immeasurable material* is the material of psychodynamic observations and theory, an attempt to make sense of ideas and imagination by attributing meaning to that which seems meaningless; attributing alternative meanings to what is said or done by the individual (so that a person behaving in a solicitous way towards someone else may be described as 'really' harbouring aggressive feelings towards him or her); by elaborating systems and mechanisms by which motives, meanings, and feelings interact; and all on the basis that a large number of the processes are beyond the individual's immediate awareness but none the less powerfully influence his or her behaviour.

The potential for elaborating such systems is infinite; the whole of mythology, art, music, and literature is concerned with people's behaviour towards each other, the motivations behind it and the consequences in the form of general lessons or morals for people to take note of. Indeed, the fairy story is one powerful way in which human feelings and relationships and their consequences for good or ill are made sense of when used for the amusement, comfort, and education of children (Bettelheim, 1976). It is easy to underrate the importance of telling stories when mythology now appears something to be safely confined to specialist libraries and overshadowed by 'common sense', but for the greater part of the period in which man has existed on earth children have been helped to make sense of their feelings of the world and their place in it, by the telling of stories; further the age-old roles are still with us: the hero, the villain, the young challenger, the motherly person, the fatherly person, the rescuer, the magician.

Meanwhile the new mythologies of those imaginative people who have linked the personal stories of their patients to systems and structures drawn from aspects of technology, science, religion, and philosophy (for example Freud, Jung, Klein, Adler, and others) have themselves become categorized as heroes or villains, gods or demons, to an extent that makes it quite difficult for some to think clearly about them.

These clinical mythologies have their well-documented inperfections; the point is that they provide conceptual models for dealing with aspects of individual development, intrapsychic functioning and relationships for which there is no other language. They are considered further on page 80 *et seq*.

Emotional functioning is difficult to separate from physiological and behavioural and social data. Psychosexual development, for example, includes important components of all three. For the purposes of this section the following will be briefly considered. The literature is very large and areas of particular relevance to clinical practice are emphasized.

1. Temperamental and affective development.
2. Behavioural models of emotional development.
3. Psychodynamic models of development.
4. Psychosocial models of development including external influences.

1. Temperamental and affective development

A large number of studies (see, for example, Thomas *et al.*, 1968; Rutter, 1977c; Dunn, 1980) have demonstrated the considerable differences in such temperamental attributes as activity, aggressiveness, sleep and arousal patterns, regularity of habits, adaptability and competence and sensitivity to others' feelings from child to child. Although it is not surprising that this should be so, social and psychodynamic theorists have taken relatively little account of it. The emerging pattern of personality development already outlined is influenced by the child's temperamental attributes; but what is equally important is the way in which the child's temperament influences what happens to it. An irritable, restless child, slow to adapt and slow to learn, will elicit a different atmosphere around itself, among peers, parents and teachers, than will a placid, adaptable fast-learner. This atmosphere in turn will affect the child. It is this emerging pattern which shapes a child's personality, behaviour, interaction with parents and circumstances for good or ill (Dunn and Kendrick, 1980). This developmental model is more in accord with the facts of normal and abnormal development than the notion of the 'traumatic incident in infancy' causing later problems. It would be unlikely that an uncharacteristic physical assault on a child by a depressed parent would alone 'cause' later depression or delinquency. But a parent depressed in the context of marital discord, behaving erratically and inconsistently towards a child, sometimes negligently and sometimes overindulgently, would be likely to raise the child's anxiety, cause unhappiness and result in poor social learning; and if in addition the child was temperamentally labile and slow to adapt, this pattern of parental behaviour towards the child would: (a) be likely to persist and worsen; (b) not help the child to change for the better; but (c) make the child's problems worse. It is this unfolding story of individual development interacting in a two-way process with relationships and other circumstances that makes the most sense of our knowledge of children's growth. It explains the inexorable move towards difficulty, shaped by multiple individual and environmental processes, and it also allows for at least the possibility of change for the better if one or more of these influences can be improved.

Individual temperamental differences of the sort discussed have been shown to be associated with other problems. For example impulsiveness, restlessness, poor concentration in general and reading difficulties in particular are associated with each other, which is not the same as saying that one causes the other (Malmquist, 1958; Rutter et al., 1970; Kagan, 1965), while irregular eating, sleeping, bladder and bowel habits and non-adaptability have been associated with intense and negative moods and psychiatric behaviour problems at home and at school (Graham et al., 1973).

Other studies have shown the persistence of individual characteristics such as destructiveness, demandingness, jealousy, shyness and other peer-relationship problems from middle childhood (around six to seven years) into adolescence (Macfarlane et al., 1954; Robins 1966, 1979; Roff et al., 1973; Graham and Rutter 1973; Rutter 1976; Zax et al., 1968), while studies in the Isle of Wight (Graham and Rutter, 1973) and London (Rutter, 1976) have demonstrated the persistence in adolescence of problems in a large proportion of children who had emotional problems at age 10.

The persistence of fears varies considerably with the type of fear. While younger children may fear the dark, strange noises and strangers, the fears that affect older children and adolescents tend to be associated with social occasions and behaviour such as attending school (Rodriquez et al., 1959; Hersov, 1960a, b; Hersov and Berg, 1980). Temper tantrums became less frequent in older children and adolescents, the decrease in girls coming a little later (Shepherd et al., 1971).

The capacity for feeling and showing depression is an interesting example of the way the experience and expression of emotion depends on several aspects of developmental progress, and also illustrates the clinical problem of diagnosing mood disorders in young people.

Depression as it occurs most characteristically in adults with ideas of guilt and self-blame and thoughts and acts of self-destruction requires a capacity for abstract thinking, verbal self-expression, and social sophistication (for example the organization of an act of suicide) that is beyond the smallest children. There is no doubt that very young children show distress in certain circumstances, for example in separation from familiar people, and that the phenomena seen after acute distress such as reduction in activity, withdrawal from making demands on others, monotonous crying and (in older children) downcast facial expression and aimless play (Bowlby, 1969) could very likely go with self-report of sad feelings in older, more articulate people. This physiological and behavioural state, accompanied presumably by pre-verbal imagery of uncertain significance and persistence, may well be the biological template for the most highly organized psychosocial phenomena of depressive states as seen in older children, adolescents, and adults, but the relationship between the two is not clear.

In older children and through adolescence the capacity to feel and express despair and hopelessness verbally makes it easier to describe what is being experienced as depressive. We can assume that the feeling state and its meaning are subjectively different too. Verbal and intellectual development and the development of a concept of self (and hence also loss of self and personal mortality), the capacity for more elaborate social behaviour and wider social opportunities all conspire to make feasible and recognizable the depressive state of the relatively mature person. There may be something common to the distressed and abandoned infant on the one hand and the angry, despairing, guilt-laden adolescent whose boy friend had let her down, going to the supermarket to buy some aspirins, but there are such considerable differences too that it is hard to be clear how far the clinician can extrapolate from one predicament to the other, in diagnosis or in treatment. In addition to such charges at psychological and psychosocial levels, there may be development and change in biochemical terms too, perhaps underlying normal sadness and perhaps underlying abnormal affective states. Certainly adult-type major affective illness with its physiological symptomatology is rare in childhood, appears in adolescence, and then increases in incidence into adulthood (Anthony and Scott, 1960; Winoker et al., 1969; Steinberg, 1980 and Chapter 13 of this volume) as do feelings of sadness including self-depreciation and suicidal ideas (Shepherd et al., 1971; Pearce, 1978; Graham and Rutter, 1973; Rutter et al., 1976). Attempts at suicide and suicide too are both rare in early childhood and rise during adolescence (Shaffer, 1974; Rutter 1979a; Hawton et al., 1982b).

The picture that emerges, then, is of progressive changes in the capacity to feel and express the moods of adulthood, including those associated with adult symptomatology, as part of overall maturation.

2. Behavioural models of emotional development

Rutter (1980c) has reviewed briefly and helpfully the difficulties of applying conditioning and learning theory to emotional development. Classical observations, such as Watson's induction of fear of white rats in an infant, have not been replicated by other workers and these theoretical models do not account for either the enormous variation from individual to individual in the transformation of a particular situation or stimulus into a lasting fear, or the variation in the types of fear seen at different ages. There is plenty of evidence that the mechanism of conditioning works; what is unclear is how and in what circumstances the experience of a particular event becomes incorporated into the lasting emotional and behavioural repertoire of a developing individual. This will be discussed again in the section of aetiology (page 120); meanwhile our understanding so far of conditioning is that it must take its place among the many other external circumstances and internal processes, from the biochemical through the psychodynamic to the social, that contribute to the developing personality. Perhaps at certain times, in certain circumstantial sets and in certain moods a pattern of mood or behaviour may be acquired, but what exactly is acquired is likely to depend on its meaning to the child (which means its meaning to his or her parents too) and whether it persists will depend on the presence or absence of factors to sustain it. Thus anxiety in a particular situation, for example on attending school, is less likely to result directly from a bad experience on the first day than from fearfulness being maintained by the pattern of mutual behaviour of parent and child.

Much effective work with the families and parents of disturbed children recognizes how patterns of behaviour in relationships and families as in small groups maintain a member of the dyad or group in a particular position, for example lack of confidence, low self-esteem, inactivity, or misbehaviour. This may not be the whole explanation of aetiology in any particular case, but may be overlooked if the clinician is seeing aetiology and abnormality only 'in' the presenting patient.

On the other hand it does seem that at some point in the development of child and problem the latter does become part of the individual's repertoire. The child, for example, who has been maintained in a state of anxiety by the parents' behaviour towards him now becomes anxious in other circumstances. In behavioural terms the problem becomes generalized, which means that the individual now carries with him the potential to react in similar ways in circumstances other than those which caused the difficulty. Symptoms and disabilities may therefore become self-perpetuating, regardless of origin whether the origin is without or within. In psychodynamic terms this seems very much the equivalent of a problem or relationship being described as 'internalized'.

3. Psychodynamic models of development

The specific value of art for man is that it is closer to reality than science; that it is not dominated, as science must be, by logic and reason ... some scientists say that man's most precise tool is the mathematical symbol; semantically some equations and theorems appear to have a very austere and genuine poetry. But their precision is a precision in a special domain, abstracted, for perfectly good practical reasons, from the complexity of reality.

John Fowles, in *The Aristos*, 1981

It is not surprising that psychoanalysis causes controversy, because the style of work and thinking required by the intuitive, divergent, speculative approach of the psychodynamicist is so different from the methodical painstaking measurements and cautious, heavily qualified hypotheses of the more mathematically inclined scientific worker. Further, they are asking different questions.

For the psychodynamic approach it may be said that it deals, sometimes brilliantly, with an area of life for which hard, measurable data are completely inadequate, and that it has proved a most fruitful source of ideas leading, for example, to many developments in work with families, groups, and organizations, particularly where the creative, diversely imaginative approach of psychodynamic thinking has been allowed to inform anthropological and biological science as in the work of Bateson (1973), Hinde (1976, 1979), and Bowlby (1979). Psychodynamic theory and practice has also proved vulnerable to misuse and application without wisdom, and the charge that it is entirely subjective. On the other hand it is worth noting again Ey's conception of the content of consciousness as being neither wholly subjective nor wholly objective, but as a third modality of existence: 'consciousness has an object; one is conscious of something' (see Evans, 1972). In this sense some psychodynamic observations, both introspective and the observations of other people, are approximately equivalent to the early descriptive work of natural science, and making equivalent advances and mistakes. They are also heavily influenced by the technology and symbolism of the day; thus Freudian theory is heavily influenced by the impressive technology of the nineteenth century, while much modern work takes its conceptual framework from cybernetics (see Von Bertalanffy, 1968; Bateson, 1971). Jung characteristically searched for the origins of his own ideas and found them in gnosticism, mythology, and anthropology (Jung, 1963).

The psychodynamic perspective gives us a tentative way of dealing with important aspects of growing children (and the adults among whom they grow) which cannot be described in other terms. It is true that the terminology and concepts of psychodynamic language, symbolism, and metaphor are nebulous, elusive, and changeable but then so are the unconscious or part-conscious meanings and feelings they attempt to describe. We may refine and perfect ways of measuring the physiological or behavioural expression of anxiety or enjoyment, say, just as we can technically perfect a thermometer, but we would still be dealing with physics, chemistry, muscular movement, and social signals, not feelings. The subjective feelings of a boy of 13 about, for example, a family trip to the seaside, cannot be captured by such measures, but the partial feelings, ideas, and attitudes at this ultimately unmeasurable level, whether about small matters or large, fleeting or transient, are the material of individuality and relationships and help to determine attitudes to relatives, to friends, to authority, to career, to interests, to the personal style of reaction to challenges arising from within or without, and thereby to ways of dealing with problems, which is a direct link with the pathway to patient status.

Freudian theory Ellenberger (1970) has demonstrated how psychodynamic thinking predated Freud, but Freud brought together a number of concepts into a more or less coherent and consistent system which is both a theory of development and a method of treatment.

These concepts included the idea of an emerging sense of self, the ego which is powerfully influenced by its primitive, biological origins (the id) on the one hand and by the parental values and strictures which it incorporates on the other (the super ego). The notion of incorporating external parental and therefore cultural values recurs in one form or another in many theories of development. In Freudian theory the primitive id instincts, perhaps conveniently conceived as equivalent to the mental processes of cat or dog, have to come to terms with demands of the super ego, loosely equivalent to the conscience, the effects of social experience.

In addition, Freudian theory includes the idea of unconscious motivation affecting conscious thoughts and behaviour. The idea of the unconscious has been the subject of considerable controversy of varying sophistication (see Eysenck, 1953, 1957; Brown, 1961) but whatever its nature it is useful in clinical practice to accept that what patients say and do and how we respond is influenced by, among other things, mental processes which are not noticed and not verbalized although later on some of what motivated a particular attitude, decision or piece of behaviour may be evinced (see Freud, 1922; Brown, 1961; Stafford Clark, 1967; Wyss, 1966; Dare, 1977).

According to Freudian theory one of the first great challenges to the id is a dawning consciousness that the child cannot have his mother to himself because of the third person he now begins to notice, his father. The child must make some personal adaptation to being pulled in three directions; an instinctive intense and greedy love for his mother, furious anger at the intrusive outsider, and anxiety about the possible consequences of asserting himself in either direction.

This classical Oedipal conflict, like much else in psychodynamic theory, is subject both to vehement support and to ridicule. One of the problems is the linguistic and conceptual difficulty of discussing primitive pre-verbal feelings and intuitions and fantasies which are presumably part-formed, chaotic and just grasped as a part of emerging consciousness. There is a tendency to consider these developmental mechanisms as if they were being played out by sophisti-cated adults shrunk to baby-size with all their concepts of 'sex', mother, father, and 'punishment' intact, so that the mature adult finds it ridiculous to suppose that he or she 'would conceivably have felt like that' at that age; but this informed retrospective view tends to mislead both supporters and critics about the dimly perceived but powerful emotions an infant is likely to experience.

According to the Freudian model ego development proceeds from birth, with super ego development (the conscience; self-control) shaped by unconscious processes such as those concerned with the individual coming to terms with Oedipal conflict. Ego development and super ego development are charged with sexuality but in the five or six years preceding puberty this is supposedly largely latent although Rutter (1971c) has pointed out the increasing sexual talk and play during this period. In adolescence, according to Freudian theory there is a resurgence of sexual drive with a tendency to recapitulate infantile preoccupations but now with a more powerfully somatic basis that enables sexual fantasy to be fulfilled. Possibly this potential for fulfilment adds to the danger and therefore the anxiety associated with incestuous desires, the barrier against which, Freud considered, is mysterious (S. Freud, 1905).

Two patterns of behaviour are seen in clinical work with children which support the idea expressed earlier of the human potential to behave (or experience anxiety) in ways which are consistent with Freudian theory, even if not all children and adolescents invariably act in this way. One is the anxiety, misconduct, and mixed feelings about authority seen in some children who have experienced serious marital discord and violent rows between parents, followed by the sudden loss of the father by separation or, less commonly, bereavement. We know that children are particularly vulnerable to loss of a parent, particularly the loss by death of a parent when a child is aged three or four years (Rutter, 1966), which is also the age at which, according to Freud, genital sexuality and Oedipal conflict are reaching their height, and it may be assumed that there is the greatest need for the same-sexed parent to remain alive and well while the child works out his personal resolution of the anxieties referred to earlier. Of course such observations do not confirm the theory but they are not inconsistent with aspects of it.

The other clinical observation is of the child growing up in a chaotic family where parental and sibling roles are not clear: a depressed mother who cannot cope; a young stepfather flirting with the eldest daughter, and so on. In such circumstances disturbed adolescents are sometimes seen who tend to confuse sexual needs for ordinary physical comforting and affection and behave sexually inappropriately with considerable accompanying tension. Again, the occasional observation does not confirm Freudian theory. But it suggests that the developing child needs to get his needs for affection, limit setting, and sexual gratification into the right places, so to speak, as part of his maturation from early family relationships through adolescent family relationships to social relationships, and confusing messages on the way about love, sex, and control result in social ineptitude, sexual misbehaviour, anxiety, or all three.

Freudian theory often appears to consist of abstractions piled upon abstraction, yet it has some consistency with animal biology. To use an evolutionary justification, it is plausible to suggest that the type of human being that has survived, in evolutionary terms (that is, like we who are alive today) is that in which there is an absolutely imperative instinct, first, to keep close to mother and suck. A child born without such an internal programme would perhaps survive in a sophisticated middle class family or an intensive care unit but not among anthropoid apes or in proto-human society as comparative zoologists have described it. Developing consciousness, self-consciousness, and the consciousness of others, one may speculate, will also evolve in such a way that in adolescence considerable anxiety would be associated even with fantasy about sexual relations with someone with a similar set of genes. Those who have survived would have done so because they have inherited both tendencies, and the complex network of constructs and feelings that have been coloured by these tendencies would be found in the clinical material we find when we talk to adolescents and families in difficulties.

Kleinian theory (Klein, 1950; Wyss, 1966) is often obscure and like other analytical theory is couched in language which tends to invite rejection (Graham, 1974). I have found aspects of the Kleinian concept of early development particularly helpful, even though Melanie Klein had little to say about adolescence.

The notion that the infant's earliest experience must be an entirely chaotic set of perceptions and feelings without any sense of self, sequence or purpose seems entirely plausible, although there is no way of confirming this. That the earliest sense of regularity (that is something that happens has happened before and is anticipated as perhaps happening again) comes from within (hunger coming and going) seems also plausible. If we believe that the third imperative human characteristic (after surviving and reproducing) is actively to make sense of what is around us (Cobb, 1977) then the infant's developing consciousness will consist in large measure of a sense of something 'out there' being good (and loved) and of something 'out there' being bad (and hated), the latter being the withdrawal of what was good, that is, the alternation of being fed and not fed. These primitive abstractions of time, goodness, and badness are the psychic representations of the periodic arrival and departure of physical attention, in the actual form of parts of the parents (for example, 'good' and 'bad' breast or part-objects). According to Kleinian theory, this world 'peopled by gods and devils' (Brown, 1961) is for the child a primitive, dangerous place full of arbitrary external events and his or her own rages (not yet recognized as part of self) and in which the child feels helpless and, often enough, threatened. Klein called this the *paranoid–schizoid position*. The theory becomes developmental with the conception of a further stage; with experience and learning over time (a few months later, according to Klein) the child realizes that the anger and wildness 'out there' comes from himself, and that the object of his hatred has turned out to be exactly the same as the object of his love.

The child's attempt to impose sense and order on these totally conflicting experiences would be, if Kleinian theory is a true commentary, a first creative act and a major step in maturity – namely an appreciation that not all is totally 'good' or 'bad' (or black and white) but that a person (or object, in Kleinian terms) can contain good and bad characteristics, as can the child himself or herself. This realization that the totally loved person and the totally hated person are one is accompanied by remorse and the first feelings of guilt, which Klein called the *depressive position*.

The Kleinian myth or model is a helpful metaphor for five emotional and behavioural patterns seen frequently in clinical practice with adolescents

1. Reversion to more primitive, tense, hypersensitive, paranoid thinking seen in emotionally immature people under stress and who perceive themselves as in danger (again, a human capacity that makes evolutionary sense).
2. The irrational division of people (for example members of a clinical team) into allies and enemies, again characteristic of distressed adolescents and people under stress or threat; even ideas (such as theoretical positions) may tend to be categorized as wholly bad and to be rejected, or wholly good and be swallowed whole.
3. The sense of maturation (or progress in psychotherapy or social therapy) when an adolescent ceases to see everything (himself and others) in black or white terms, full of idealism or hatred, and instead is thoughtful, reflective, and sad.
4. Skynner (1975) interestingly describes the development of a group of professional workers in training in similar terms; an early, paranoid stage (experienced by most people in a totally new group setting) followed by a reflective depressive stage when work can be done. Staff groups often seem to go through such stages in cycles.
5. Ambivalence, the common adolescent dilemma of attempting to hold conflicting views and feelings in a way that is only partly reconciled with consequently inconsistent or alternating attitudes and devious behaviour (see A. Freud, 1936, 1966).

Anna Freud These theories are developments of the Freudian theories, with greater emphasis on older children and adolescents and on ego development, and particularly the defensive mechanisms in the ego by which it achieves harmony between its various competing impulses. Five major defensive mechanisms described by Anna Freud, additional to the classical Freudian defences, are *denial in fantasy*, *denial in word and behaviour* (for example saying or acting as if a disliked person is admired), *restriction of the ego* (for example completely giving up an aspect of personal life because some aspect of it is too threatening), *identification with the aggressor* (for example the hurt, abused child who becomes the bully or torturer of small animals), and *altruistic behaviour* in which personal needs are satisfied by providing for others (for example the neglected adolescent who wants to work with peers or children).

Anna Freud also introduced the concept of developmental lines, derived from her observations on growing children, and described the gradual unfolding ego functions as arising from sequential interactions between ego and id. She described as a prototype a sequence beginning with mother–infant biological unity, a primitive set of relationships built upon needs and their fulfilment by part-objects (Klein 1950; page 84); a stage of inner constancy where a consistent internal image is built up and maintained, regardless of transient satisfactions and dissatisfactions; an ambivalent phase, characteristically combining closeness with anger and fear rather than warmth (for example clinging behaviour); a period of rivalry with the same-sex parent and possessiveness towards the parent of the opposite sex; a latency period when such feelings are temporarily referred to people outside the family; a pre-adolescent return to earlier more infantile behaviour with re-emphasis of need fulfilment; and an adolescent stage characterized by a return of pre-Oedipal and Oedipal internal demands and their resolution in a basically unsatisfactory way which verges on the antisocial and psychotic, so that Anna Freud's view of normal adolescence is essentially one of near-pathological turbulence (see A. Freud, 1966).

One aspect of adolescent turbulence to which A. Freud drew attention is the adolescent's tendency to use, or perhaps try, a range of alternative defensive mechanisms. This and the adolescent tendency to denial and ambivalence is among the reasons why interpretive work should be used with caution in psychotherapy with adolescents, if at all (see Chapter 17).

Peter Blos   Peter Blos (1962, 1967, 1970) has described the move towards independence of parents which is characteristic of adolescence in terms of a distinct step away from the mother. The first step is that of the child of three or four becoming bolder in his or her social experiments showing more initiative and planning and experimenting with moves away from the protective parent; in order to do this successfully, the child, according to Blos, internalizes the mother, a concept which is consistent with Freudian, Kleinian, and Eriksonian ideas and with aspects of attachment theory (see page 106). Another way of putting this is to say that to separate from mother the child needs confidence, and his or her personal experience and memory (in both cognitive and emotional terms) of the mother provides this confidence.

The second step, described by Blos as the second individuation process, requires abandonment of this security-giving internalized representation, in order to seek and use relationships in the real world which provide the means by which the adolescent continues development towards maturity. Blos considers that the powerful infantile feelings concerned with the original maternal attachment must be reactivated if they are to be surrendered, in other words some degree of emotional regression is a precondition of this developmental advance. The adolescent's idealization of selected adults (characteristically relatively remote and prominent adults such as 'television personalities') and falling in love and powerfully identifying not only with other adolescents but also with movements and philosophies are regarded by Blos as examples of this second phase. Like the reactivation of loving and hating (Klein), alternation between involvement and non-involvement, acceptance and rejection, the experiments in these new roles and relationships account at least in part for the ambivalence which is also characteristic of adolescence. What is particularly important, if Blos's viewpoint is accepted, is that these personal and social explorations involve very powerful feelings; they involve 'giving up' and 'trying out' and at a time too when the adolescent is far from sure what (in terms of his self-esteem and confidence in himself) he will be left with if what he involves (or immerses) himself in does not replace satisfactorily what he has given up. It involves major losses and uncertain gains, and therefore aspects of his developing identity are at risk; there is also a danger of activation of powerfully felt anxiety, anger and sadness, as well as high excitement, with which the boy or girl may or may not be able to cope.

D. W. Winnicott This account of emotional development (1971, 1972) contributes to the idea of its dangerous aspects, for example in that form of experimentation called play. Adults may not believe child's play is dangerous at first sight, but the anxieties and difficulties the shy child and still more the autistic child has in play, and the quite common discomfort and awkwardness many mature adults (and certainly shy adolescents) experience if asked to take part in adult 'play' (for example charades, singing in public, playing a dramatic part, 'making a fool of oneself') suggest that playing is not necessarily that easy. Like teasing, which again shy and autistic children cannot tolerate, play has a two-edged, ambiguous quality, part fun but with an aggressive component too (as with the fighting play of young predatory animals), and it requires a measure of social skill to balance the play against the roughness so that enjoyment results rather than hurt.

Winnicott's writings are themselves exploratory; he is both readable and at times obscure. It seems that through play Winnicott sees the child as experimenting, rehearsing, practising, and ultimately acquiring a group of capacities that underpin healthy development. The child's concentration in play is regarded as important: a near-withdrawal state in which the child can lose himself with preoccupied pleasure and without anxiety, and within the play time and play space which Winnicott describes as outside the individual but not the external real world (that is, it is a projected, external psychic reality) the child uses real objects to deal with inner concerns.

Playing implies trust, and belongs to the potential space between (what was at first) baby and mother-figure, with the baby in a state of near-absolute dependence and the mother-figure's adaptive function taken for granted by the baby . . . playing is inherently exciting and precarious. This characteristic derives not from instinctual arousal but from the precariousness that belongs to the interplay in the child's mind of that which is subjective (near-hallucination) and that which is objectively perceived (actual, or shared reality). (Winnicott, 1971)

In this last move towards what is real, and what is shared, is contained again the recurring concept of the child making sense of the world (page 112).

The implication of Winnicott's views is that the 'good enough' mother is the parent who is sufficiently responsive to the baby – but not too much – so that he or she develops the trust to play and 'be himself', and this 'being himself', exemplified by the ability to let go and withdraw happily (but not necessarily without anxiety) into play represents the root of a healthily developing ego. The transitional object, and transitional phenomena (about which Winnicott is again occasionally hard to follow) are objects, fragments of behaviour or later ideas and fantasies which are neither entirely subjective self, nor external reality, but a means of making a psychic transition from the one to the other. The cuddly toy is not perceived as a comforted self, nor as a comforting other, but as something important between fantasy and fact. Possibly that is a relationship between the developing level of consciousness described as being between pure subjectivity and external reality, and Ey's assertion of consciousness as being neither purely subjective nor objective (Wyss, 1966; Evans, 1972).

In adolescence Winnicott, like Anna Freud and Blos, sees a repetition of infantile problems but now with the added force of the adolescent's new physiological, psychological, and social capacities. His statements can be dramatic:

If, in the fantasy of early growth, there is contained death, then at adolescence there is contained *murder*. Even when growth at the period of puberty goes ahead without major crises, one may need to deal with acute problems of management because growing up means taking the parent's place. *It really does.* In the unconscious fantasy, growing up is inherently an aggressive act. And the child is now no longer child size. (Winnicott, 1971)

Winnicott's view is that the potential for rebelliousness is inherent in adolescence, indeed his view is that the results of parents bringing up their children well does not mean that there should be less trouble, but on the contrary, there may be more. 'If you do all you can to promote personal growth in your offspring, you will need to be able to deal with the startling results.'

Rebelliousness

How this can be reconciled with the common observation, supported by systematic study (Rutter *et al.*, 1976) that for all the serious and increasing rebelliousness and misconduct of a minority, most adolescents in fact get on well with their parents and the adult generation in general?

First, part of the apparent contradiction is in the different age groups studied. Young adolescents, for example up to age 15 or 16, are often quite conservative and tend to conform to parental standards over major personal, moral, and broadly political matters, although there are tussles over matters like hair-style, clothing, and bedtimes. Overt rebelliousness when it occurs, whether political or criminal, is more the style of the late teens and twenties. Thus if we define adolescence largely in terms of biological development (roughly 11 to 18), which is appropriate enough for psychiatric purposes, the population of young people we are concerned with are not characteristically rebellious. But that important aspect of adolescence which is the period of transition from dependence to independence has been artificially extended in the more technical cultures, because of the longer period of education and training required before young people can play a full part in the community, and the classical adolescent attitude that adult politicians and professionals 'are doing it all wrong' is less a parent–child phenomenon than one to do with people in their twenties and thirties.

This leads to the next point, which is the question of the actual social power wielded by the younger group. This is not simply a matter of legislation; cultural phenomena such as increasing earning capacity, loosening of social and moral conventions and the weakened authority of adults, wider and longer education, including political education and political propaganda, all enable real challenges to adult authority to take place. How far it may go depends on the nature of adult authority. It is reasonable to assume that if there is a widely accepted adult moral and political consensus and general agreement about the imposition of adult authority, the point of compromise between social innovation and conservatism will be less contentious than if the adult ethical code is a source of dispute, as it is, or at least appears to be, in the Western world. Social pressures and expectations help determine whether the intergenerational confrontation described by Winnicott happens or not, at what age, and where the front line is set.

Thirdly, it is not surprising that there is disagreement between what psychodynamic workers like Winnicott have described in the relatively few adolescents they have got to know in depth, and the results of large-scale but relatively superficial questionnaire studies. The former are describing what they infer as inevitable when the child generation, socially and biologically, begins to replace the parent generation. The latter studies describe the outcome in terms of observed behaviour and reported feelings. Both sorts of observation are important but they are quite different. The psychodynamic conception of adolescent–adult conflict is equivalent to the idea of dynamic physiological, homoeostatic mechanisms such as those maintaining blood pressure or blood sugar at a particular level. There is a potential for disaster in either direction which usually does not happen but may take place in ill-health or in adverse external circumstances. To understand physical development, maintain health, and treat disorder it is necessary to have a conceptual model of the many variables which maintain blood pressure or blood sugar at a certain level. Equally, it is vital that there are valid and reliable means of measuring that level.

In clinical psychology and psychiatry it is equally important that we do not confuse models which attempt to describe the components of dynamic systems, maintaining a particular state of expressed feeling and behaviour, with measuring devices that tell us what that state is. Both are necessary.

Fourthly, it is in disordered individual and family states that this dynamic equilibrium goes awry. In clinical practice with adolescents extremes of aggression or overcompliance are commonly seen in children and in the parents.

C. G. Jung   Jung's teaching is difficult to incorporate into other theories of child and adolescent development; it stands by itself as a philosophical system which has more to say about the nature of humanity and creativity than about normal and abnormal development (Wyss, 1966). His advice that children should not be analysed, but rather be allowed to grow up is characteristic, and the world into which the child grows, including its history, arts, and beliefs, is more his concern. It is not that Jung is not concerned with children and adolescents, but rather that his theoretical position is about the whole of life, including people's biological and anthropological ancestry and their individual deaths. His approach, often castigated as merely mystical, in fact has biological roots. He is most misunderstood in his concept of the collective unconscious, in which he sometimes appears to say that individuals inherit what their ancestors have experienced. What he also says and appears primarily to mean is that individuals inherit a nervous system and system of psychophysiological functioning that shapes what they perceive.

It is in my view a great mistake to suppose that the psyche of a new born child is a *tabula rasa* in the sense that there is absolutely nothing in it. In so far as the child is born with a differentiated brain that is predetermined by heredity and therefore individualised, it meets sensory stimuli coming from outside not with *any* aptitudes but with *specific* ones and this necessarily results in a particular, individual choice and pattern of apperception...their presence gives the world of the child and the dreamer its anthropomorphic stamp...it is not, therefore, a question of inherited *ideas* but of inherited *possibilities* of ideas (Jung, 1936).

The capacity to take part in the world (initially by what seems to be a crucial reciprocal relationship between child and parent) may depend on an inherited potential to attach certain primitive feelings to elementary perceptions, such as the configuration of the human face. One may speculate that this too is of evolutionary significance, those infants without this capacity failing to survive, a handicap possibly represented among some victims of child abuse and neglect (Ounsted, 1972).

It is in a style of psychotherapy rather than in its theoretical or technical detail that Jung's approach is of interest in clinical work with adolescents. First, his approach to self-indivuation, while concerned with self-development in the whole of life, and not only in adolescence, is pertinent to adolescence. Second, his method is a natural one, often described as conversational in style rather than as directive or passive, more flexible and adaptable, and seems to have more regard for the patient's individuality and autonomy. The Jungian approach is also more directed to the present and the future rather than the past. Jung believed that the cause of neurosis was to be found in the present, not in the past; as far as the origin of what became neurotic behaviour was concerned, he tended to agree broadly with Freud (Storr, 1973), but work needed to be done with what the patient was doing now, problems in the present causing regression to past fixations, rather than past fixations causing problems in the present. He also paid considerable attention to the patient's artistic productions, and the use of painting and music and other forms of creativity (regardless of aesthetic merit), and was suspicious of special technical method in psychotherapy. Anything which suggested that the psychotherapist was seeing the patient in terms of dogmatic, mechanistic theory or technique made him doubt the efficacy of the approach and perhaps even its ethics. 'So much is said in the literature about the resistance of the patient that it would almost seem as if the doctor were trying to put something over on him' (Jung, 1963).

The Jungian recommendations for a conversational, non-didactic therapeutic style, its sense of wit rather than pomp, its doubt about dogma and its emphasis on the present and future and in particular on creative activities, come close to much of the advice given about psychotherapy with adolescents.

Jungian theory is important in another sense too; Winnicott considered that healthy adolescent development required considerable strength and integrity among adults, who would stand firm by their principles even though the adolescent in turn was right to attack them, and the confrontation, in excellent understatement, might not be 'nice' (Winnicott, 1971). Jung's theories are about the whole of life, and about the confidence and integrity of adults whose failings, evasions, difficulties, and poor example, major and minor, are so often behind the problems of their children.

Erik Erikson   Erikson (1964, 1965, 1968) also deals with the whole of life, and again the emphasis in his theory on periods of crisis and development not only in childhood and adolescence, but through middle age and to death, puts the crises of adolescents into perspective; other age groups have their crises too. His approach helps us see what we often find in practice, that the child's move from 10 to 20 is usually paralleled by his or her parents moving from, say, youthful mid-thirties to middle age, and with a natural rising incidence of ill-health, disability, and death in the extended family.

Erikson's approach emphasizes: (a) the whole life span; (b) epigenetic development, that is to say each stage growing out of that reached so far; (c) the critical nature of each stage, that is, the nature of each advance depends on the way in which a crisis special to that stage of life is resolved; and (d) the links between personal psychological development and social tasks.

Erikson emphasizes the epigenetic nature of his scheme by presenting it as a series of rising steps rather than as a simple linear progression. Implicit in this is the idea that each stage depends on the developmental achievement of those that went before. For example, less than adequate development at one stage does not prevent developmental passage through subsequent stages, but it does leave an area of vulnerability, for example in the individual's sense of trust, or autonomy. Also implied is that progression need not be a straight diagonal across the chart, but development may vary in timing and intensity so that the individual spends longer, for example, in the oral sensory stage.

It is important to note that the chart represents not only individual development; the social culture in which that individual grows is so constituted, in Erikson's words, 'as to meet and invite this succession of potentialities for interaction and attempts to safeguard and to encourage the proper rate and the proper sequence of their unfolding. Thus developmental conflicts require the supportive response of cultural institutions if they are to be productive, creative and therefore truly maturational.' (See, for example, Table 4, page 98.)

Each of the stages represents a psychosocial task, or crisis, equivalent to the stage of physiological development reached, thus the oral sensory stage of maturity in physiological and psychoanalytic terms is represented psychosocially by the task for the child of trust achieving what Erikson calls a favourable ratio with mistrust, and resulting in an outcome in the form of an enduring strength, or 'basic virtue'. Failure to achieve a 'favourable outcome' results in a persisting vulnerability.

Erikson has stressed that his scheme is no more than a conceptual tool; like much else in psychodynamic thinking, as a model it invites rejection on the one hand or too literal acceptance on the other. As a frame for drawing together a number of psychodynamic, social, and anthropological aspects of development it is helpful. Erikson has also warned against using it as a guide for child training and psychotherapy, nevertheless the author and colleagues have found it a useful framework for setting goals in small group work with adolescents (see page 300).

Figure 14 illustrates Erikson's scheme in outline, but his own account should be read (Erikson, 1965) to convey his meaning about each stage. Figure 15 represents the crisis at each stage, with the outcome seen rather as the resultant of a parallelogram of forces or, in neurological terms (Sherrington, 1906), a 'final common path'. Taylor (1972) has suggested modifications of Erikson's scheme in relation to the development of children with epilepsy. Some of his phraseology is particularly helpful and included in Figure 14.

Erikson's descriptions helpfully categorize patterns of ideas, feelings, and circumstances regularly seen in work with adolescents. The extent to which they can be linked together in an epigenetic, developmental, cumulative sequence is

Erikson's epigenetic chart								
Maturity (mature age)								Ego-integrity v. despair*
Adulthood (adulthood +)						Generativity (including productivity, care) v. stagnation*		
Young adulthood (young adult +)					Intimacy v. isolation*			
Puberty and adolescence				Identity v. role confusion*				
Latency (school age +)			Industry v. inferiority*					
Locomotor-genital (play age +)		Initiative v. guilt*						
Muscular-anal (early childhood +)	Autonomy v. shame and doubt*							
Oral-sensory (infancy +)	Basic trust v. mistrust*							
	1	2	3	4	5	6	7	8

Psychoanalytic / physiological stages of maturity

Time ——→

* Elaborated in columns (2) and (3), pages 94,95

Figure 14   Erikson's developmental scheme (1965) incorporating some modifications suggested by Taylor (1972)

	Erikson's elaboration of each critical stage (1965)	Modifications suggested by Taylor (1972)	Enduring strengths or basic virtues (Erikson, 1965)
8	Post-narcissistic love of the human ego – not of the self – as an experience which conveys some world order and spiritual sense, no matter how dearly paid for . . . it is the acceptance of one's one and only life cycle as something that had to be . . . renewed love of one's parents ; failure is signified by fear of death and despair and disgust.	We have been v. We have been robbed	Renunciation and wisdom
7	Man the teaching and instituting as well as the learning animal. Concern in establishing and guiding the next generation. Loss of self in meeting of bodies (sexual) and minds (intellectual) leads to enrichment. When it fails, leads to personal impoverishment, pseudo-intimacy, stagnation.	I can create and give v. I must hold on.	Production and care
6	Readiness for committing self to sharing affiliations and partnerships; the individual becomes trustworthy, reliable, develops ethical strength to abide by commitments; able to face fear of ego loss in situations (e.g. sex, conflict, intuition) which call for self-abandon. The avoidance of such experiences because of fear of ego loss results in isolation and self-absorption.	We are; you are v. I am not; self-absorption.	Affiliation and love
5	Comparison of how boy or girl appears to be in the eyes of others with what he (she) feels he (she) is; questions of how to connect roles and skills cultivated with the social and occupational roles available. Adopt idols and ideals as 'guardians of a final identity,' and appoint others as adversaries for personal social experiments which cause confusion when they fail.	I am v. I am not	Devotion and fidelity

4	Stage in all culture of systematic instruction in skills and the use of tools; with specialization comes confusion about the goals of initiative; with more complex social realities comes confusion about parental roles in it. Danger at this stage is of sense of inadequacy and inferiority.	I can v. I can not	Method and competence
3	Characteristically the child resolves a crisis 'more or less beset with fumbling and fear' after which he is more loving, relaxed, brighter in judgement, more activated and activating. Initiative adds to autonomy the qualities of undertaking and planning. It also invokes anticipatory rivalry and competition which, with failure, leads to resignation, anxiety, guilt.	I will v. I will not	Direction and purpose
2	Muscular maturation enables experimentation with holding on and letting go. Either can be positive (holding on, letting be) or negative (retaining; letting loose). Reassuring outer control enables the child to learn to hold on or let go with discretion. Lack of competent outside guidance leads to obsessiveness, self-consciousness, shame, and doubt 'the brother of shame'.	I am free v. I am a dependent part	Self-control and will-power
1	The experience of mutual (mother and child) regulation of needs and maternal provision produces familiarity with comfort and discomfort; consistency, continuity, and sameness of experience provide a rudimentary sense of ego identity depending on an inner population of remembered and anticipated sensations firmly correlated with an outer population of familiar and predictable things and people.	I am loved v. I am not loved. Experience of mother's joy' warmth and feeling	Drive and hope

Figure 14   Erikson's developmental scheme (1965) incorporating some modifications suggested by Taylor (1972)

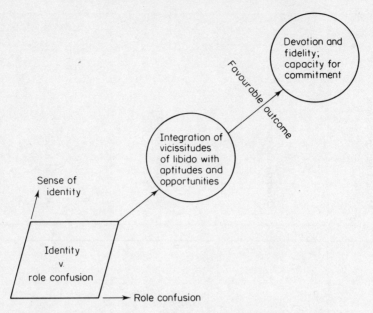

Figure 15   'Favourable outcome' of each critical stage: example

not proven, although they seem roughly to approximate to successive levels of social and personal maturity.

4. Psychosocial models of development including external influences

Much of the development described so far takes account of external events but in considering psychosocial models we take a further step away from the individual child as the focus to the psychology and sociology of the groups and networks of which the child becomes a member and in which he or she grows up. It is an extremely wide field, and three aspects will be considered, starting from the outside:

(a) *External cultural, social, and legal factors: the world into which the adolescent is growing.*
(b) *Community, school, peer, and family influences.*
(c) *Attachment theory: the making, use, and breaking of social bonds and resulting influences on development.*

(a) External cultural, social, and legal factors

As has already been pointed out, while there are many different aspects to the story of adolescent development, the common denominator is the move from dependence to independence. The power to think and argue coherently, to influence others in an articulate way, to conduct social experiments and play risky games, to reproduce whether responsibly or irresponsibly, to organize and administrate and take physical action represent together an extraordinary change in circumstances and possibilities over the relatively few years from, say, 12 to 18. The significance of this shift of position and power is not lost on the adult world which has a necessarily ambivalent relationship to the developing child and adolescents it needs, but whose judgement and skills emerge variably and unreliably, and whose wishes and needs may not coincide with its own. The legal 'milestones' in the United Kingdom (Table 4) give official expression to the way the reins are held. For clinical purposes, it will be noticed that important legal changes take place at the age of 16, such as the ability of an adolescent to withhold consent to medical treatment (and therefore discharge himself or herself from hospital). Every right that the mature adult can exercise in relation to accepting or rejecting psychiatric help is acquired in full by the adolescent on his 16th birthday. Adults are very much concerned with what young people are doing; the contents of newspapers show this preoccupation, and from time to time conduct more or less casual surveys of what adolescents feel about delinquency, sex, parents, politics, etc. These surveys tend to coincide, often it seems to the journalists' surprise and relief, with systematic studies of adolescent attitudes and behaviour: that overt attitudes and behaviour (see page 88) do not show the massive gap between generations in ethical, moral, and political attitudes that is sometimes feared (see, for example, Rutter's review, 1979a). On the other hand, since the 1920s, there has been a steady increase in the occurrence of sexual intercourse among the young, and greater acceptance of pre-marital sex and homosexual relationships. In considering such surveys it is important to remember how variable the lives of adolescents are, despite the relatively few years encompassed; the 18-year-old American college student, the 13-year-old girl living at home in middle-class England, the sixth-former at a British public school, and the unemployed inner-city 16-year-old will have very different backgrounds, experiences, opportunities and attitudes, and be exposed to quite different influences. Delinquency and vandalism have both increased, but in his review Rutter (1979a) points out the caution that has to be exercised in interpreting statistics that vary so much with how a problem is defined, the extent to which it is officially reported, area-to-area variation, and of course changes in the law which can criminalize or de-criminalize behaviour overnight.

All these areas represent trends in adolescent behaviour which will in turn influence how the rising generation of older children behave. While changing fashions have shifted the issue of responsibility for undesirable behaviour back and forth between younger generation and older generation, it can hardly be denied that the weight of ultimate responsibility for how children and adolescents behave must be with those who have the most official and unofficial power, which is generally on the side of adults. There may be good reasons for

Table 4   Legal milestones from birth to maturity

Age	Individual and family matters	Legal and medico-legal proceedings
From birth	May have own bank or building society account and passport, and hold premium bonds	May be taken into the care of the Local Authority; may be detained under the Mental Health Act; and admitted under s.26 for subnormality or psychopathic disorder up to the age of 20 (that is, not if 21 or older)
From 5	Must have full-time education; may drink alcohol in private; may see U or A films	
From 7	May draw money from post office account	
From 10		May be convicted of a criminal offence if prosecution can prove the child knows right from wrong
From 12	May buy a pet without a parent being present	
From 13	May have a part-time job for not more than 2 hours a day (and not on Sundays)	
From 14		May be held fully responsible for a crime; can be sent to a detention centre; can see an AA film; own an air gun; go into a pub but not drink or buy alcohol there; may be finger-printed; boys may be found guilty of rape
From 15		May be sent to borstal, or (boys) to prison on remand
From 16	May leave school, get full-time job, join a union, marry with the consent of one parent, a guardian or a court; leave home with a parent's consent; consent to sexual intercourse (girls). Claim supplementary and social security benefits.* Buy cigarettes and tobacco; drink beer, wine cider or perry in a pub, hotel or restaurant if with a meal. Choose own doctor; consent to medical treatment (and withhold or withdraw consent) have to pay*	If married, cannot be made the subject of a Care Order

*If left school

Table 4   (*contd.*)

Age	Individual and family matters	Legal and medico-legal proceedings
	prescription charges; hold a licence to drive a moped, motorcycle, or invalid carriage. Buy fireworks and Premium Bonds Join the armed forces with parents' consent (boys)	
From 17	Join the armed forces with parents' consent (girls)	Be sent to prison if convicted of a serious crime.
From 18	Leave home, marry, join armed forces, get passport without parental consent. Get cheque or credit cards, buy or hire purchase, get a mortgage and own land, property or shares, sign contracts and be sued. Vote, sit on a jury, make a will, act as executor for someone else's will. Buy alcohol and drink in a pub, work in a bar and use betting shops. See birth certificate if adopted. See an X film; give blood	Can no longer be taken into care; and existing Care Orders normally end, but may last until age 19
From 21	Adopt a child; stand for council or Parliament; engage in homosexual activity in private if a man and partner over 21 is consenting. Hold a licence to drive a heavy vehicle or bus, or to sell alcohol	Be sentenced to life imprisonment

adults to be reappraising their views of what is right and wrong, or desirable and undesirable, and certainly middle-aged adults are experimenting openly with new sexual and social mores in a way which received less publicity in Victorian times. Adolescents perceive this adult uncertainty at every level: parental hesitation over matters which were once moral certainties; educational methods shifting with different political and educational approaches; the law, for example on sex, drugs, abortion, and responses to crime being something not given from on high but open to public debate and often acrimonious dispute. There is now good evidence that violent behaviour, whether fictional or factual reporting, on television (Surgeon-General, 1972; Lefkowitz *et al.*, 1977; Belson, 1978; Rutter, 1979a) or in the press (Barraclough *et al.*, 1977) can result in imitative behaviour. Man's earlier styles of culture had relatively rigid rules by which to live, backed up for formidable social pressure and, if necessary, severe physical measure of control (for example female circumcision in African countries, binding women's feet in China, execution for transgressors nearly everywhere). At the end of childhood the pubertal boy or girl has been ritually received into the accepted culture, and given adult status. As pointed out earlier, what is accepted or desirable, particularly in Western cultures, is open to dispute, while the adolescent is legally, educationally, and socially enabled to take part in that dispute.

Major social upheaval, for good or ill, certainly seems to produce an upheaval and turbulence which is particularly marked among the adolescent population; there have been interesting accounts of the impact of major cultural changes in young people in Zambia (Mwanalushi, 1979) the People's Republic of China (Dixon, 1981) and in Northern Ireland (McLachlan, 1981). Whether or not this results in improved social systems is hard to predict; developments around the world are not encouraging. However, man is an experimental animal who plays and finds things out for himself, and it would be arrogant to suppose that natural selection is no longer operating albeit at a more clearly social level; perhaps the next stage of sociobiological evolution will determine the amount of immature radical experimentation a youthful culture can contain while maintaining sufficient homoeostasis to provide for basic physical needs.

This sociopolitical consideration is not so far removed either from the psychodynamic views of Winnicott (see page 88), from Berlin's dictum that history is the story of parricide, and from the sociobiological necessity of the parental generation handing over authority and responsibility to the rising generation. The rules, then, are important, in their making, their challenging, their defence, their breaking and in the reaction to their being broken, and part of the adolescent's transition is from being someone with little influence on the rules to someone who can be in a position to challenge, break, or defend them. Keesing and Keesing (1971) have elaborated the theme of man as creator of rules, sometimes on a more or less arbitrary basis along with myths and rituals (Levi-Strauss, 1966) but also as one version of ecological adaption. Bringing together work by Bateson (1958), Scheffler (1965), and Allen (1967) they suggest that rules about rights, duties, and authority, constantly being made and broken, negotiated, revised, and elaborated, tend to be about the following themes: the relative states of men versus women; the relative importance of husband–wife and brother–sister ties; the relative importance of collective versus individual rights; the conflict between competition for resources versus the need for uniting in achieving common goals; the unity of peers from different families versus the ties within their families; and competition and conflict between generations over authority, rights and access to resources, sometimes leading to an alliance of alternate generations.

In many cultures it is the grandparental generation that can quite strikingly exert a moderating, stimulating, or provocative effect on the young, with the middle-age group happily or unhappily in between – a pattern that may be seen in international affairs as well as in the clinic. 'The tyrant and the mob, the grandfather and the grandchild, are natural allies' (Schopenhauer).

(b) Community, school, peer, and family influences

We know that both the family and the wider cultural environment are both influential in child and adolescent development; which is the stronger influence will depend on such things as the nature of the child–family pattern of feeling, mutual regard and communication, characteristically impaired where there is disturbance in a child (Rutter, 1977), and on the particular issue in question. Further, the family as well as the child is influenced by the external culture. Thus Mead (1928, 1930, 1953) and other anthropologists have emphasized how patterns of child upbringing are expressions of society along with its artistic, educational, and cultural activities, rather than its determinants. Nevertheless, to return to an earlier theme, in late adolescence and as adulthood approaches the boy or girl begins to see how he or she may in turn have some influence on that culture. A society's influence on its developing adolescent population may therefore be seen in terms of:

(i)   the effect of more or less enduring factors (for example its rules and resources);

(ii) the effect of compliance with or resistance to its rules and acceptance or rejection of its resources;

(iii) the effect of the rules and resources changing.

One may take, as measures of a given community's effect on its children, the rates among them of delinquency and psychiatric disorder (as defined on page 10). Studies have consistently shown large and persisting differences between areas, with the highest rates in overcrowded, poor industrial city centres, lower rates in country towns, and the lowest rates in rural communities and affluent, spacious areas (see Rutter and Madge, 1977; Rutter, 1979a; Quinton, 1980). The nature of the problem makes it difficult to clarify the causes of this. Thus Rutter and Quinton (1977) were able to demonstrate that the higher rate for psychiatric disorder among London children compared with those in the Isle of Wight was entirely attributable to the higher incidence of family disadvantage in London, but why this should be the case in cities like London is not clear and seems not to be explicable in terms of lack of family support, poor housing, or overcrowding (Rutter, 1979a).

Within the family there is good evidence that certain constellations of difficulty and behavioural and emotional problems in the children are closely related, but not in the simplistic notion of 'early childhood trauma' causing later psychiatric problems, which remains a myth. Rather the evidence points in the direction of individual predisposition, the overlaid and cumulative family factors influencing each other and thereby shaping normal and abnormal aspects of the child's development.

Hinde (1980) has summarized some of the issues involved as follows (slightly modified);* his review and discussion of the complexities involved need to be read.

1. Children differ at birth as a result of genetic and prenatal influences and these differences include varying susceptibility to *later* environmental influences (Dunn, 1980).

2. Each characteristic of feeling and behaviour depends on multiple influences, some widespread in effects and some of which affect one or a few types of behaviour (Bateson, 1976).

3. The ways in which factors influence behaviour and their interaction are themselves variable. To take one example, a pattern of behaviour *or* vulnerability may depend on not one experience (for example loss of a parent in early life) but on a pattern of experiences (for example loss of a parent with whom there was a troubled relationship and followed by low social status).

4. The nature of the interaction between a parent and a child and its effects depend also on other family relationships. For example, the quality and severity of a child's failure to respond to a mother's attempts at control may depend also on the relationship (for example jealousy) between the child and a sibling and that between mother and father (for example hostility, lack of regard, lack of support, competition for one or other child's favour).

5. Individuals and relationships change over time in their properties and in the susceptibiliy to influences. And even if a particular pattern of interaction has a degree of consistency over time and maintains certain characteristics the overt behaviour through which those characteristics are experienced may change with time. For example, hostility of a child towards his or her mother could be expressed successively as obsessional behaviour, school refusal, and conduct disorder, depending on the further individual, psychological, and social development of the child, changes in family response, and changes in social opportunities and expectations. Rutter (1979a) has discussed the concept of the 'sleeper' effect by which particular circumstances have an effect leading to disorder some years later. There is little evidence for submerged problems, later resurfacing, to use a different metaphor. When adolescents present with difficulties, however, there are commonly current as well as early stresses in the history, although the relationship between them may not be evident.

6. The already complex interrelationships described are themselves subject to influences from outside the family. For example a mother's anxiety about the normality or otherwise of her daughter's sexual development and behaviour will be influenced by neighbourhood, school, and cultural attitudes and responses to sexual behaviour as well as her own. A problem which may seem to be due primarily to individual or family anxiety or misinformation about sexual development may also, or instead, be formulated as a problem of

---

* The brief clinical vignettes are those of the author.

parental control or confidence in the face of pressures, expectations or anxieties from outside.

7. The effect of these influences may be slight, moderate or marked, because: (a) their effect depends on their association with other factors at different times; (b) individuals are not passively responsive to all potential influences but select actively from those they encounter (for example choice of spouse often seems related to the individual's experiences of his or her parents and as a result tends to reproduce old problems or strengths in the family that results); (c) most influences do not have a continuous effect but operate only when above a threshold value; (d) relationships have certain self-regulatory properties. An influence that seems important in the short term may be unimportant in the long term.

With regard to the last point, Hinde points out that regulatory properties may protect against 'abnormality' but not against differences 'within the normal range'. This is of particular significance for clinical work, where the issue of what is abnormal (unusual, disordered or undesirable) is open to dispute and a normally functioning individual or family may have anxieties (or have anxiety thrust upon them from outside) because of uncertainty about normal variation. It also means that the clinician must be aware of all the individual's and family's strengths as well as the possibly relatively minor failure in regulation that has tipped the balance. Anxiety in an apparently out of control adolescent, bursting out of his or her family's trust and controls, may be immense, but a relatively small change may redress the balance, for example helping to reassert parental confidence.

The lesson for clinical diagnosis is that the clinician must be aware of (and assess) an extremely wide range of possibilities and must try to construct a reasonably economic diagnostic formulation that does not contain an un-manageable number of alternatives or too much speculative cement between the factual bricks. The clinician must be prepared for the *probability* that while the process of making a diagnosis is difficult and complex, the nature of what has gone wrong for this particular child in this particular family may be stated in quite simple operational terms. Unfortunately it is the number of alternatives in people's lives and in theoretical positions that pose a vast dilemma for clinical diagnosis, and a way of dealing with this is discussed in Chapters 6 and 7.

What can be said about family factors that disrupt development and those that are protective?

Rutter (1979a) tentatively mentions as *positive* or *ameliorating* influences in the family the importance of the child developing a sense of achievement, the protective value of strict parental supervision, and the maintenance of at least one good relationship preferably in, but if necessary outside, the home throughout periods of discord and disharmony. The lesson for the clinician is that he may forget to remind child and family of what they *have* achieved and of the strengths and advantages that they have already made available for themselves;

such things need to be said, in addition to pointing out painful realities (which must also be faced) to a family whose members may already be feeling guilty and regarding themselves as failures. In bringing into the discussion 'bad' things and 'good' things in a balanced and friendly way the clinician can also present a helpful model for a family which has managed to muddle discipline with hostility, supervision with intrusiveness, and encouragement with overindulgence.

Disruptive influences include the accumulation of adverse factors as opposed to the occurrence of a single stressor: loss of a parent by divorce or separation which is almost certainly a result of loss plus disharmony rather than loss alone; childhood bereavement, although again the relationship between this form of loss and its consequences is complex: parental death may have slight or no pathological consequences for the child (Rutter, 1971b), greater long-term effects if the loss was at age two or three years, or it may predispose to depressive disorders in later years (Bowlby, 1973; Brown *et al.*, 1975). Death of the parent of the same sex appears to increase the risk for the child, which may represent loss of an important adult model for childhood and adolescent development (Rutter, 1975) and is also consistent with some psychodynamic viewpoints (see page 80) in that the child needs time to work out ways of dealing with angry, jealous, loving, and anxious feelings towards his parents, and loss of the parent may give the child a frightening sense of his or her power to cause damage. A perhaps oversimplified impression, drawn from such studies and clinical evidence, is that there is a tendency for conduct problems to be related to family discord, whether or not the latter resulted in a broken home by the time the adolescent presents, and emotional problems, particularly sadness, to be more related to loss. Again, the relationship is a complex one. A child who has lost his or her father may in another sense experience loss of the surviving mother because of her prolonged grief, withdrawal, and preoccupation, particularly if there is lack also of the family and social supports necessary for effective grieving which again brings in extra-family influences. It also seems that other parental emotional problems, particularly chronic depression, increase the risk of similar problems in children, while antisocial or personality problems in parents tend to be associated with conduct problems in their children (Rutter, 1966, 1975).

Much the same considerations apply to the question of separation which seems not particularly damaging in itself but can be so against a background of family discord or pathology, which tends to be true also of childhood experience of major disasters (earthquakes, floods). If children are properly looked after and cared for by reasonably confident, consistent secure adults who help the child face painful realities and contain his or her distress (without discouraging its expression), children can be remarkably resilient.

Separation should be seen not as a single active event but as an interruption in the positive aspects of the child's upbringing and therefore representing removal of part of the developing links in continuity in a child's development. Similarly, 'deprivation' is not a simple concept, but is a general rubric for a multiplicity of quite different experiences (Rutter, 1972b). Separation that results in rearing of the child in an unsatisfactory institution with multiple and changing caretakers is fraught with risks to the child's development. These risks are likely to be due partly to the experience of that institution's pattern of care and partly to the experiences which took the child into institutional care in the first place (Wolkind and Rutter, 1973; Wolkind and Renton, 1979).

The second major environmental influence on a child's development is the school. The work of Rutter and his colleagues has demonstrated very large differences between schools in attendance, behaviour, academic achievement, and delinquency rates which persisted even when account was taken of differences in the type of pupil making up the schools' intake (Rutter et al., 1979), although the study did not go in depth into the family qualities that may have characterized socially and academically successful children. School factors which did not seem particularly significant in differentiating broadly successful schools from others were their size or age, and nor did a particular academic or pastoral approach appear significant. Eight key factors which did affect children were: (i) a reasonable balance of intellectual ability among the children; (ii) the ample use of rewards, praise, appreciation, and encouragement of children; (iii) good, comfortable working conditions and responsiveness to children's needs; (iv) adequate opportunities for children to take responsibilities in running aspects of their lives at school; (v) an adequate academic focus, with good use of homework and clearly set goals; (vi) good behaviour among the teachers such as punctuality, responsiveness to pupils, and generally courteous behaviour as opposed to the slapping and pushing about of pupils; (vii) care and skill in the preparation for and attention to work, with swift action to deal with disruptive behaviour; and (viii) firm leadership among the teachers but combined with all teachers' views represented in decision-making.

It has long seemed that the physical environment, whether of school, home, or play area, influenced children's and adolescents' behaviour, but since family discord and other problems, poverty, poor schooling, poor physical resources, vandalism and other forms of delinquency tend to cluster it is difficult to tease out causes from effects. The overall impression from a number of studies is that vandalism is an indicator of lack of supervision (including indirect factors in supervision such as the nature of street lighting); lack of a sense of personal territory and personal ownership, for example of front doors, corridors, and play areas; lack of flowers, trees, and grass; and lack of repair, repainting, and other maintenance work (Newman, 1975; Clarke 1978). Of course the old argument is that if nice facilities are provided they will soon be wrecked. What tends to happen is a token provision of pleasant surroundings in the form of the odd skimpy young tree or patch of grass and perhaps a bit of artwork from the local technical college, and these are soon attacked by children and not replaced by 'the authorities'. What is required is a sense of choice and ownership of such things, their more generous and thoughtful provision, more thought given to how they will be supervised and protected, and more persistence with repair and replacement when damage does occur. Certainly this policy works in children's homes and adolescent units.

(c) Attachment theory: the making, use, and breaking of social bonds and resulting influences on development

Bowlby's attachment theories (and related concepts which his work has stimulated) are of special interest because they provide a general model for behaviour and development which is compatible with a number of quite different observations and theoretical positions; and because it encompasses psychological (including psychodynamic), social, and biological ideas and data.

The general usefulness of the attachment model can be seen in clearer perspective if we first consider briefly some other work related to it, and in particular studies of the challenge and problems of coping with change.

Parkes (1969, 1971) has described as *psychosocial transitions* major changes in individuals' perceptions of themselves and their personal worlds, giving as examples major losses, for example of close companions, relatives, or parts of the body. The sense of a personal world is an important one, which is related to the self-image of a person but is more than this since it includes not only a sense of self but of 'possessions' (my father, my mother, my wife, my home, my eyesight, my limbs) and also of more abstract conceptions, composed of memory and feelings, of the world 'as it probably will be', including both ideal and feared possibilities. This *assumptive world* (Parkes, 1971) is a modification of a related concept of Cantril (1950), and an adaptation of what Lewin (1935) has termed the 'life space' and what Bowlby calls the 'world model'. Parkes considers that we are closely tied by affectional bonds to those things and feelings which constitute the assumptive world, and since change consists of losses and gains it requires something akin to grieving and something akin to exploration and experimentation, both of which can generate feelings that may be hard to cope with. Reorientation and readaptation to changed circumstances, people, feelings and ideas is therefore a challenge, and although Parkes does not include developmental maturation among these challenges the model throws light on the changes required in adolescent growth. Coleman (1978, 1979, 1980) while not drawing on Parkes's model, has suggested that the majority of adolescents cope with the necessary major changes in the transition from childhood to adulthood, and largely without turmoil and turbulence, by dealing with potentially stressful social relationships (for example conflict with parents, sexual relationships with peers) at different times, hence spreading their adaptation to change over a time span of years. Problems are likely to occur when for whatever reason (for example personal skills or circumstances) more than one issue at a time has to be coped with.

The concept of social challenges and the individual's sense of mastery, autonomy, and control are important factors in establishing self-esteem and a sense of personal competence and confidence (White, 1959, 1960; Lazarus 1966, 1969; and reviewed in Steinberg, 1972). Brown and Harris have taken this and attachment concepts further in a model for the development of vulnerability to depression in women (Brown and Harris, 1978). Like Parkes (1971) they explain how loss can be understood in terms of loss of value or reward, for example lost capacities, roles, and ideas as well as lost relationships, which results in a feeling of hopelessness which may generalize to feeling hopeless about wider aspects of life and becoming depressed. Thus an adolescent who finds she has not the interest or aptitude to meet a particular academic expectation or who loses a boy friend, may feel a general sense of despair and self-deprecation that is not warranted on purely intellectual grounds. Brown and Harris see the challenge of coping with significant loss as a factor in personality development, with successful resolution of the period of difficulty helping the individual deal with future losses; in this sense the model is compatible with the form of Erikson's developmental theory (page 91) if not its content.

The development of a capacity for anxiety, anger, and even paranoid feelings (page 85) can be seen as having some evolutionary advantage. Can the same be true of depression? The fact that a mood state which in one way or another can end in isolation and self-destruction is still part of the human repertoire suggests that it had some protective value during human evolution. Evolutionary models serve to draw attention to individual behaviour in social groups which is of interest from both general and clinical points of view, and provides an opportunity to match psychodynamic hypotheses with historical and behavioural evidence as to what man and the higher primates actually do. There are a number of intriguing views which will be mentioned briefly because of their possible links with the attachment model.

First, Storr (1972), among others, has drawn attention to the connections between creativity and the manic-depressive temperament, Lewis (1934) considered the depressive state as a paradigm of adaptation to intolerable situations, while psychoanalysts have regarded manic and hypomanic states as a defence against feelings of disappointment, and depression as related to the selective inhibition of aggression. Would a cyclothymic anthropoid ape have had survival and reproductive advantages over his contemporaries?

Second, Heymann (1965), pointing out that four great glacial eras separate us from early man, has speculated that the inheritance of a hibernation trait (lowered metabolism, lowered appetite, social withdrawal, changes in sleep rhythm, and phasic nature of mood states, all features which as Lange (1928) pointed out are shared with some depressive states) may have been a biological development consonant with surviving long, hard winters.

Third, Price (1978) drawing upon observations of baboons and macaque monkeys which, like man, rely for survival on a stable group dominance hierarchy, suggests that a depressive-like state in the senior individual allows him to finally withdraw without bloodshed when it is time for a younger, fitter male to take over; just as the equivalent submissive state allows the younger challenger to withdraw, again without bloodshed or disturbance of the social hierarchy, when the time is right.

Aggression and irritability characterize behaviour to subordinates, who are constantly reminded of their position by acts of minor threats and provocation, such as the direct gaze. The subordinate responds with anxiety and withdrawal; he grins or looks away from the direct gaze, gets out of the way when a superior approaches, or presents his hindquarters in a gesture of submission. (Price, 1968)

There is considerable compatibility of such observations with Winnicott's conceptions of fantasies of murder being just below the surface in the adolescent challenge and the adult response (see page 88), and with Erikson's model of the dangers and difficulties inherent in achieving self-assertion and initiative in the social group (page 91).

Fourth, Bowlby (1961) and Parkes (1969) have shown how many of the characteristics of grief, long regarded in largely abstract terms by psychoanalysts as the loss of a loved object, have much in common with the actual behaviour of animals and young children who become separated. For the human baby who is totally dependent on the parent for so long, and who would in primitive conditions soon die if lost, there is a biological imperative to stay close. The pining for the missing person; the preoccupied urge to recover his or her company; the crying, agitated, restless searching and angry protesting; the heightened perceptive set that makes an ambiguous image seem like that of the lost person – all convey the profound pressure for parent and child to get together again as a matter of urgency, and the behaviour and depth of feeling seen in grief reactions.

Bowlby's work on the concept of attachment, and his development of theories and hypotheses about attachment behaviour, brings a number of psychoanalytic and biological ideas together in a control systems model which will be outlined here, although the wide range of observations and inferences on which it is based, and wider implications of his approach, should themselves be read (Bowlby, 1969, 1973, 1980). For the relatively simplified control-systems model described below I am grateful to Dr Dorothy Heard, one of Bowlby's collaborators, who has applied the model to crisis-intervention methods, family therapy, and other aspects of child psychiatry and described its relationships to object relations theory (Heard, 1974, 1978, 1981), and with whom the author developed a tentative model for social interaction in treatment organisations which is discussed on page 131 (Steinberg and Heard, 1976).

Bowlby's attachment theory is based on five principal propositions.
1. An individual must have *an internal working model of his environment* if he is to find his way about, in a metaphorical as well as a literal sense, frame effective

plans, and know his own capabilities. This is not a simple static plan (although some such plan serves for lower animals) but an immensely complex picture of the world and the individual in it (see assumptive world, etc., page 106). Also 'the idea of a model in the brain is that it constitutes a toy that is yet a tool, an imitation world which we can manipulate in the way that will suit us best, and so find out how to manipulate the real world, which it is supposed to represent' (Young, 1964).

This inner world-model is one which develops over time, and has affective and cognitive aspects.

2. The developing individual needs to *maintain proximity to its parent*; for the human child, this need is particularly long-lasting. The parent meets the child's needs for warmth, food (through the child's inbuilt propensity to suck the breast), and to cling to a human being (see page 108).

3. The corresponding behaviour by which the parent responds to the child is *care-taking behaviour*; one important form seen in primates is retrieval behaviour, when the mother gathers the infant into her arms and holds him there.

4. The developing infant needs also to *explore the environment* which requires moving away from the parent figure. Initiative for breaking and resuming contact lies partly with mother and partly with infant, and the balance changes as the infant gets older.

5. These four components of the model (*elaboration of an internalized working model of the environment; proximity-seeking attachment* behaviour (PSAB); *care-taking behaviour (CB)*; *exploratory behaviour*) are arranged together in a dynamic control system.

Exploratory behaviour and the building of an internal model are open parts of the system while exploratory behaviour and proximity-seeking attachment behaviour (PSAB) are necessarily antithetical to each other. PSAB such as arm-raising, crying, following, clinging, 'switches on' care-taking behaviour (CB), to develop the cybernetic model, while adequate care-taking behaviour 'switches off' PSAB and this enables the infant to explore its environment. Experience of the environment and of close attachment both contribute to elaboration of the internal model of the world. These four components of the basic attachment model operate together as in Figure 16.

This model can be elaborated in a number of ways. First, it is compatible with many broad tenets of psychodynamic theories of development, as outlined earlier in this chapter. The critics of psychodynamic theory have sometimes been over-preoccupied with some of the odd things psychoanalysts have said and the mistakes they have made over the past 80 years and not recognized the extraordinary and quite revolutionary change in psychological thinking brought about by Freud and his successors. At its simplest, and stated broadly in terms of attachment theory, normal emotional development can be described as the child steadily accumulating inner feelings and memories of past achievements

Parent achieves perceptive, responsive finely-tuned balance between encouragement and protectiveness at a point which enables child to explore confidently with manageable anxiety and sure of parental backing

Child adds to its 'backing' the part-affective and part-cognitive recollection of past challenges, past explorations, and past care-taking. A sense of what he or she can/cannot do, and where help comes from, forms the core of growing self-image, self-confidence and self-esteem (S)

The older child and young adolescent now needs actual care-taking less, though may need occasional 'boost' when the boy or girl has over-reached himself or herself. Much more self-reliance and S begins to contain images not of parents but of future supportive relationships

Mature individual, now self-reliant but able to recognize occasional need for support (which may be emotional, intellectual or physical) and willing to seek and use it but also to recognize this need in others and give it without being over-protective or negligent. Perceptive, responsive, finely-tuned balance forms the core of mature peer–peer behaviour

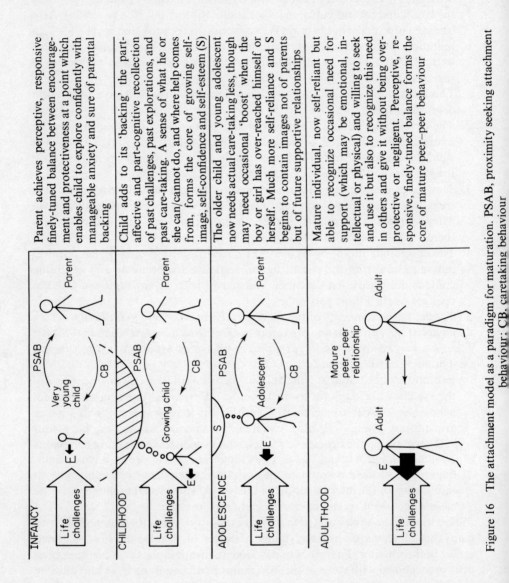

Figure 16   The attachment model as a paradigm for maturation. PSAB, proximity seeking attachment behaviour; CB, caretaking behaviour

(including both good experiences and bad experiences survived) most of which cannot be put into words or even thought about very precisely, but which becomes a core of self-esteem and trust which enables the making of sound judgements, and this in turn permits the safe experimentation and exploration by which new relationships, knowledge, and skills are acquired. So much of our thinking and feeling seem based on the dynamic outcome between opposing forces (good and bad; left and right; up and down; trust versus mistrust; conscious versus unconscious; attachment versus exploration; the binary system) that it could well be that the way we perceive and make sense of the world is strongly influenced by the way our nervous system develops, a notion detectable, if sometimes rather obscurely, in the work of Bateson (1973, 1979) and Jung (page 90).

Second, the attachment dynamic that Bowlby describes does not apply only to infancy. An adolescent or adult in a new and potentially challenging situation (which can include roles and relationships lost and gained, new environments and atmospheres to operate in, even ideas and new concepts to assimilate and relate to long-held, treasured ones) relies on (a) his internal assumptive world of self-image and belief as a safe base from which to explore; but in so far as the safe base may be seriously challenged, he relies also on (b) real relationships such as those of relatives, friends, colleagues and, if necessary, professional helpers (see pages 129 and 131). Henderson (1974), following Bowlby's conception of attachment as affectional bonding throughout life (Bowlby, 1977), has described the individual's repertoire of care-eliciting behaviour as developing throughout childhood, adolescence, and into adult life in ways which may be normal or pathological. The continuation of the relevance of the attachment model for adult life has three important clinical and practical implications.

1. The individual (adolescent or adult) under more stress than he can cope with himself and with existing supports increasingly expresses behaviour designed to elicit help and, if it fails to work, resorts to behaviour which *used to work* (as an 'childish' behaviour, or regression). Meyerburg and Post (1979) have suggested ways in which the facts of neurological development can account for a return to more primitive responses when under stress, including those of psychodynamic significance.

2. The fine balance of mutual social signals which elicit care and support and respond to the need for care and support is ordinarily unobstrusive and is the equivalent of a physiological potential space. A healthy child in a circumstances in which he or she can cope cannot be seen showing dramatic care-eliciting gestures and the mother responding massively; on the contrary, except in crises, this might be evidence of the attachment dynamic failing. Correspondingly, normal social behaviour between, for example, husband and wife, or professional colleagues, will include unobtrusive and near-unconscious mutual regard and responsiveness which is the basis of mature friendship and collaboration in work. By the same token, among mature

adults care- or support-eliciting and responding roles should quite readily be exchangeable, perhaps several times during the same interaction.

3. Perceptiveness and responsiveness are the key attributes of whoever is in the role of the attachment figure because finely tuned responsiveness maintains the care-eliciting figure in the 'ideal' state of comfortable exploration.

Exploration is not only the real exploration of physical topography but an inner creative process of model-making too. Intellectual and imaginative exercises, the various psychodynamic and cognitive theories of defence (Festinger, 1957) 'playing with ideas', 'coming to terms' with difficult realities, new learning and self-reappraisal are all examples of intrapsychic creative activity which can be understood as exploratory in nature. The individual who copes with difficult circumstances primarily by changing how things are in reality may be, or be regarded, as a psychopathic manipulator, a radical reformer, or a creative innovator, depending on factors too complex to be argued here. The individual who copes primarily by internal psychic manoeuvrings may become, or be regarded, as psychotic, neurotic, unrealistic, a 'dreamer', or someone with strong 'inner reserves of strength', with the happy, self-sufficient meditator being the archetype. If part of exploration is perceived as keeping the inner 'world models' consonant with outer reality, and outer support systems, the individual becomes increasingly self-moderating, becoming increasingly adept at handling new situations, his judgement of them and of his own capacity to cope, and his judgement of what he needs of other people and how they will respond develops; moreover, he is increasingly confident of his capacity to manage when his predictions about reality or other people's responsiveness go temporarily wrong. Achievement of this fine balance between reality facing (reality testing) and inner planning, and autonomy without isolation, is one way of conceiving the foundations of mature self-esteem and optimism, mature peer–peer relationships, and therefore a firm foundation for such adult relationships as marriage, professional teamwork and interprofessional collaboration. (see Chapter 20).

Attachment theory can be criticized on the grounds that it is, as presented by Bowlby too broad a perspective for detailed and specific understanding and testing, and it does not take sufficient account of individual differences in attachment behaviour. However, as Ainsworth et al. (1978) and Heard (1981) have pointed out, that is the sort of theory it is, an open-ended model and explanatory theory rather than a rigid mesh of propositions. Certainly more specific propositions from other frames of reference such as regression, introjection, mutual social signalling, selective reinforcement, and individual differences in child and caretaker remain testable, and both the confirmation or refutation of specific hypotheses are more worth while and indeed make more sense against the background of a general and in some ways quite simple model for the way in which the developing individual learns from experience of the world, experience of relationships, and experience of himself.

Chapter 5

The Emergence of Problems:
II. The Referral Process

INTRODUCTION

The types of adolescent referrals made to psychiatrists fall very broadly into the following categories (see also Figure 17):

1. The adolescent needs psychiatric help as described earlier (page 51). There are also young people in the community who might benefit from psychiatric assessment or treatment but who for some reason are not referred.
2. There is a problem, but consultation with the referring agent clarifies that an alternative to psychiatry is desirable and appropriate.
3. The adolescent may be the focus of a problem which clearly needs help of the sort which a psychiatric team *or an alternative service* could provide. Whether the adolescent psychiatric team takes the problem on or helps explore alternatives in consultation depends on how it sees its functions and the alternatives available locally.
4. Occasionally there is no perceived (or agreed) problem at all by the time of the appointment, which may be cancelled or not kept by the adolescent and family or referring agent. The referral may have been a misunderstanding, or a crisis has proved transient and resolved itself.

ADOLESCENT PROBLEMS IN THE COMMUNITY

Goldberg and Huxley (1980) have described psychiatric problems in the general, largely adult community as existing at five levels, each level described in terms of the particular population of which the psychiatric observer is aware.

113

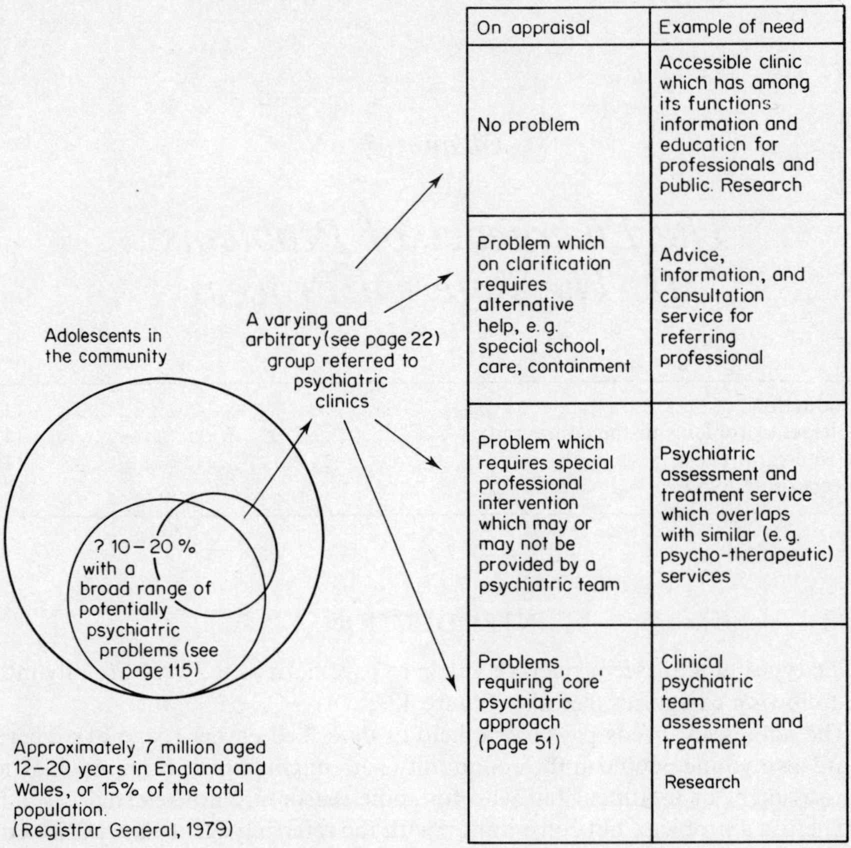

On appraisal	Example of need
No problem	Accessible clinic which has among its functions information and education for professionals and public. Research
Problem which on clarification requires alternative help, e. g. special school, care, containment	Advice, information, and consultation service for referring professional
Problem which requires special professional intervention which may or may not be provided by a psychiatric team	Psychiatric assessment and treatment service which overlaps with similar (e. g. psycho-therapeutic) services
Problems requiring 'core' psychiatric approach (page 51)	Clinical psychiatric team assessment and treatment Research

Adolescents in the community

A varying and arbitrary (see page 22) group referred to psychiatric clinics

? 10 – 20 % with a broad range of potentially psychiatric problems (see page 115)

Approximately 7 million aged 12–20 years in England and Wales, or 15% of the total population.
(Registrar General, 1979)

Figure 17   Adolescents in the community: a broad spectrum of psychiatric and non-psychiatric needs and responses

Level 1: psychiatric morbidity in the community.

Level 2: psychiatric morbidity among those patients attending general practitioners.

Level 3: those patients attending general practitioners who are identified as psychiatrically disordered.

Level 4: those attending psychiatric out-patient clinics.

Level 5: those admitted to hospital.

Goldberg and Huxley suggest that 'psychiatric illness proper' begins at Level 4 because psychiatrists 'seldom send patients away undiagnosed'. This sequential pathway from domestic setting through general practitioner to out-patient and then in-patient hospital setting has more in common with the referral route of the child with meningitis (page 20) than with the more kaleidoscopic 'Rubic cube'

Table 5   Comparison of Goldberg and Huxley's levels of psychiatric presentation with adolescent psychiatric practice

Level	Goldberg and Huxley (1980)	Approximate equivalent in adolescent psychiatric practice
1	Psychiatric morbidity in the community	Psychiatric morbidity among adolescents in the community
2	Psychiatric morbidity among patients attending GPs	Psychiatric morbidity among those referred for special help, e.g. to special education, counselling services, GPs, the courts
3	Psychiatric morbidity among patients identified as psychiatrically disordered by GPs	Psychiatric morbidity among those regarded by special teachers counsellors, GPs, the courts *et al.* as being possibly/probably psychiatrically disordered
4	Psychiatric morbidity among those patients attending psychiatric out-patient clinics	Psychiatric morbidity among those referred to child and adolescent psychiatric clinics
5	Psychiatric morbidity among those admitted to hospital	Psychiatric morbidity among those taken on by psychiatric clinics for treatment or admitted to psychiatric units

model of how disturbed children and adolescents present via many alternative and randomly crossing pathways. Table 5 suggests the approximate equivalents in child and adolescent psychiatric practice to the levels proposed by Goldberg and Huxley, and will be referred to again later (see below). From what has been said already it will be clear that in child and adolescent psychiatry the incidence of psychiatric disorder from Levels 2 to 5 in Table 5 are heavily dependent on the attitudes of parents, of professionals involved on an intermediate basis, and of the 'receiving' psychiatrists and their colleagues. However, a useful way into this question can be made at Level 1, the epidemiology of psychiatric disorder in the adolescent population.

Epidemiology of adolescent psychiatric disorder

Incidence of relatively clearly defined psychiatric disorders

The schizophrenic disorders, manic-depressive and depressive illnesses, anorexia nervosa, hyperkinetic disorder (when persistent beyond puberty) and seriously handicapping anxiety, phobic and obsessional disorders with adult-type symptomatology begin to make their appearance in late childhood and early adolescence, while autism and related disorders, present from early infancy, of course, continue into adolescence when they may present with renewed difficulties (see Chapter 14). These conditions tend to be more clearly recognized as individual disorders by the community and professional workers alike, and their referral to psychiatrists more readily follows the traditional routes to specialist medical care.

They are also relatively rare. The prevalence of schizophrenic disorders in mid-adolescence is about 1 : 1,000 (Rutter, 1979a) and that of manic-depressive illness and depressive psychosis probably of a similar order. Autism as broadly defined is found in about 1 in 2,500 children, with about half, 1 in 5,000, showing more specific autistic characteristics (Lotter, 1976). Anorexia nervosa varies in prevalence, depending on age and social class and probably other factors in the shifting sands of social circumstances, from 1 in 100 girls in high risk groups to 1 in 300 in those less at risk (Crisp *et al.*, 1976; Crisp, 1978, 1980). It also occurs in boys. Obsessional disorders were found in only seven children (1 in 500) by Rutter and his colleagues (1970) in the Isle of Wight study of children up to age 12, and none had the fully developed adult-type disorder, although it would be found more frequently in an adolescent population. (See Chapter 10, and Bolton *et al.*, 1983.)

Less well-defined psychiatric disorder

Those childhood and adolescent problems categorized as emotional disorder, conduct disorder, or mixed disorders of emotions and conduct are particularly difficult to delineate clearly as psychiatric disorders. Thus an unknown proportion will prove responsive to changes in social (for example housing and educational) policy, and improvements in the general level of child upbringing ability in the general population; of the remainder many children and adolescents designated as having special difficulties are likely to be helped by means which are not primarily psychiatric, for example by improved social and special educational services. Moreover, we do not know how many problems of this sort will prove adequately responsive to family therapeutic approaches; very likely a large proportion will. On the one hand it could be argued that this does not make these children's problems non-psychiatric, any more than widespread infection and malnutrition at the turn of the century were primarily non-medical because what ultimately put such disorders right was not clinical treatment but changes in the law regarding sanitation, water supply, housing, and the general care of children. On the other hand, that facet of psychiatry which in due course may most help very many conduct disordered and emotionally disordered children may prove to be epidemiological and preventative psychiatry, rather than clinical treatment.

Of the 500 adolescents referred to a regional adolescent service over a two year period, about 80% were diagnosed as being within this group of relatively ill-defined disorders (Steinberg *et al.*, 1981), and this group probably constitutes a still greater proportion of the out-patient population of child and adolescent psychiatric clinics. This number could probably be reduced not only by making alternative and more precise individual diagnoses, but by diagnosing 'no individual disorder present' more often. In the adolescent population in general estimates suggest that some 10–15% of boys and girls have psychiatric disturbance mostly of mood and conduct (Chapter 10), a figure which rises to around 21% depending on the age group and area surveyed, and of course on where the diagnostic line is drawn (Graham and Rutter, 1973; Leslie, 1974; Rutter et al., 1976; Rutter and Madge, 1977; Graham and Rutter, 1977). Rutter and his co-workers point out that the presence of psychiatric disorder as operationally defined does not necessarily mean that help from a psychiatrist was needed, even when special help of some sort is indicated.

Adolescent mood problems not referred to psychiatrists

Another perspective on adolescent problems at large is the concept of emotional turbulence in adolescence. Much of the literature on adolescence has stressed that the 'inner turmoil' of adolescence is so widespread as to be the norm (Hall, 1904; Geleerd, 1961; Eissler, 1958; Anna Freud, 1958, 1966; Blos 1970). Rutter and his colleagues have confirmed that feelings of misery, self-depreciation, and ideas of reference occur quite commonly, often as transient experiences, among 14-year-olds, and were found to be causing appreciable personal distress in 20–40% (depending on the symptom) of a general population sample of 96 boys and 88 girls. Thus over 40% of both sexes reported feelings of misery, problems of sleeping and early waking occurred in 20%, ideas of reference in about 30%, self-depreciation in about 20% and just under 8% reported suicidal ideas. The adults in contact with these young people tended not to know about these feelings.

The significance of these findings in terms of the existence or prediction of psychiatric disorder in these young people remained uncertain (Rutter et al., 1976). What can be said, pursuing the theme that psychiatric disorder in this age group is often a matter of opinion, is that if primarily social circumstances should bring a boy or girl to the attention of an adolescent psychiatric clinic, the finding of symptoms such as those listed above does not itself confirm that the boy or girl was correctly regarded as being psychiatrically disordered. Certainly the clinician must consider the boy's or girl's distress as an important factor in making a diagnostic assessment and planning help, but this particular clinical finding does not make out, say, an underachieving, misbehaving, or uncommunicative adolescent as being psychiatrically abnormal.

Adolescent behaviour problems

Finally, problems of misconduct among teenage boys and girls attract considerably publicity, and are particularly open to varying interpretations as social, family, or psychiatric problems. Absconding from home, promiscuity, violence, theft and vandalism, and the abuse of alcohol, drugs and other substances are increasing, although Rutter (1979a) advises caution on how statistics of increasing crime and vandalism should be interpreted. A related group of disadvantaged young people are those in the long-term residential care of local authorities, and who include among their numbers a high proportion with persisting emotional and behaviour problems (Wolkind and Renton, 1979). In general none of these groups is coped with well, from the adolescents' point of view nor from that of the community; they remain a large, perplexing assemblage, probably growing in number and including more girls, and more pre-adolescent children among their number.

THE REFERRAL PROCESS

In Chapter 1 (pages 13 to 15) the range of reasons (by no means mutually exclusive) for the referral of an adolescent to a psychiatrist were listed as: *distress, disability, disturbing behaviour, presumed diagnosis, and administrative routine*.

Leaving aside the last, which is a special case, two fundamental motives are involved in referrals:

1. The largely logical, rational request for the technical expertise of the specialist team to whom the boy or girl is referred. (Not, incidentally, immensely highly regarded in the case of psychiatry and related services.)
2. The feelings involved, for example hope, trust, confidence, friendliness, caution, suspicion, ambivalence, competitive feelings, anxiety, anger, wish for help. (See also page 131).

The rational aspect of referrals is the most readily acknowledged, but the feelings associated with the referral of children and adolescents at all points in the referral chain (parents, teachers, primary care professionals, adolescent psychiatric team) can directly affect the decisions that are made and how they are responded to.

Whether or not a boy or girl is referred to psychiatric care may depend as much on the confidence and attitudes towards the adolescent of the parents (or the staff of a school or a children's home) as on the state of the child himself or herself. This does not make the parents' (or staff members') intellectual decision any less important, and nor does it deny the importance of the mental state of the individual boy or girl. There are four aspects of the emotional component of the referral to be considered:

1. *Response to the adults involved in the referral*
   The feelings of those involved in the referral (parents and professional workers) need recognition and responding to, because they can be very painful feelings indeed.
2. *Diagnostic assessment*
   Assessment of how disturbed or abnormal the child may be requires some

measure of how normal are the feelings in the group from which he or she has been referred. For example, the referral of an 'unmanageable' child from a confident, competent children's home is a different matter to referral from a children's home in chronic disarray. Equally, parental anxiety about a 'misbehaving' or 'underachieving' child needs to be assessed against some idea of whether the family's expectations are high, normal or low, ordinary or extraordinary.

3. *Collaborative work*

Collaboration with at least some of those involved in the referral will be needed. There are of course many variations and alternatives; a family doctor or another child psychiatrist, for example, may very much wish to remain involved or may prefer to hand the child's case entirely to the new clinical team. On the other hand, those involved directly with the child's care and education must remain involved to some extent, either totally (in family therapy) or partially (for example in collaborating with parents and teachers over an adolescent's progress and future schooling). If admission to an in-patient unit is required, feelings to do with separation, collaboration in treatment, visits, the return home (and the possibility in some cases of not returning home), must all be worked with.

It is important to note that this aspect is not only a matter of coping with areas of vulnerability and difficulty, it requires recognizing and encouraging strengths and skills, and avoiding their being undermined.

4. *The clinical team*

Finally, the feelings of the receiving clinical team must be taken into account by those leading and supervising its work.

In the attachment model discussed in Chapter 4, it was pointed out that some feelings occupy a potential space, in the sense that an important parenting skill is knowing the child well enough to respond very early to the signal of anxiety or, alternatively, to respond appropriately if the child does need 'stretching' in order to learn to cope with new things and with feelings of anxiety, yet not pushed too far.

Equally, adult peer–peer relationships and mature social skills require sensitive perception on both sides as to what can be coped with or should be coped with, which requires mutual understanding and sharing of feelings, without great heat needing to be generated in order to put a point across (see page 110). Among the professional worker's tasks, in diagnosis as well as in continuing treatment, is the need for perceptive recognition of what the adults involved so far with the adolescent can contribute to the adolescent's care and to the demands of treatment.

Very powerful feelings can become overt in work with adolescents: a family, children's home or school may be at their wits' end over a particular adolescent, and highly anxious, angry or despairing. The psychiatric team can also become overstretched with equally strong feelings. From time to time the two peaks of feeling will coincide, with an imperative, urgent demand to take on (or admit) a very demanding adolescent coming at the same time the clinical team has gone beyond its limits with its existing clientele. Again, someone must deal with and reconcile these feelings too, in order to respond with a sensible decision.

Overt or covert feelings, minor or major, in the family, in the intermediate professionals involved, and in the 'receiving' team are part of the assessment of the adolescent and his circumstances.

ASPECTS OF AETIOLOGY

To summarize, the process by which a boy or girl becomes a psychiatric patient depends on three approximately sequential but overlapping processes:
1. The young person's development, which is primarily a matter of individual maturation within the family and, later, outside relationships.

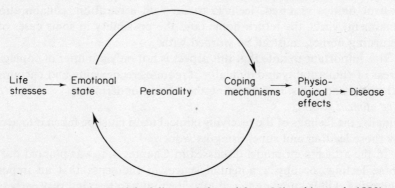
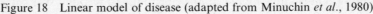

Figure 18   Linear model of disease (adapted from Minuchin *et al.*, 1980)

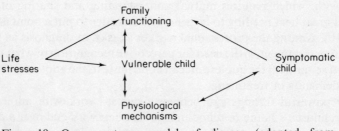

Figure 19   Open systems model of disease (adapted from Minuchin *et al.*, 1980)

2. Adult attitudes to the child and his or her development, for example concern about difficulties, anxiety about behaviour, and how they are responded to; this is primarily a matter of how the family copes with problems.

3. The selection of certain sorts of problems as specifically requiring psychiatric assessment or care, that is the referral process, which is primarily socially determined.

The referral process therefore takes its place among the areas of the adolescent's life which need to be explored for aetiological factors; not aetiology of disorder, but aetiology of patient status.

Aetiological factors in child and adolescent psychiatry tend to be multiple; causative factors quite often cluster (for example the emotional, conduct, family, educational, and neighbourhood problems outlined above); they interact with each other, with some having a cumulative effect and making matters worse, others (sometimes unknown) having ameliorating or protective effects (Rutter and Madge, 1976; Rutter, 1979a); some cause problems, some account for disorders, and some are influential in the referral process.

One therefore has to 'pin down' what constitutes a disordered state or situation before asking about its aetiology. From what has already been said, it can be seen that disturbed behaviour in a child may be a presenting problem or a contribution to continuing family discord. One psychiatrist may see the problem in terms of individual conduct disorder, caused by family disruption; another may see it as a family problem in which the child's misbehaviour is an aetiological factor. Thus Minuchin *et al.* (1980), in relation to psychosomatic disorder, have distinguished between the *linear model* (Figure 18) in which individual disorder is seen as a final common path, emerging from the interaction between social, psychological, and biological processes and the *open systems model* (Figure 19) of functioning, maintaining family members in various positions, roles and mood and behavioural states, including the selected child with his or her symptoms.

The two models are not incompatible. From the complex interaction between different levels of functioning already described (for example pages 64 to 69) it is reasonable to believe that what is described in Figure 19 is simply that which would be going on *at any time during development* if one were to take a cross-section so to speak, for example at the time of referral.

To understand how things have developed, the history will consist of a detailed and chronological life story, a biography (Ounsted, 1972) beginning with grandparents, parents' lives, and marriage. It is also necessary to understand what is going on *now*, also in physiological, psychological, family dynamic or social terms.

It is also helpful to think of causes in terms of four sets of ways in which they can operate:

(a) *The power of an aetiological factor*; a cause may be *necessary*, in the sense that disorder will not develop in its absence, but alone it may not be sufficient to cause disorder. Or a cause may be *sufficient* in that alone it can account for disorder. Variable penetrance in genetics is an example. A schizophrenic illness may develop in one individual come what may, and in another with less biochemical vulnerability, because of external factors.

(b) *The timing of the effect of aetiological factors*; for example, suppose a hypothetical biochemical or family dynamic influence made a child highly aroused when under certain conditions of social stress. The child might have tantrums in infancy, persistent bed-wetting in later childhood, become quiet, withdrawn and tense early in adolescence, and aggressive in late adolescence. He might be considered at the successive stages naughty, emotionally disturbed, normal, and then delinquent, the expression of each manifestation of the underlying aetiological factor depending on how and when the child is vulnerable, for example in bladder control at one stage, in terms of aggressive self-assertion at a later stage.

(c) *Precipitation or maintenance of problems*; one set of internal and external aetiological factors may *predispose* to a disordered state, that is the boy, girl or family is all the time or recurrently vulnerable. Another set of factors may *precipitate* disorder. Other factors may *maintain disorders or problems*. A schizophrenic illness, for example, may begin as an inherited predisposition (page 233), be precipitated by social factors (page 234), and possibly be maintained by family circumstances (page 234).

Table 6   Different perspectives of aetiology

General models for development of disorder	1. Multifactorial 2. Multifactorial and interacting 3. Linear interaction 4. Systems interaction 5. Developmental model including { linear interaction / systems interaction / individual maturation
Mode of influence of aetiological factors	1. The power of aetiological factors < necessary / sufficient 2. The timing of aetiological factors in relation to individual maturation and external circumstances 3. Aetiological factors < predisposing to / precipitating / maintaining } problems
Concept of disorder	1. As a single psychological, psychodynamic, family or neuropsychiatric entity 2. As a cluster of processes, events and phenomena that with varying appropriateness may be regarded as psychiatric disorder, depending on the nature of the problem and on external social and cultural circumstances

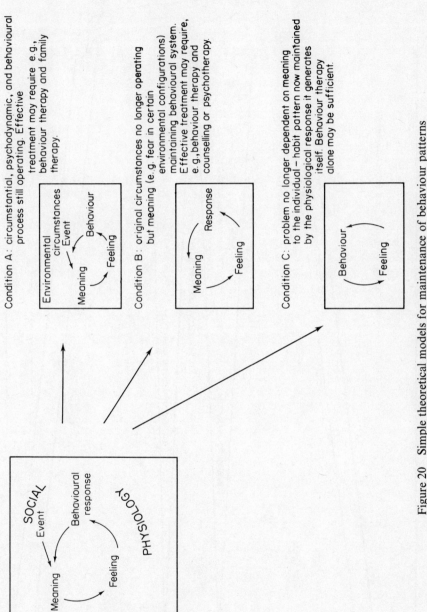

Condition A: circumstantial, psychodynamic, and behavioural process still operating. Effective treatment may require e.g., behaviour therapy and family therapy.

Environmental circumstances Event, Behaviour, Feeling, Meaning

Condition B: original circumstances no longer operating but meaning (e.g. fear in certain environmental configurations) maintaining behavioural system. Effective treatment may require, e.g., behaviour therapy and counselling or psychotherapy.

Response, Feeling, Meaning

Condition C: problem no longer dependent on meaning to the individual – habit pattern now maintained by the physiological response it generates itself. Behaviour therapy alone may be sufficient.

Behaviour, Feeling

SOCIAL Event, Behavioural response, PHYSIOLOGY, Feeling, Meaning, PSYCHOLOGY

Figure 20 Simple theoretical models for maintenance of behaviour patterns

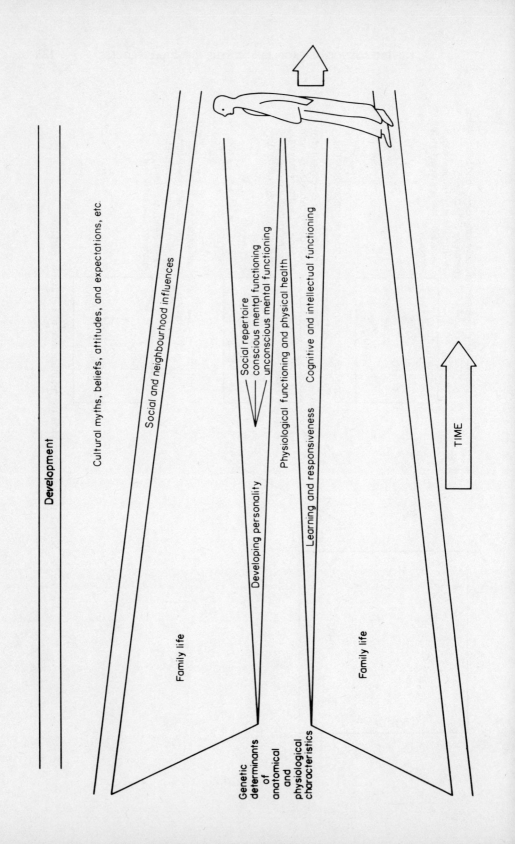

Development

Cultural myths, beliefs, attitudes, and expectations, etc.

Social and neighbourhood influences

Family life

Developing personality

Social repertoire
conscious mental functioning
unconscious mental functioning

Physiological functioning and physical health

Learning and responsiveness

Cognitive and intellectual functioning

Family life

Genetic determinants of anatomical and physiological characteristics

TIME

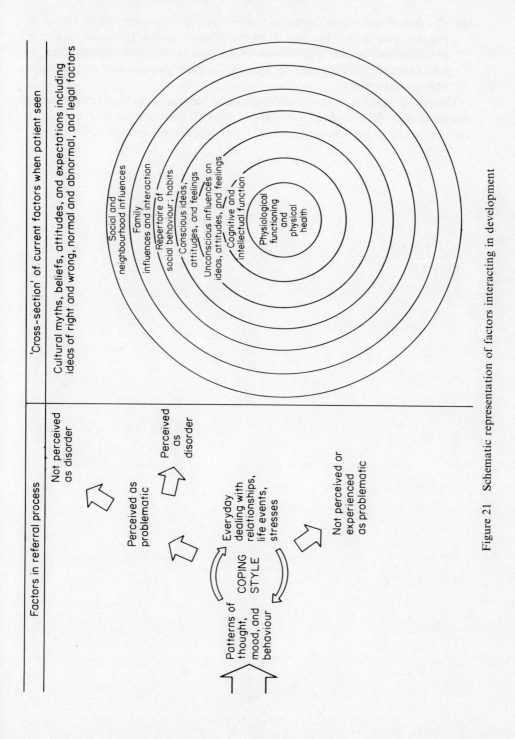

Figure 21   Schematic representation of factors interacting in development

Factors in referral process

Not perceived as disorder

Perceived as disorder

Perceived as problematic

'Cross-section' of current factors when patient seen

Cultural myths, beliefs, attitudes, and expectations including ideas of right and wrong, normal and abnormal, and legal factors

Social and neighbourhood influences

Family influences and interaction

Repertoire of social behaviour; habits

Conscious ideas, attitudes, and feelings

Unconscious influences on ideas, attitudes, and feelings

Cognitive and intellectual function

Physiological functioning and physical health

Everyday dealing with relationships, life events, stresses

COPING STYLE

Not perceived or experienced as problematic

Patterns of thought, mood, and behaviour

(d) *Problems becoming self perpetuating*. Finally, maintaining factors (social or behavioural) may take over from the original causes (psychodynamic or physiological) which then become redundant as far as treatment is concerned. (Figure 20). This may happen in, for example, enuresis or phobic or obsessional states.

Figure 21 combines the aetiological and developmental models already discussed, a model modified from Rahe *et al.* (1974), and the place of the referral process, into a single scheme. Table 6 shows different perspectives of aetiology.

Chapter 6

A System for Assessment

INTRODUCTION: GATHERING INFORMATION

Three broad categories of information are needed (see also figure 22).

1. *Diagnostic assessment of the adolescent and the current situation, of particular importance for prognosis, treatment plans, and monitoring progress.*
2. *Historical and recent information, throwing, light on aetiology.*
3. *Historical and current information about the availability, attitudes, feelings, methods, and capacities of adults (parents and professionals) who are already involved with the adolescent, or who could usefully be.*

The contribution made by people outside the clinical team falls broadly into two categories:

(a) *Maintenance of care and help already under way.* As already pointed out, all children need care and education whether or not they also need treatment. Accordingly, part of the task of the clinical team is to sustain and encourage that care and education that is already functioning reasonably well, throughout and after a period spent in treatment. There is therefore always work to be done with parents* and to a more variable extent (depending on the problem) with teachers, and accordingly the clinical team must get to know them, and about them. This requires an exchange of information, too; up to the point of referral, parents, teachers, and others may not be sure what a psychiatric team can and cannot do.

Sometimes it emerges after consultation alone, or after clinical examination, that the professional workers already involved in, say, special teaching, social casework or treatment are able and willing to carry on.

---

* To avoid repetition, parents will refer equally to professional people such as residential child care workers who for some children are in close contact with them as surrogate parents.

127

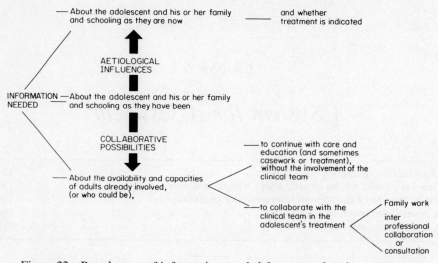

Figure 22   Broad areas of information needed for comprehensive assessment

Again, an exchange of information is required to establish that this is a possible way of proceeding.

(b) *Additional help from the clinical team.* The clinical team will often want to offer help in addition to the care and help already under way. At the minimum (for example an acutely ill adolescent admitted to hospital for investigation) it comes to a matter of keeping others informed of progress and supporting the rest of the family, or it could mean systematic work, for example with the parents, with the family as a whole, or with school teachers with a boy's or girl's conduct as the focus. Again, an exchange of information and the beginning of building up trusting relationships is needed in order to proceed in any such direction.

As Dare (1975) has pointed out, the overall strategy of a clinical team is itself an intervention, and of course this applies to the way in which the team discusses the presenting problems with patient, family, and referring professionals from the start; its whole style of approach in establishing contact and collecting necessary information can prove influential and sometimes crucial for what follows, whether it is simply the offering of advice or a matter of sustaining a demanding therapeutic programme. Seeing the adolescent separately, or with the family as a whole, will be taken as a comment (not necessarily an enduring one) on how the clinician perceives the problems.

GENERAL POINTS: WHOM TO SEE, WHEN, WHERE, AND HOW

Before discussing assessment systematically, some general points which commonly cause difficulty will be mentioned:

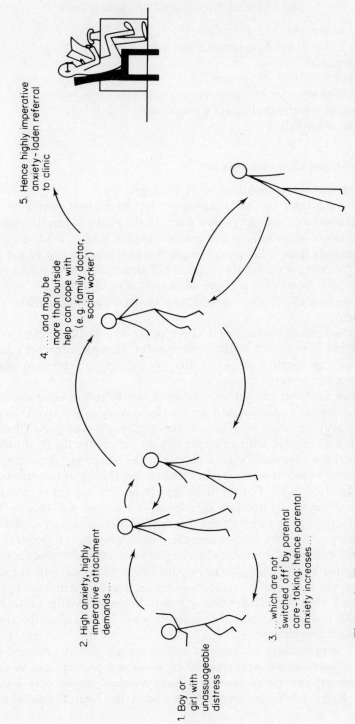

2. High anxiety, highly imperative attachment demands ...

1. Boy or girl with unassuageable distress

3. ...which are not switched off by parental care-taking: hence parental anxiety increases ...

4. ... and may be more than outside help can cope with (e.g. family doctor, social worker)

5. Hence highly imperative anxiety-laden referral to clinic

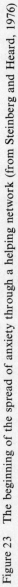

Figure 23   The beginning of the spread of anxiety through a helping network (from Steinberg and Heard, 1976)

1. Whom to contact for information
2. Whom to see at the assessment interview
3. Confidentiality
4. Urgency
5. Where to meet
6. Consultation without clinical examination
7. Physical examination

1. Whom to contact for information

It is important to establish at an early stage:

(a) Who other than the referring agent and immediate family may have information that will help throw light on the problem and its background (for example schools, past and present; clinics; distant relatives).

(b) Who among these other people ought to know that the boy or girl is being seen (for example the family doctor, if not already involved; the adolescent's school; the social worker if the adolescent is in care).

(c) Who among these other people may be in a position to help with the problem.

It can be surprising how different a perspective on a particular child's case can be once other information begins to arrive, for example a teacher's or a past psychiatrist's perspective or what the young person's brother, sister, or grandparent has to say.

A balance has to be reached between involving the people listed above, in the referred adolescent's interests, and the need for privacy (which is not the same as confidentiality). My own view is that the only people who *must* know about psychiatric consultation with an under 16-year-old are the family doctor, both parents, and the adolescent's social worker if the boy or girl is in care; indeed their approval would be necessary for offering a psychiatric appointment, if they were not involved so far. For someone aged 16 or over and not in care, I would always want the family doctor's agreement; if a boy or girl does not have a general practitioner to turn to then that is an aspect of neglect or self-neglect which needs putting right. If there are other people who ought to be involved (for example the parents of a 16-year-old living at home) then the psychiatrist must decide whether he is in a position to help the boy or girl or not without access to them; except in the most unusual circumstances it would be difficult to proceed sensibly with most difficulties without at least some involvement with parents. Such issues, and many others (for example when parents disagree about the referral) need consultation.

Finally, on grounds of efficiency as well as privacy, the involvement of large numbers of professional workers is to be avoided if possible, but in the most difficult, anxiety-provoking cases very large numbers indeed may want to be involved. Every adolescent psychiatrist knows the referral that has a premonitory aura of letters from solicitor, member of parliament, action groups, head teachers ('most disturbed case in all my years of experience . . . strange look in his eyes . . . will consider return to the school when you can guarantee him cured'), psychotherapists and counsellors, and then twice-daily telephone calls from the adolescent's parents. The parents are characteristically highly anxious, often with good reason, and have allowed a large accumulation of experts and helpers to become partly involved before they have lost confidence in them and sought second opinions without quite relinquishing those involved so far. In terms of the attachment model (page 129), parenting and 'care-taking' having failed to cope with the adolescent's distress, the parents and other adults themselves become anxious, turn to others for help, are unable to receive or to use it, and anxiety and feelings of despair and loss of competence spread. Such feelings, to a minor or major degree, are common in the referrals of adolescents for specialist care (see figure 23, also page 119).

2. Whom to see at the assessment interview

The discussion above is a guide to this decision too; the general principle being to balance what the clinician needs to find out in order to make a consequent assessment, whom he will need to work with to undertake effective treatment, and the feelings of the adolescent and the family. In the cases of most adolescents living at home, it is important to see both parents and it is advisable to see the adolescent's brothers and sisters too, again at least for the initial assessment because of the important contribution they usually make, and their right to hear an explanation of what has gone wrong and what help can be offered.

Sometimes a parent demurs. A family doctor will say 'You'll never get the father along', or a mother will say 'He's too busy, he can't get a day off work', or 'He's not interested'. Or the brighter, more successful siblings are not expected to miss a morning's schooling to go along to their 'stupid' brother's session at the clinic. Sometimes, too, an adolescent will not want a sibling to attend.

The trainee in child and adolescent psychiatry will hear two confidently expressed and totally conflicting views. The first is to see whoever is willing to turn up and take it from there. The advantage of this view is that it is realistic and respects the wishes of the referred adolescent and at least one parent. The disadvantage is that it may give a grossly distorted picture of what is going on.

The second view is that the whole family, including all siblings, must *always* be seen; that is if they will not all come they will not be seen. This approach has the advantage of affirming the importance of the whole family as a group which has a most important part to play in a child's care and development; all its members have a right to understand what is going on, and an important role in sustaining treatment. Further, if a clinic's approach is primarily or entirely family therapeutic, it can no more help half a family than a surgeon can help someone who will not agree to be examined. This is, of course, fundamental to family work, and its particular relationship to assessment and decision making is discussed for example by Bruggen *et al.* (1973), Skynner (1976a, b), Hildebrand *et al.* (1981), and Bentovim and Gilmour (1981). On the other hand, and particularly where family therapy's proponents are fighting innovatory battles or where the family approach is uncritically taken on as the correct approach, there can develop an ideological commitment, to total family assessment or nothing, that can become rigid and institutionalized.

The family approach has been developing for quite a long time since gestation in Pao Alto and elsewhere in the 1950s but its growth spurt is relatively recent. The time has been too short for its practitioners to do more than experiment with taxonomy (Dare, 1975) and tentative metaphors and hypotheses (Skynner, 1976a, b) and there is relatively little systematic information on the ways in which the family approach may usefully be used (see, for example, review by Walrond-Skinner, 1978) or its effectiveness as a treatment (Wells *et al.*, 1972; Lask, 1979). Moreover, family work appears time-consuming for staff (including training and supervision time and the widespread use of co-therapists rather than single practitioners), and some family members may find it stressful (Slipp *et al.*, 1974; Shapiro and Budman, 1973). Nevertheless carefully supervised and staff-intensive methods can save time in the long run, and attempts have been made to evaluate the effectiveness of brief, focal family therapy (Bentovim and Kinston, 1978; Kinston and Bentovim, 1978).

Many child and adolescent psychiatrists can see the value of the family approach for some aspects of diagnosis and treatment (see Cox and Rutter, 1977) while others see the family approach as a matter of principle, a particular orientation, in which all assessment and most or all treatment *must* involve all participants, that is the whole family. Moreover, the position is sometimes taken that even to see some members of the family separately in advance of considering family therapy as a way of proceeding immediately begins to undermine the latter. It is a complex debate with, for some practitioners, its roots in strongly held personal beliefs. The area requires research; one way of beginning might be to recognize the distinction between the family approach as a means of assessment; as a means of treating a problem of the whole family system; as a means of using the family to treat an individual member's problem; and as a particular ideological style of professional–client engagement which is simply considered correct. These are not the same things, and each view has its proponents.

My own practice is to *invite* the whole family to the assessment, explaining the value of everyone attending; and if the whole family do not attend, explain the position if any decisions and plans cannot be made in some members' absence. For example, the admission to an adolescent unit of a young person with major conduct problems, sibling rivalry, and a history of absconding can be so much wasted time and lead to disappointment unless both parents appreciate the difficulties involved for staff and themselves and work out a family strategy together, while a 'failed' admission (for example the boy hurries home and father cannot persuade mother to allow him back) can actually put an already muddled, troubled boy at greater risk than had admission not been attempted at all. Another example would be the difficulty of working on an out-patient behavioural programme for an obsessional adolescent who has involved the whole family in his rituals, without the whole family being involved in the therapeutic work. However, there are many adolescent problems where it is not a *Sine qua non* for everyone to attend, and I would not insist. My own rule is not to have a rule about it in advance of making an assessment, but people taking this approach will upset some family therapists. Similarly, unless one works in a totally family-therapy-orientated team, the boy or girl should always be seen by himself or herself for part of the interview. The proportion of time spent with the family (or adolescent and parents) together, and separately, will be a matter of judgement guided by what emerges in the family part of the assessment, and by what the referring agent wants, which may be a clinical opinion on the adolescent's mental state. Nevertheless the family therapeutic view is a cogent one (see for example, page 296); to make family therapy a viable possibility in an eclectic team may require separation of the assessment process from assessment for family therapy.

3. Confidentiality

Medical ethics permit doctors to share information about a referred patient freely, and one should do so and tell the adolescent and family. For example, although in my own unit referrals are accepted from any source, the support of the family doctor is invariably sought and he or she, of course, receives a letter explaining what we have found and what we are doing.

Obtaining medical information about other family members is, I feel, a different matter and permission should be sought for this (from the person concerned) as it should be for any other report, for example from a school. Withheld permission is of course a problem; the family are entitled to know why it is wanted, how it will be used, and how important it is. If permission is still refused, this is likely to be far from the only problem of trust in that family, and dealing sensitively, courteously, and openly with the issue almost always provides a way forward and achieves some useful work along the way. If an impasse is reached, then the clinician can console himself in the knowledge that impasses are not unknown in adolescent psychiatry.

4. Urgency

Some referrals of adolescents are presented as extremely urgent. It is worth finding out what is meant by urgency; sometimes one telephones back, prepared to explain in detail how difficult it is going to be to see the boy or girl in less than a day or two to find that the referrer simply wants the adolescent seen in a week or two rather than a month or two.

Extreme urgency should usually be taken to mean that without the clinic's speedy intervention (that day or the next day at the latest) serious harm is likely to befall the adolescent or someone else. Threatened or feared suicide comes into this category, as do some cases of violent behaviour (that is if there seems to be primarily psychiatric reasons for it, which may need medical and nursing methods of control), and high levels of anxiety about an acutely ill (for example schizophrenic or depressed or pathologically anxious) adolescent, where there may be something a psychiatric team can do that no one else can. But in practice if a clinic were to try to see *every* very urgently referred case very urgently, it would not have time to undertake its routine work unless it was able to put people and time specially aside for a crisis intervention service. It is a matter of economics and logistics; even the most acutely anxious parents and referring agents expect adequate time to be spent dealing with an adolescent's case properly, and (particularly for the anxious) this may take not less than an hour and perhaps far longer. Most important, in practice so high a proportion of 'extremely urgent' referrals turn out not to be extremely urgent as defined above, but more a matter of high levels of anxiety on the part of the involved adults, that unless a team operates a primarily crisis intervention approach (Bruggen *et al.*, 1973), making effective therapeutic use of the high levels of concern being expressed, it will actually waste time (including that of people waiting for appointments) to try to fit in full assessments with great speed.

The nature of most referral problems (page 118) and the fact that adult anger and anxiety may be the main factor in urgency (page 129), point to the correct approach to urgent referrals being urgent consultation. This means one team member putting time aside, to discuss with the person making the referral (by telephone if convenient) what he or she fears is going to happen, and alternative ways of dealing with these areas of concern which, of course, still include the possibility of seeing the boy or girl very urgently if necessary.

Sometimes this becomes a specific piece of work:

Example 5
A family and the family doctor are anxious because an anorexic girl is losing weight rapidly; it emerges that she has just been discharged home by her parents against medical advice because of her unhappiness with the treatment programme offered by a hospital. It further emerges that this also represents the second admission that has ended this way, and the fifth contact with a psychiatrist in a year. The anxiety is that the girl may die if nothing is done; as well she may. The question is, however, is she less likely to die if admitted very urgently (the request is for admission now) with perhaps the adolescent unit becoming the third admission and the sixth psychiatric team abandoned, or if the

psychiatric team first puts time aside to meet the girl and her whole family to deal with the family's experiences of treatment so far, their justified or unjustified mistrust of professional help, and their difficulty in balancing what help the girl needs against the painful aspects of providing it? It depends on her weight, and the rate at which she is losing weight. If she is in acute physical danger she would in any case need to be in a general hospital. Again, it is a matter of balanced judgement, but the important thing to bear in mind is that an emergency admission accepted over the telephone, without dealing with whatever has undermined treatment so many times before, may result in yet another failure, and be far more dangerous, raising the risk of death, than 'holding' the family's and referring agents' anxiety as best one can, and arranging an appointment at which the adolescent's and family's anxieties and problems about treatment can be discussed, and a sustainable treatment strategy planned.

The issue of dealing with different types of emergency has been dealt with at some length, and is discussed further in subsequent chapters; it is one of the most important aspects of day-to-day work in adolescent psychiatry and clinical teams need systems for responding to it helpfully but appropriately. It also needs to be said that anxiety about adolescents is not the sole prerogative of 'outside' referring workers. Adolescent problems can cause high levels of anxiety in those working with them, and understanding the reasons for it, and its consequence is important for reasons other than dealing with new referrals. Meanwhile the efficiency and economy of different strategies of response need evaluation.

5. Where to meet

This too can be a contentious issue. As Bentovim and Gilmour (1981) point out, a clinical rather than domestic setting, as well as having necessary resources at hand, also helps establish the clinical team's role and boundaries, although it can also be anxiety provoking, which may be helpful or unhelpful.

That choice depends partly on mutual convenience and partly on the nature of the work. A routine clinical assessment with a view to taking a boy or girl on for treatment is perhaps best carried out at the clinic; a meeting with a social worker or teacher and with adolescent and family, to decide whether the social work department or school can deal with a particular problem largely by themselves may best be conducted in the social work office or at the school. An urgent pre-assessment consultation to discuss the reason for high levels of concern may best be carried out at the family's home or in the family doctor's surgery. A home visit at some stage is useful particularly since we know that families behave differently in different settings (Hatfield et al., 1967) and in any case a home visit gives a better view of what life is like at home than can any history.

On the subject of work settings, it is a pity that more administrators and even some psychiatrists do not give higher priority to the needs in this respect of a therapeutic team. Place as well as time are important in psychiatric work. Neglected, noisy, ill-ventilated, badly decorated, impersonal premises with excessive room-swapping and room-sharing is a false economy, and tends to undermine many basic social, psychodynamic, and behavioural principles as well as defying common sense.

6. Consultation without clinical examination

For reasons already given it is helpful for the psychiatrist to be available to people wishing to discuss possible referrals, for example, on the telephone. Some of these will quite properly result in routine appointments as opposed to urgent ones, and some may equally properly result in referral to a non-psychiatric service. For example, it may be quite clear from a child's behaviour that the first step is to establish control, whether treatment is needed or not.

Example 6
A family doctor requests an urgent second opinion and domiciliary visit for a misbehaving 15-year-old boy who will not attend either his surgery or an out-patient appointment. He has not seen him recently. He adds that the boy has threatened to run away from home for the day if a psychiatrist calls, and has done so each time a previous psychiatrist tried to see him. The aggressive nature of the boy's behaviour and the parents' combined inability to cope means that they are unable to keep him in the house against his will. Indeed, the reason for referral is that he stays out half the night, possibly takes drugs, is mixing with delinquent company, and is verbally abusive and physically threatening to his parents when they try to do something about it. On the other hand he attends school frequently enough for the education department to feel that they have no complaint to make. The psychiatrist is invited to offer advice; discussing the boy with the family doctor reveals no psychiatric or physical symptomatology that the doctor knows of, but he has not seen the boy for over a year. Clearly it is *possible* that the boy is depressed; he could conceivably have a cerebral disorder. Either way, the psychiatrist is not going to find out unless he sees him, which may prove impossible on a voluntary basis; it may be worth an attempted visit, but valuable time is passing. There is no justification at all for admitting him to hospital against his will. The parents are seen to clarify their responsibilities and powers in this situation; either they manage, together, to insist that their son stays to see the psychiatrist, or, if this looks or proves impossible, they are advised to meet with a social worker to explore how they can insist on asserting normal parental authority, which includes obtaining medical

(including psychiatric) opinions on their child if they consider it necessary. The process of consultation with a psychiatrist would also leave room for clarification of alternative approaches if any could be found, for example involving the help of a mutually trusted relative or friend. But the boy may need to be taken into care.

Many consultations are less dramatic and the issues less clear. Advice may be sought, for example from a social worker or probation officer, about whether a boy or girl needs a psychiatric assessment or not, and it is unfair and unreasonable to book such adolescents in for a detailed assessment the psychiatrist believes is not needed 'just to be on the safe side'. Two strategies are possible.

First, the clinician will know that a great deal can be learned about a boy or girl from those closely involved. This does not replace clinical examination, but questioning about history, peer relationships, mood, appetite, sleep, and behaviour will be a guide as to whether the adolescent ought to be seen.

Second, it is important to make it clear to the caller whether the clinician is trying to establish something about the adolescent's clinical state or whether true consultation (see Chapter 20) is being undertaken, in which the clinician is simply trying to help the caller decide for himself or herself what the problem is and what alternative decisions are possible.

These two tasks are different, and the clinician should try to be clear about which he is doing, and make it explicit. The second approach – consultation – is the one to begin with. It helps establish what the referrer can do, and what information is already available for the decisions he or she has to make, and therefore what, if anything, is left which requires clinical examination.

7. Physical examination

This is a particularly difficult issue and must take account of the following:
(a) Psychiatrists working along primarily psychotherapeutic lines quite often believe that physical examination is contraindicated, either because it distracts from the psychosocial nature of the problem, or because it brings mutually unwelcome physical intimacy into the relationship which will interfere with transference.
(b) Some psychiatrists take the view that every patient must have a general physical examination because he or she may be harbouring a physical illness (an atavistic anxiety for all doctors). One risk of this approach, however, is that the physical examination then becomes a routine with the risk of it being rather casually performed without the real expectation of finding anything abnormal.
(c) Physical maturity, nutritional state, general physical robustness and health, height, weight, sight, hearing and neurodevelopmental state are most

important aspects of child development and the clinician should have a reasonably clear view of whether all is well in these areas. Equally important is evidence of abuse (for example assaults, self-injury, misuse of toxic substances).

Early or delayed puberty (Brook, 1981) may be due to normal variation in the population or be indicative of endocrine anomaly, but in either case it may cause distress to the adolescent and family and requires diagnosis and prognosis.

Physical health problems may be relatively minor but troublesome (for example acne) or seriously disabling; and while adolescents are generally physically fit as a group, the incidence of chronic disorders such as diabetes mellitus, epilepsy, and chronic neurological conditions is more common than is sometimes recognized (Mattson, 1972; Shevin and Jones, 1979). Brain injury has a number of complicated associations with psychiatric disorder (see, for example, review by Shaffer, 1977) while Rivinus et al. (1975) and Corbett et al. (1977) have warned of serious neurological disorder presenting with psychiatric symptoms. (see also Chapter 15.)

(d) The general medical skills of a psychiatrist vary considerably depending on his or her interests, experience, and usual clientele, and may be limited. Nevertheless (i) the psychiatrist is the doctor in the multidisciplinary team, (ii) boys and girls are referred who quite often are not well known to another doctor or who have not been recently seen by another doctor, and (iii) a family doctor who has referred an adolescent to a psychiatrist may not expect a detailed physical examination to be carried out, but he may assume the assessment of the adolescent's general health as well as mental state to be within the psychiatrist's area of interest and competence. If not, he could not, for example, seriously expect the psychiatrist to order physical investigations or prescribe drugs. Moreover, many neurodevelopmental matters (reading skills and coordination) are equally physical and mental matters.

As a general principle, all adolescents should have their general physical health and maturity and their neurodevelopmental state assessed by the psychiatrist as outlined on page 149. This need not be a lengthy or elaborate exercise, and can be conducted with the adolescent having to take off no more clothes than shoes and socks.

However, a variable number of referred cases, depending on the nature of the clinic, will be young people with problems the psychiatrist regards confidently as entirely social in origin, with his formulation leaving no room for doubt. Many child psychiatrists would not examine a healthy-looking, symptom-free adolescent if this is the case, but if so they should mention this to the family doctor when they write.

Whatever the psychiatrist's practice it is most important that he or she maintains a high level of awareness of major and minor physical problems, disorders, and handicaps; collaborates freely and frequently with general practitioners, paediatricians, and neurologists for his own continuing education as well as for the sake of his patients; and finally he or she should be sensitive to the need for full and if necessary repeated physical investigation on any case of doubtful aetiology, which includes all adolescents with psychotic and atypical disorders, including severe depressive illness. (see Chapter 15.)

OTHER ASPECTS OF THE CLINICAL INTERVIEW AND EXAMINATION

Rutter and Cox (1981) point out how little psychiatric interviewing techniques for clinical purposes have been studied, and in a series of detailed studies they and their colleagues showed that non-directive, 'open' interviews led to almost as much symptomatic and family information as did systematic questioning, but the latter approach was far more effective in eliciting such qualities of symptoms and problems as their severity, frequency, context, and duration (Cox *et al.* 1981b). They also found that eliciting expression of feelings as opposed to factual information was favoured by an open style of interview (including open-ended questions and questions about feelings), few interruptions by the interviewer, and the use of interpretations and expressions of sympathy (Hopkinson *et al.*, 1981).

Different clinicians, they reported, could be trained in different clinical skills by relatively simple short-term means to use different approaches and thereby elicit different sorts of information, although this seemed to be more straightforward for fact-eliciting techniques than for approaches aimed at eliciting feelings (Ruter, and Cox, 1981). Overall Rutter and his colleagues favoured an approach adaptable to the needs and preferences of clinicians and informants and with an active style for eliciting both fact and feelings; all of which encourages versatility and flexibility in interview techniques (Cox *et al.*, 1981c; Cox *et al.*, 1981a).

Within the limited time at his (and his clientele's) disposal, the psychiatrist has to undertake a formidable task; he or she must gather an extraordinarily wide range of factual information about the family, normal and abnormal aspects of development, school and social performance, and about the facts of the presenting problems; and at the same time the psychiatrist must respond to the feelings of family and adolescent about these topics and, indeed, about the referral itself and the clinical workers too. Most important, a therapeutic relationship within which work can be done must be encouraged to develop while eliciting information.

As far as encouraging the expression of feelings is concerned, for both diagnostic and therapeutic purposes, several studies have affirmed the value of warmth, empathy, genuineness, understanding (Truax and Carkhuff, 1967; Mitchell *et al.*, 1977) and also verbal activity and directness (Shapiro and Budman, 1973). In concluding how little there has been in the way of systematic studies of clinical evaluation, Rutter, Cox and their colleagues are in agreement with similar views expressed 15 years before and as long ago as 1937 (McDonald, 1965; Greenacre, 1937). There have been a number of illuminating personal accounts in practical terms of establishing relationships with adolescents (Meeks, 1971; Cohen 1976); some helpful accounts of practical aspects of general principles to adopt in psychotherapeutic working relationships with this age group, and which are discussed in Chapter 17 (Stranahan *et al.*, 1957; Evans, 1965, 1966, 1980; Miller, 1969; Acton, 1970; Bruce, 1975, 1978; Bruggen, 1979; Berkowitz, 1972); and a small number of practical accounts of clinical evaluation (Schwartzberg, 1979; Slaff, 1980; Heacock, 1980b). Which approach achieves what has not received much study.

A GENERAL APPROACH TO ASSESSMENT

Many writers comment on the special difficulties of establishing relationships with disturbed adolescents because of their ambivalence to authority and to any attempt to help them, which may make them either uncooperative and resistive or unduly compliant and sensitive. They may have unclear and indeed changing relationships to their parents and others, and difficulty in establishing how they really feel about themselves, their families, and their problems.

In addition to any special difficulties of working with adolescents (which it may be added is perfectly true of some boys and girls, but not particularly so for most), there is the issue already mentioned of the many adults already involved as parents or professional workers; responding to their various needs and wishes and eliciting helpful information from them can be the greater challenge.

Where the psychiatrist's involvement proceeds beyond consultation alone to full clinical assessment, the total task may be outlined as follows:

1. To clarify what problems have led to the referral and why.
2. To assess the adolescent ⎱ as they are now, as they have
      his or her family, and ⎰changed and developed over the
      his or her social circumstances⎰ years, and in terms of facts and feelings.
3. To establish helpful working relationships with those involved.

Figure 24 outlines a general strategy for approaching each newly referred case, in terms of possible areas of enquiry, the groups of people involved, and the type of work needed at different stages. The diagnosis represents a chronological sequence and in this sense develops out of Figure 21 on page 125; as far as the clinical team is concerned, the first clinical intervention is in the middle: consultation about the nature of the problem.

As to detailed styles of work, these are so numerous, so variable and each is so hotly defended that they cannot be reviewed or summarized here. Instead, an approach developed from the guidelines for history-taking used in the Children's

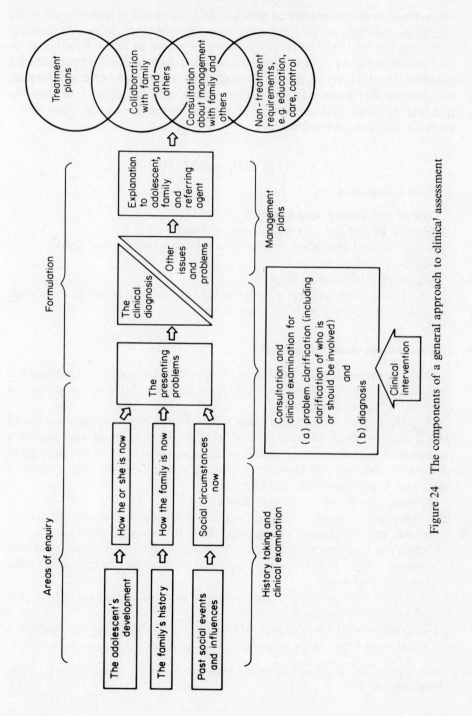

Figure 24 The components of a general approach to clinical assessment

Department at the Maudsley and Bethlem, and elaborated to take account of the principles outlined in the previous pages, is presented below. It broadly represents the approach taken at the Adolescent Unit at Bethlem, although of course it is modified to meet different needs and situations.* Organizational procedures and qualifying notes are occasionally added for clarity, and because the unit has day-patient and in-patient as well as out-patient functions the questions of admission is often an issue. It is an outline and a guide, not a checklist, nor comprehensive.

A SYSTEM FOR ASSESSMENT

1. Basic information

Date of first contact and interview
Referred boy or girl – name and date of birth
Family address and other details; or social worker if in care. School
General practitioner
Any other professionals involved
> This basic information is recorded at the first contact made with the clinical team, for example with the team secretary.

2. Consultation about the referral

The focus at this stage is as much the reasons for referral (that is the difficulties the family or current professional workers are having with the boy or girl) as the problems of the adolescent.

The nature of the consultation varies widely, from a brief telephone discussion with a decision about the adolescent reached at once, to the arrangement of a meeting with the referring professional or other involved workers to discuss what to do next, and how the clinical team can best help. Occasionally a series of consultative meetings is mutually agreed.

Decisions about the boy or girl include:

(a) *Appointment* (urgent or routine); with the family doctor's agreement and the adolescent's and family's knowledge about the referral, information is sent about the interview procedure and permission sought for obtaining school reports. One or two involved professional workers may be invited to attend the case conference.

(b) *Admission*; rarely so urgent that a prior meeting as above cannot be set up, which is to be preferred.

(c) *Alternative help*; it may emerge in consultation that referral to, for example, a social work department or special educational setting is more appropriate.

---

* *Unit teachers* refer to the staff of the Adolescent Unit's school. *School-teachers* refer to outside schools' staff.

3. Clinical assessment: sequence

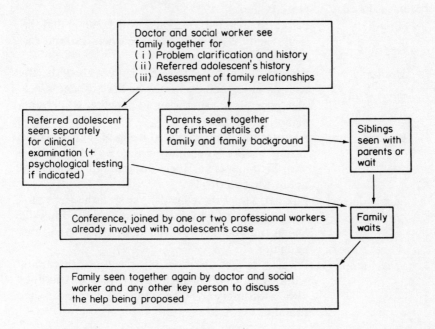

The main modification lies in how much time is spent with the whole family and how much with the boy or girl alone. This is decided by the clinical team before the appointment, but with clinical co-workers able to adapt the timing depending on what emerges. For some problems (for example some conduct problems, school non-attendance) the whole family are seen together for most of the time. For others (for example boy or girl with prominent clinical symptoms or referred for 'second opinion') a larger proportion of the time is spent with the adolescent alone.

If admission is contemplated, adolescent and family meet senior nurse and unit teacher who subsequently join the conference.

4. Clinical assessment: areas covered

BASIC DATA

REASONS FOR REFERRAL AND PROBLEMS ELABORATED: who is concerned about what? why?

Referred Adolescent's problems

Problems for members of family

Problems for referring agents

Problems for other people involved

Example 7

Referred girl:	No problems
Father:	Perplexed, irritated. He agrees with daughter that she is all right. Wife and school teachers making unnecessary fuss.
Mother:	Anxious about school teachers' concern about daughter, and angry and frustrated by her husband's lack of support. Is not sure whether daughter is 'all right' or not.
Brother:	Angry with his sister, and at being brought to clinic saying 'there's something wrong with her'; angry with his parents for their dispute and uncertainty about what to do.
Family doctor:	Puzzled. Supports referral – has seen the girl's mother for recurring physical complaints and knows she has a number of worries about husband and daughter.
School teachers:	Puzzled. Bright girl who either will not or cannot work. 'Can't get through to her' and find mother always too angry and in too much hurry to talk to her usefully.

Details of main areas of concern

These details include the exact nature of the problem, how long it has been present, how it first began, and how it changes or has changed over time. In what circumstances it changes, what the family and others have tried, and with what success. What members of the family think/fear will happen without or with the clinic's help.

How do the family cope with having different views about the problem?

How does the referred girl feel about being here but with no problems she wishes to complain about?

With these and similar direct questions, but allowing plenty of time for all members of the family to talk freely around the issue of the girl's problems and attendance at the clinic, a picture is built up of what exactly has been going on; what all feel about it, and how they think things will develop; how they feel about psychiatric involvement, acknowledging anxiety and mixed feelings, if and how they would like to use the clinic's help, and how differences (for example about the latter issue) will be resolved. This is an immediate practical issue, but also is a helpful focus for seeing how the family works together on a problem and how to help them do so.

Family and developmental history

The most helpful history is a chronological story of events beginning with genes and family circumstances, and describing how members of the family anticipated the referred child's birth and responded to this and other events, and to each other. This is a difficult history to take quickly, but once collated makes more sense than a series of 'short stories' about development, physical health, etc.

The first sketch is intended to help as a diagrammatic mnemonic for the main areas that need to be considered.

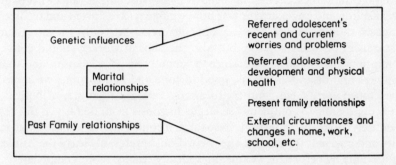

The second sketch is a reminder that drawing out a family tree is a helpful joint activity for the family, and a helpful way to record information clearly in the notes. (Miscarriages and other details should be recorded.) Names, ages, jobs, illnesses, etc., can easily be written into a diagram like the one shown.

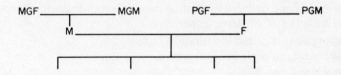

(i) Genetic influences Psychiatrists dispute the relative strengths of genetic and environmental factors; in many families there may not be the slightest doubt that something is 'in the blood', or that one or other sibling has qualities 'just like his father'. The facts of mental and physical illness, developmental difficulties (reading problems, enuresis) and prominent personality traits (obsessional, moody, always in trouble) should be recorded, as should the myths, feelings, and fears about what may have been inherited.

(ii) Family and marital relationships constitute a complex story which can be immensely time-consuming. It helps at this stage to focus on three areas:
(a) The influences of the families from which each parent comes and in particular his or her experiences of adolescence.

(b) Marital and wider family relationships and events during the referred adolescent's early years, for example early separations, starting school, changes for the parents at home and work.
(c) Recent and current relationships and events.

(iii) Current family relationships, hopes, and fears This includes what the clinical worker hears and sees for himself now, as well as historical data. It should also include a detailed account of how the parents, together or separately, encourage the adolescent in some behaviour and discourage him or her in others; how affection and anger are shown; how arguments are started and resolved; the emphasis should be not only on difficult areas, nor only (in an attempt at reassurance) on what is good, but also the clinical worker should convey the assumption that family experience is composed of successes and failures, happiness and disappointments, good fortune and bad fortune, welcomed and unwelcomed events, etc., and try to discuss relevant examples of both.

It is impossible to completely separate diagnosis from therapy in this respect. An entirely 'objective' interview, in so far as it could exist, might leave the parents guilty and puzzled; the clinical interview should preferably leave them at least as able to cope as before they came, and ideally feeling more competent.

(iv)   Development and physical health of the referred adolescent Areas to consider are:

(a) Developmental milestones and progress
    Pregnancy and delivery (including parental relationships, maternal health and mood) and obstetric experience
    Eating, sleeping, and elimination habits
    Movement, strength, coordination
    Speech and reading
    Sight and hearing
    Attention and concentration
    Height and weight
    Sexual development and behaviour
(b) Physical health and medical attention
    Major and minor illnesses including allergies
    Accidents and operations
    Periods of medical treatment
    General health and well-being
        Fits, faints, headaches, dizziness, weakness
        Aches and pains
        Diarrhoea and vomiting
        Appetite, sleep, mood

      Fears, worries, sadness; ask about threatened or actual self-neglect or
      self-injury

(c) Social and personality development

      Confidence; friendships (all age groups) Interests, hobbies. Ability to play,
      relax, have fun

      Persistence with and enjoyment of tasks

      Openness, secretiveness; trusting or cautious

      Academic and social progress at school

      Misbehaviour and delinquency; alone or in groups?

      Bizarre or unusual ideas, speech, experiences

      Use of alcohol, drugs, and other toxic substances

Note that minor physical variations (height, weight, appearance) can have major influences on a child.

The family's experience of past medical (and other professional) care can profoundly influence the present clinical relationship. Life-threatening (or apparently life-threatening) illness or chronic handicap in a child (for example asthma, diabetes, epilepsy, autism, mental handicap) can result in powerfully mixed feelings on the part of a family towards past, present, and future doctors and others, compounded sometimes of unwilling dependence and mistrust.
In all the above areas, the clinician will need to know

(a) *facts of the matter* (nature, onset, better or worse, duration, periodicity, what circumstances affect it in any direction);

(b) *what the family and referred adolescent feel about them* and in particular how distressing it is;

(c) *Effect on relationships in the family and outside*;

(d) *Other effects*, for example on boy's or girl's hopes, plans, fears.

Some of these areas will be covered when the adolescent and family are seen together. Going over experiences of babyhood with the parents, with the adolescent listening, can bring a family closer together, at least temporarily. Sensitive areas, for example about sexual experience and worries, fears about madness or physical illness may be dealt with separately: the interviewer should gently approach such topics while making it clear that they can be talked about together or individually. The clinician needs carefully to balance respect for the family's and adolescent's privacy against the undoubted relief that gentle but confident exploration of a 'taboo' topic (for example is the family going to split up? Is parental health all right?) can bring.

    Secrets are a problem. They can burden the clinician if accepted. ('I'm having intercourse with my boy friend but don't tell my parents'; or 'Look what I've found in her diary, but don't tell her I know.') Whatever the clinician's views are on confidentiality (what to share with family and/or team members) they should be made clear early in the interview.

(v) External circumstances Again, facts, feelings, and effects of changes (losses and gains) such as moves of home (including near and away from friends/relatives)

Changes of school and in school
Illness, incapacity, and death among relatives, friends and acquaintances (including behavioural and psychiatric problems and other problems in children known to the family)
Changes in economic fortunes, jobs (part-time as well as major career changes), family social activities.

An external circumstance also to be considered is the family's mobility and proximity to the clinic, and any difficulties that get in the way of attendance. Motivation to attend regularly cannot be judged in isolation from flexibility and autonomy in working hours, possession of a car, and similar matters.

The referred adolescent's mental state

General appearance Dress, demeanour, spontaneity, including willingness to be seen and willingness to be seen with or separate from rest of family. Aggressive (verbal or physical) or compliant manner.

Adolescent's own conception of problem Attitude to referral, and interview, and the idea of psychiatric help, including feelings about confidentiality and privacy.

Mood State of anxiety, tension, irritability, anger, suspiciousness, apathy, sadness, excitability, elation. Depression can be hard to judge in adolescents who commonly experience mood swings, may cover up depressed feelings, or may look withdrawn and miserable when their prime emotion is anger, perhaps with the interviewer. Suicidal, self-injurious or self-neglectful behaviour, plans or attitudes are particularly important, as are feelings of being isolated, of hopelessness, despair, self-blame or guilt.

Thought form and content Perplexity, muddle, marked ambivalence about important topics (those on which decisions may have to be reached). Preoccupations, misinterpretations, overvalued ideas, delusions; hallucinations, depersonalization, derealization, *deja vu*. Wishes and ambitions and sense of judgement; balance between introspection and concern with external realities. (Realistic or a day-dreamer.)

Cognitive functions   General information, including neighbourhood knowledge and interests appropriate for age (bus routes, TV programmes, musical groups, where to look for information/supplies for hobbies and interests, etc.). Memory, attention, concentration. Capacity for reflection. General impression of intelligence, liveliness, and imagination. Reading, writing, and ability to copy simple drawing. Arousal.

The style of the interview and methods adopted will clearly vary with the interviewer's preferences and the adolescent's ability and age. A 12-year-old will need a different approach from a 19-year-old. Age-appropriate play and activity materials can be helpful for younger adolescents; even those up to 14 or 15 may enjoy, or at least be more comfortable, scribbling with pencil or crayons, and this can also provide helpful talking points.

Physical state

General appearance   Facial expression; impressions of general health (including skin lesions, cuts, bruises); evidence of drug abuse; nutrition; physical and sexual maturity; sight and hearing; height and weight.

Neurodevelopmental state   Cranial nerves; coordination of fingers and limbs; right or left handedness; constructional skills: copying simple drawing (diamond, star), drawing a man, writing name and address. Ability to write: (as above). Use of language: length of sentences and syntax; use of words; descriptive ability. Ability to read. Speech: dysarthria, dysphasia, stutter. Involuntary movements. Limb tone, power, reflexes, plantar responses.

General physical examination   Pulse, thyroid, rest of cardiovascular, endocrine, respiratory systems, and abdomen, and temperature, if indicated by clinical symptoms or other findings, or if admitted to hospital.

See discussion of the physical examination on page 137. It is important to know if puberty has been reached, and a history of seminal emission in boys and menarche in girls confirms this.

5. Conclusions and action

(a) *Diagnosis* of adolescent's problem. This is made using the multi-axial classification system; see page 170.
(b) *Diagnostic formulation*: see Chapter 7, page 151.
(c) *Management plans*, which include:
  (i) What else needs to be learned in order to proceed, from adolescent and family; from other sources; and by special tests for example psychological and physical investigations).

(ii) With what authority can management proceed? How much needs to be
—the referred adolescent's authority?
—his or her parents' authority?
—medical authority?
This is most important and is discussed in Chapter 16, page 265.

(d) *Explanation* to the family of the clinical team's conclusions and recommendations in simple, clear terms; and arrangement of appointments, etc. This is done by not more than two or three of the key workers who have taken part in the assessment.

(e) *Information* to family doctor and to other professionals involved in the referral, again with family's agreement.

6. Management

Further investigation, clinical treatment, and other aspects of management are discussed in Part Three, beginning with Chapter 16 which discusses general strategies of management. The intervening chapters deal with some prominent clinical problems and diagnostic categories.

Chapter 7

The Diagnostic Formulation

INTRODUCTION: DIAGNOSIS AND CLASSIFICATION

Diagnosis means, literally, to perceive thoroughly, to know through. Traditional clinical diagnoses include the purely descriptive (for example erythema multiforma, epilepsy) and those that reflect knowledge about disease in general or the disorder in a particular patient's case (for example cerebellar astrocytoma, phenylketonuria). Our knowledge of the nature of the psychiatric disorders, however, is scanty, and although epidemiological and other large-scale studies have now provided quite a lot of useful information about factors associated with child psychiatric disorder, the way they interact with each other and their relative importance in the case of the individual boy or girl is largely a matter of clinical judgement and informed guesswork.

Diagnosis of disorder in child and adolescent psychiatry remains a largely provisional exercise. The process of diagnosis should be aimed at identifying those aspects of an adolescent's predicament which, because of their similarities with other adolescents' cases (a few or very many) tell us what else to look for, what to expect, and what forms of intervention (psychiatric or otherwise) may be helpful. Those aspects of mood and behaviour which more or less consistently recur have been given names (autism, obsessional disorder, depression, phobia, etc.) by which clinicians and researchers can communicate with each other. As Rutter (1965) has pointed out, it is the disorder which is labelled, not the individual and it is right that we should recognize and remember that the diagnosis is a convenient and possibly temporary abstraction, open to re-appraisal, redefinition, regrouping, even abandonment.

With the possible exception of some forms of depressive illness, there is practically no category of psychiatric disorder where we can add to the descriptive diagnosis a reasonably full account of the probable processes that lie behind it and their relative weights in terms of importance. Thus a psychiatrist can make as certain a diagnosis of acute schizophrenia or phobic disorder as a general physician can of diabetes mellitus or hyperthyroidism. But while the general physician can be reasonably sure about many of the metabolic abnormalities he will find and which will have to be corrected, the psychiatrist can only know *in general* what sort of family circumstances, psychological attributes, etc., most people with schizophrenia or phobic disorders will have. He will have an idea in the particular patient's case, and this hypothesis about the nature of the individual's problem and the social, psychological, and biological factors that contribute to it is the diagnostic formulation. Descriptive clinical diagnoses are used in classification schemes but the diagnostic formulation remains an individual exercise for each patient's particular case.

But there is more to diagnosis in child and adolescent psychiatry than the diagnosis of clinical disorder. The multi-axial classification scheme developed by Rutter and his colleagues (Rutter *et al.*, 1975b; Rutter *et al.*, 1975a), and used in this book, extends description beyond naming the clinical psychiatric disorder, if there is one, to also describing characteristics of the boy or girl which are not statements about psychiatric disorders, but about aspects of the child and his or her life relevant to disorders and problems. These are his or her developmental state, intellectual level, physical health and social circumstances, and the diagnosis of each adolescent's case is made with a simple statement, which can be coded, for each dimension of problems or axis, including, of course, the absence of a problem. This five-part diagnostic statement is not a *diagnostic formulation* but provides a framework upon which one can be based (see Table 7).

The diagnostic and classification system in use in the United States uses the American Psychiatric Association's Diagnostic and Statistical Manual III (DSM III) (American Psychiatric Association, 1979; Rapoport and Gittelman, 1979; Spitzer and Cantwell, 1980). Like the British multi-axial classification, DSM III emphasizes the importance of grouping phenomena by as objective, reliable and valid means as possible to enable clinical and scientific workers to communicate with each other, and of distinguishing between different dimensions of disturbance, for example neurological disorder and mental retardation. In a recent review Rutter and Shaffer (1980) concluded the DSM III system to be a significant step forward from DSM II, but criticized among other things its lack of explanation of the principles of using a multi-axial scheme and the importance of coding of all axes in all cases; including mental retardation in the same category as psychiatric disorder; apparently indicating that developmental disorders tend to remain much the same throughout childhood, which is not the case; and, in the psychosocial axis, of not clearly differentiating between independent external influences of the environment and those arising as a consequence of the individual's own behaviour. Rutter and Shaffer concluded that DSM III was an undoubted and valuable advance, but had many conceptual and taxonomic flaws, and they looked forward to DSM IV.

The diagnostic formulation is composed of these factors but more, in an attempt to state in a few sentences the particular problems the adolescent is

Table 7   Outline of the multi-axial classification scheme

Multi-axial classification scheme: outline		
Axis	Category	Examples (with code)
1	Clinical psychiatric syndrome	Unsocialized disturbance of conduct (312.0) Socialized disturbance of conduct (312.1) Disturbance of emotions with anxiety and fearfulness (313.0) Disturbance of emotions with misery and unhappiness (313.1) Anorexia nervosa (307.1) Tics (307.2) Infantile autism (299.0) Schizophrenic disorders of adult type (295.0–295.8) Affective psychosis, depressed type (296.1) Obsessive–compulsive disorder (300.3)
2	Specific delays in development	No specific delay (0) Specific reading retardation (1) Specific arithmetical retardation (2) Other specific learning difficulties (3) Developmental speech/language disorder (4) Specific motor retardation (5) Mixed developmental disorder (6)
3	Intellectual level	Normal variation (0) Mild mental retardation: IQ 50–70 (1) Moderate mental retardation: IQ 35–49 (2) Severe mental retardation: IQ 20–34 (3) Profound mental retardation: IQ under 20 (4)
4	Medical conditions	For example: epilepsy: diabetes mellitus; asthma; cerebral palsy; Down's syndrome; etc.
5	Abnormal psychosocial situations	No significant distortions or inadequacy of psychosocial environment (00) Mental disturbance in other family members (01) Discordant intrafamilial relationship (02) Inadequate or inconsistent parental control (05) Inadequate social, linguistic or perceptual stimulation (06) Inadequate living conditions (07) Inadequate or distorted intrafamilial communication (08) Natural disaster (12) Persecution or adverse discrimination (15)

experiencing and causing, how they might have come about, and how they might be helped. Diagnostic formulations are not easy to put together; often, statements in case-notes described as diagnostic formulations are in fact summaries of the history and findings, which is different. It is worth making an effort to construct a worthwhile formulation because the exercise requires the clinician to think carefully about what he sees for himself, what he has inferred, how various facts and hypotheses about the adolescent's life and circumstances may have affected each other, what may happen next, and what the clinician is going to do. A useful formulation should be in as plain English as possible, and as short as possible, not because there is some natural virtue in brevity, but because psychiatry is complex enough without wordy elaboration of obscure aspects of a case. Discretion must be used regarding which normal findings to include; in most cases it is helpful to mention the adolescent's intelligence.

THE DIAGNOSTIC FORMULATION

The skeleton of a formulation is composed of the following four components: (see also Figure 25):

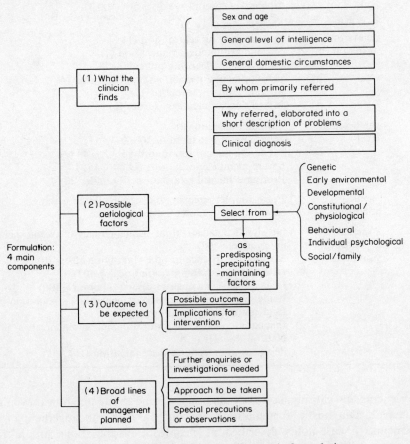

Figure 25   The components of a diagnostic formulation

1. What is going on, in terms of description and diagnosis.
2. How it may have come about.
3. What is likely to happen.
4. What the clinician is going to do.

The first step is purely descriptive. It should be a statement of facts, and should contain the diagnosis, or provisional diagnoses, which while not exactly in the same category as factual observations nevertheless should represent an honest attempt to give a name to any syndrome that may be present.

The second step (2) is essentially speculative. An adolescent's behaviour problems may seem understandable in terms of his temperamental character-istics in infancy and now, and his anger towards a father who has a poor relationship with his mother. But we cannot say, with certainty, what relative weight to attach to these factors. In one young person a tendency towards im-pulsive outbursts many have been readily exposed by the ordinary stresses and strains of family life; in another, a vulnerability to emotional outbursts may have required quite severe stress to provoke problematic behaviour. And in each case, what is 'ordinary' and what is 'severe' will depend in part on the personal meaning of family disputes to the adolescent in question. Again, in either case a clinician might be able to find the ingredients of Oedipal conflict as indeed we would have in ordinary, non-referred families too. Whether this particular psychodynamic constellation is causing sufficient individual strain in this particular case to account for the child's stress cannot be known. On the other hand it is usually possible to put the facts, possibilities, and hypotheses about aetiology in reasonable order which is in an approximately developmental sequence; approximately, because many developmental interactions are in parallel with each other and changing as they go, and an attempt to make a perfect formulation would risk ending up with the clinician writing a short novel about the patient when what is needed is a potted biography. Figure 26 is a guide to this procedure. It is important to remember that it represents *areas to consider*, not areas that must always have a genetic, psychodynamic or family dynamic statement made about them. The formulation should be as economic a working guide as the complexities of psychiatry and development allow.

Adding a prognosis is not a matter of hazarding a guess at whether or not the adolescent and his situation is going to change. It should be a short statement of what may happen with and without intervention; a clear statement that includes alternatives to be considered is what is needed for competent patient care; and if aspects turn out to be wrong the clinician will learn more from this than from a statement so general in nature that it cannot be falsified.

The management recommendations should be briefly outlined in the for-mulation, not described as a detailed plan of campaign. The latter is needed in the case-notes after the diagnostic formulation (see Table 8).

Letters to referring professionals may be mentioned here. They should be

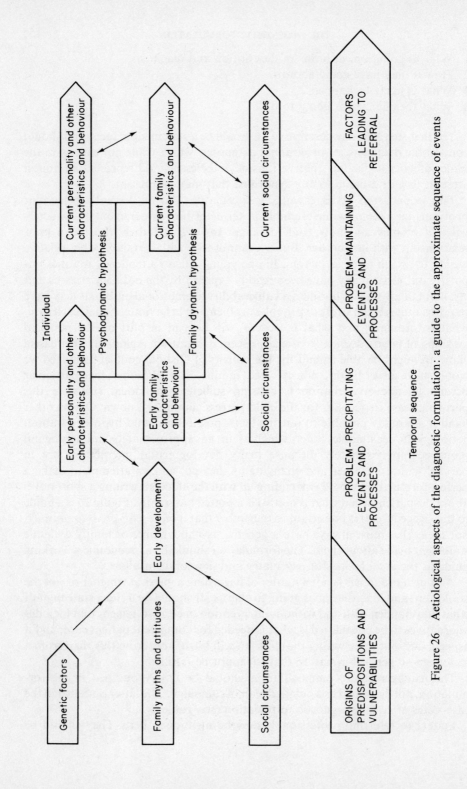

Figure 26   Aetiological aspects of the diagnostic formulation: a guide to the approximate sequence of events

Table 8:   Two diagnostic formulations

Example

A 14-year-old boy of normal intelligence living at home and referred by the school doctor for obsessional rituals in which the whole family have become involved, and which are preventing him functioning at school. The diagnosis is obsessive–compulsive disorder but the boy is so very slow and sometimes immobile that neurological disorder is possible, if unlikely. The experience of serious marital discord in his early years, replaced now by a distant, unhappy relationship between all family members, may have played a part in the cause of his problems, encouraged by the extreme rigid orderliness of current family life, which now includes lengthy assistance with his rituals at breakfast and bedtime, and may be perpetuated by fears in the family of expressing overt anger. Without intervention, which is likely to generate considerable anxiety, he is likely to remain profoundly handicapped socially and educationally. Initially one or two family meetings should be held to explore how far J. and his parents would be able and willing to cope with the demands of a behavioural programme at home, and whether they will accept his admission to hospital if necessary. Neurological investigations should be carried out early, and the reasons explained to the family.

Example

A 17-year-old girl of low average intelligence in care in a local authority children's home and cause of very great anxiety there, where she is a leader among a group of children abusing alcohol and injuring themselves. She seems angry and distressed rather than depressed. She has a long history of parental discord and rejection, followed by many failed attempts to settle down, each time challenging the security of her placement beyond its limits by aggressive behaviour to staff. Her present misbehaviour, following a relatively quiescent period, may be due to the fact that several older girls have left, and as she approaches the age of 18 she will have to leave too and has no job, no occupational skills, poor emotional capacity for coping with difficulties, and few friends. She is challenging the children's home to look after her, but in any case will soon have to leave. Meeting her long-standing need for sustained care and helping with her social and occupational skills is going to prove extremely difficult, and the first step will be to identify and meet her with present and future people in her life (e.g. social worker, careers adviser) with whose help some medium- to long-term plans can be made. Against this background it will be possible to see what treatment is required or feasible.

reasonably brief, outlining the diagnostic formulation and detailing practical plans for management such as the frequency of appointments, and including what has been explained to the patient and family. I do not believe a four or five page history is needed nor welcomed in such letters, unless particularly important incidents of which the referrer may not be aware have emerged such as recent suicide attempts or a previously unknown history of drug abuse. A simple page of four or five paragraphs should be adequate in the majority of cases, and will take two or three times as long to plan and dictate as a two or three page letter. (Shaw is supposed to have written to a friend, apologizing for the length of a letter 'because I did not have time to write a short one'.)

Part II
Problems

Chapter 8

Categories of Problem

INTRODUCTION: RESPONSIBILITY AND AUTHORITY IN PROBLEM CLASSIFICATION

Adolescent development, disturbance, and management involve a vast multiplicity of factors. In order to proceed to helpful management the clinician must have some way of bringing this enormous breadth and depth of cultural, social, psychological, and biological factors together in the service of the boy or girl before him in the consulting room. This requires a particular standpoint, and the point of view from which to begin is the social one of responsibility and authority, the first representing what any individual involved should be doing, and the latter what he can do. This has been a recurring theme in the first part of this book: what the developing adolescent has been expected and able to do from birth to maturity; what his or her family do or should do with him and for him; and what the wider community (including the clinical psychiatric team) can and should do. To bring the point into sharper focus, perhaps the common denominator of mature, fit adults is their authority and responsibility; their strengths, capacity to act, and willingness and ability to take and be given responsibility. The most striking and sad characteristic of the most incapacitated men and women in a long-stay psychiatric hospital or other institution is the authority and responsibility they cannot take or are denied.

Professional intervention is usually a process spread over weeks, months, or even years, rather than a brief event. During this period it is important that the clinical help the adolescent in difficulties receives must not undermine, and on the contrary must actively encourage, his or her relationships with non-clinicians, and even more important with his or her family and friends; that is normal life.

The point of the consultative–diagnostic approach (page 15) is to differen-

161

tiate those aspects of the presenting problem for which the clinical psychiatrist can and should take responsibility from those for which others can and should take responsibility. It is not a sequential approach but a dual approach; in the same individual or family interview the conversation should include what we (the clinical team) should and will decide and contribute, what the adolescent and family should decide and contribute, and what others (for example the school) should decide and contribute.

Possibly this seems uncontroversial. In practice it is by no means generally agreed that this line is the best way of proceeding. Some styles of crisis intervention, family work, and psychotherapy require the clinician's authority and responsibility to be limited to setting up the meeting and pressing or helping the client or clientele to make their own decisions. The traditional medical approach, taken by many psychiatrists, is to make a diagnostic appraisal and prescribe management with authority. The two styles of approach are not in principle incompatible, *but* clinicians and their teams, for reasons of personality, background, and connections quite often favour one or the other, tend to develop their work in such directions, and to accumulate a clientele who can be worked with in one or other alternative way. Indeed, this is a natural occupational developmental process, and for a team to sustain a deliberately dual consultative–diagnostic approach is problematic and requires active maintenance.

Why is this important in practice?

Example 8

A 15-year-old schoolboy develops a second acute schizoaffective illness. After a few days when the worst of his distress is over he decides to leave the hospital because he wants to return to his school and friends, and wants no further psychiatric contact. His parents cannot make up their minds about this; they are very upset at his illness and averse to his being in a psychiatric unit, but equally perturbed at the prospect of treatment ceasing. The boy is not so ill or at risk to justify use of the Mental Health Act to detain him against his will; the most that is happening is that he is behaving in an uncharacteristically embarrassing and bizarre way in the neighbourhood, and occasionally turning up at school. He is rapidly losing his friends, but seems quite happy and is not in danger. Attempts at family work fail to persuade the parents (whose undercurrent of discord is a factor in the formulation) into insisting on his return to treatment. Attempts at keeping things on an even keel by out-patient, day-patient, and domiciliary visits by a community nurse rapidly fail; he is not strongly averse to medication or attending a clinic but is simply too disorganized and does not bother. The family doctor finds he too is put in a helpless position. At a case conference the Social Service Department insists that he is a mentally ill boy who should be in hospital receiving treatment, and should be detained if necessary on a section of the Mental Health Act. The parents do not want him in hospital, certainly not compulsorily. The psychiatrist points out that the boy never refuses treatment when it is patiently encouraged, and is quite friendly and cooperative when, more by accident than by design, he comes into contact with a professional worker.

It is a controversial matter whether he is so ill and at risk to justify detention under the Mental Health Act's provisions. This is a second illness and the boy is vulnerable to a series of possibly preventable illnesses and managing the crises alone is not adequate; most important of all if his parents were to act firmly and together in insisting that he accepts treatment (as they should if he needed, for example, an appendicectomy) there is no doubt that the boy would return to the adolescent unit, cooperate in treatment, have his weekends at home and return when expected, and indeed do so reasonably happily.

Diagnosing and treating the illness is the responsibility of the clinician; but the child's age and circumstances make the acceptance of treatment the responsibility of the parents. It is agreed to consider, in consultation with the family, whether care proceedings are justifiable (including the parents seeking voluntary care for their son if they feel they cannot together generate the necessary mutual strength and consistency without outside help); the grounds are that the boy's emotional development is being avoidably impaired by the parents' failure to insist on the treatment he needs. In the event, looking at *their* responsibilities in this way galvanizes them into action; they insist on their son returning to treatment (which turns out to be effective, with the boy gaining considerably from the social and educational experience of admission too) and, having thought through their earlier mixed and muddled feelings about acting in concert, they also decide to seek some advice for themselves too. As a result the boy's discharge is possible sooner rather than later, and out-patient follow-up proceeds unimpeded by parental ambivalence.

It is important to note that in this example the family were not being misled; the boy's clinical state and general demeanour (including his ready response to consistent adult behaviour) did not justify use of the Mental Health Act. Had the parents not come together in the way they did, the alternatives would have been a Care Order, or no treatment at all, until such time as he became acutely psychotic again and at serious risk.

What would have made insistence on the boy's treatment more of a medical responsibility? First, had he been more clearly at immediate risk, for example behaving dangerously and, second, had he been actively refusing treatment when in hospital; the latter is important because unlike when in hospital at parental insistence, the authority of a Care Order may not justify treatment against a young person's will. The law is unclear here, as well it might be. After all, what constitutes treatment? Medication? Attending group therapy? Merely being in a 'therapeutic setting'? Parents or a social worker are allowed to determine a young person's address, but what treatment he can accept or reject there is less clear under a Care Order than under parental authority.

This example was a particularly difficult one. Less controversial ones commonly arise. Treatment for school refusal or conduct disorder, if resisted, does not justify the use of the Mental Health Act. Trusted parental authority (or the authority of a Care Order), the adolescent's own motivation, or some workable combination of these perhaps in the form of an agreed treatment contract needs clarifying in advance.

What must be emphasized again is that clarification of responsibility and authority is not only in order to sustain an agreed management policy. It is most important also to remind adolescent and family of their own authority and responsibilities, and what authority and responsibility they may aspire to.

Problem clarification, then, is an exercise in clarifying who is responsible for which aspects of a presenting problem. The clinician's responsibilities are primarily in the area of individual psychiatric, physical, and developmental disorder. The other problems are the responsibility of other people, and here the clinician's responsibility is to help clarify what they are.

CATEGORIES OF PROBLEMS

The *problem* is that which the referring agents, and other people involved, can see for themselves; they do not need a psychiatrist to tell them that the problem a boy or girl is presenting is that of misbehaviour, drug abuse, attempted suicide, or school non-attendance, which are descriptions of situations rather than clinical diagnoses. But taking problem clarification a step further (from *who is complaining of what* into *why*; page 143), the problem can be elaborated and then reveals underlying problems and clinical diagnosis if any.

To take the example given on page 162. The presenting problem was the concern felt by a school teacher because of a boy's uncharacteristically bizarre behaviour at school; not only could school work not proceed, but the child's relationships and reputation were being profoundly undermined. The elaborated problems were: (a) acute schizoaffective illness, a problem for the psychiatrist; (b) lack of parental resolve to insist that the child receives treatment; (c) marital discord making it impossible to get together on any important issue because any emotive discussion threatened their fragile alliance. The community's authority (that children *will* be cared for properly) insisted that the parents face this issue together, while professional authority insisted the same but, as a positive decision, opposed the inappropriate 'escape route' of sending the child to

Problems for the adolescent	Bizarre experiences and odd behaviour jeopardizing emotional, educational, and social development

Problems for the teacher	Class work impossible; behaviour and problems beyond his experience and skill

Problems for the clinician	(i) Recurrent schizo-affective illness (ii) Inability to implement treatment

Problems for the parents	(i) Anxiety and distress about their son (ii) Cannot agree on action to follow or advice to accept (iii) Fear about sharing an emotive, difficult decision and following it through

Elaborated problem	Marital difficulties

Figure 27   Problems in example

hospital on a section of the Mental Health Act. This in turn made the parents face how their marital difficulties were jeopardizing the care of their son and enabled them to see that they had to sort out some of their difficulties in order to cooperate properly over their son's care. They got together enough of their mutual parental rights and responsibilities to ensure that their child used the clinical care available. (see figure 27 for problems in example.)

This example also illustrates the importance of the clinician knowing where to stop; The task of the clinician in this case is to put it to the parents *not* that they must seek marital guidance but that if they want to use his help they must agree on what to do for their son. He can help them see how their problem in sharing or agreeing on anything is getting in the way of their child's proper care and treatment; and he may go further in explaining how their difficulties seem to him and what help is available if they want it. But the focus for the clinician in this case remains getting the boy the help he needs, not marital therapy. This aspect of his professional relationship with the family remains consultative.

THE RANGE OF PROBLEMS

Table 9 gives examples of common problems and permutations of problems seen in adolescent psychiatry, and is developed from a study of 500 referrals to a

Table 9 Problems commonly presenting to adolescent units (Steinberg *et al.*, 1981)

1. Presenting problem	Frequency among 500* referrals	2. Related or secondary problems	3. Further problems often found	4. Clinical diagnostic aspects
Unmanageably disruptive and violent behaviour Absconding/risk taking Drug/alcohol abuse Delinquency Need for court report	18%	No satisfactory or acceptable place to stay; either removed from last home, or removal threatened, usually with future home uncertain	(a) Adults responsible for adolescent's care often anxious and helpless in face of his/her challenges and demands. (b) This emerges as a long-term pattern in the adolescent's history. (c) Authority, care and control hard to sustain and 'treatment' sought as a supposed alternative	Usually problems categorized clinically as emotional and/or conduct disorder, with major problems of personality development, and understandable in terms of column 3(a) and (b). Possibility of treatment precarious without control being established first
School non-attendance	11%	Uncertainty on part of parents as to whether adolescent is 'sick' or 'naughty,' whether school is 'good' or 'bad', and what advice to take: differences of view between parents encouraged by adolescent	(a) Professional workers (e.g. teachers, educational welfare officers, home tutors, family and school doctors, social workers) contributing but with different views and responses to adolescent, as in column 2. (b) Problem often well established by time of referral (e.g. 6–18 months)	Usually long-term family problems and problems of personality development, rather than phobic or other illness; occasional 'normal' crisis, rapidly resolved

Threatened or attempted self-injury	10%	(a) Urgency/anxiety among professional workers may not be related to clinical needs (see column 4). Prognosis problematic and very variable. (b) Expectation that supervision should be primarily medical, that is in hospital	(a) Family and social problems often similar to 3(a), top of column and with implications for supervision and care required. (b) Major interruption in school and family life	Family and social problems and problems of personality development prominent and may be very severe. Depressive or other illness unusual. Frequency and urgency of referral to in-patient unit low when medico-psychiatric liaison good.
Opinion on intractable and handicapping psychiatric or neuro-psychiatric disorder	10%	Difficult and complex problem, e.g. of brian injury, mental retardation, epilepsy or other neuropsychiatric disorder, autism, or a combination of these, with either major conduct problems or grossly disabling symptoms (e.g. psychotic or obsessional symptoms). Request often for period of in-patient assessment, which may not seem helpful	(a) Many different sources of professional advice, past and present, with further 'second opinions' already in parents' minds. (b) Long-standing guilt, anxiety, sadness, recrimination, and uncertainty about the future on part of parents, who often have not been helped with these feelings. Instead maintain hope of major recovery in their child. (c) Or, parents accept nature of problem but find no suitable educational & supportive day or residential setting	Frequently multiple diagnosis appropriate (e.g. epilepsy + mental retardation + conduct disorder + family problems + educational problems), but not fully recognized or responded to by a succession of professional workers over the years, and compounded by 3(a)

*NB Problems not mutually exclusive

general psychiatric adolescent in-patient unit made over a two year period (Steinberg *et al.*, 1981); the overall picture is very much the same as that seen among referrals to the Unit at Bethlem Royal Hospital over the succeeding six years. It is not intended to be an exhaustive classification, and nor are the categories mutually exclusive: they are examples of problems that commonly present.

Chapter 9

Categories of Disorder

INTRODUCTION

This short chapter is intended only to link the past three chapters and the next eight. Any sort of categorization has its risks as well as its advantages. The clear advantage is that classification is essential unless making sense of people's problems, taking about them, predicting what may be the outcome and trying to help them is to be an entirely random process. The risk is that classifying problems and disorders may be mistaken for classifying people, which Rutter, who with his colleagues has demonstrated the value of classification (Rutter, 1965, and page 151) has emphatically warned against.

Nevertheless the risk is real, and it is quite possible for professional workers to convince themselves that they are seeing the uniqueness and individuality of child and family, while professional training, whether as doctor, psychotherapist, psychologist or social worker really does persuade us to focus on the *case*, the somewhat odd, somewhat alienated child and family who act as repositories for whatever psychiatric, psychological, or sociological system of interests and convictions we have. It is better to be aware of this insistent, professional predisposition than to wish it away; and the tendency can be at its most insidious when the frame of reference is socially orientated and apparently progressive and libertarian.

Two anecdotes: Wilfrid Warren, hearing his junior colleagues extolling the normality, social acceptability and indeed virtues of an adolescent whom he felt was socially disadvantaged and disabled would enquire if the speaker would be happy about the adolescent marrying his son (or daughter); a question which aroused feeling and reflection. Second, the parents' evenings at the Bethlem Unit school, where patients and their families mingle with hospital and school staff with the focus on the school curriculum and the children's work, prove powerful antidotes to the attitudes and feelings, however kindly and caring, that arise in family meetings, clinical interviews, and when parents visit the ward. In general it is very difficult indeed for professionals really to perceive their clientele as they perceive their friends and neighbours and their children, and to do so requires vigilance and imagination, not only for ethical reasons, but to retain a grasp of how things really are.

CATEGORIES OF DISORDER

The multi-axial classification system already referred to (page 152; Table 7) is the system broadly adopted in this book, and the main psychiatric syndromes (Axis I) are listed in Table 10. It includes disorders of younger children, for example the hyperkinetic syndromes, as well as adult-type disorders, such as manic-depressive psychosis, which begin to make their appearance in adolescence.

Table 10   Clinical psychiatric syndromes seen in adolescent units

Syndrome	Reference to multi-axial scheme (Rutter *et al.*, 1976
Disturbance of emotions specific to childhood and adolescence	313
with anxiety and fearfulness*	.0
with misery and unhappiness	.1
with sensitivity, shyness, and social withdrawal*	.2
with relationship problems	.3
Disturbance of conduct not elsewhere classified	312
unsocialized disturbance of conduct	.0
socialized disturbance of conduct	.1
compulsive conduct disorder	.2
mixed disturbance of conduct and emotions	.3
Acute reactions to stress*	308
Adjustment reactions with depression, anxiety or conduct problems*	309
Hyperkinetic syndrome of childhood	314
simple disturbance of activity and attention	.0
hyperkinesis with developmental delay	.1
hyperkinetic conduct disorder	.2
Psychoses with origin specific to childhood	299
infantile autism	.0
disintegrative psychosis	.1
Schizophrenic psychoses	295
simple schizophrenia	.0
hebephrenic schizophrenia	.1
catatonic schizophrenia	.2
paranoid schizophrenia	.3
acute schizophrenic episode	.4

Table 10 (*contd.*)

Syndrome	Reference to multi-axial scheme (Rutter *et al.*, 1976)
Affective psychoses	296
manic-depressive psychosis, manic type	.0
manic-depressive psychosis, depressed type (which includes psychotic depression)	.1
Neurotic disorders	300
anxiety states	.0
hysteria	.1
phobic state	.2
obsessive–compulsive disorder	.3
neurotic ('reactive') depression	.4
neurasthenia	.5
depersonalization syndrome	.6
hypochondriasis	.7
Personality disorders	301
paranoid	.0
affective	.1
schizoid	.2
explosive	.3
anankastic	.4
hysterical	.5
asthenic	.6
asocial	.7
Special syndromes not elsewhere classified	307
stammering and stuttering	.0
anorexia nervosa	.1
tics	.2
stereotyped repetitive movements	.3
specific disorders of sleep	.4
enuresis	.6
encopresis	.7

* Elective mutism may be in any of these categories

As already mentioned, the principle of the scheme is that it is based on description rather than aetiology, in which context Rutter (1977d) refers to Stengel's distinction between public and private classification schemes, the former for communicating between professionals who may well have different theoretical views, and the latter for testing new ideas (Stengel, 1959) a principle which applies to clinical work as well as research since the state of psychiatry and the reality of people's lives means that every piece of clinical work is in the nature of an experiment.

The headings of Chapters 10–15 represent convenient groupings, and are not intended to detract from the multi-axial classification scheme, which is recommended for recording and communicating clinical diagnoses.

Problems of feeling and behaviour (Chapter 10) are grouped together because of the particular prominence of social and family influences in their presentation, management, and aetiology; such variegated problems as conduct disorder and drug abuse, overdoses and absconding, school non-attendance and anxiety states or unhappiness have as many similarities as differences. They represent a group of patterns of feeling and behaviour which include many problems only on the fringe of psychiatry. We do not yet know what proportion could ultimately yield to developments in social and educational policy and social and family work: probably it would be high.

To a lesser extent this could be true of some forms of *anorexia nervosa* too (Chapter 11) although the influence of physiological vulnerability to this particular pattern of symptoms is probably stronger, and the need for special skills in psychotherapeutic intervention greater. The emphasis on eating and weight and the threat to health and life influence aspects of its clinical management and link it to other eating problems.

Enuresis, encopresis, and tics (Chapter 12), while quite different disorders, have similarities in the relatively circumscribed patterns of behavioural anomaly with which they present, and in approaches to their treatment too.

The major disorders of mood (Chapter 13), depressive and manic-depressive illnesses, have particularly important physiological components to their aetiology and treatment and are considered together with *schizophrenic illnesses and some similar major disorders of personality*. These again represent a wide range of quite different disorders, but with some similarities in presentation which, particularly in adolescence, can make differential diagnosis difficult.

Autism and related disorders (Chapter 14) have in recent years become a relatively well-defined group of disorders, with strong evidence for a fundamental neurodevelopmental abnormality profoundly affecting language development.

In *learning disabilities* and *mental retardation* (also in Chapter 14) biological influences on intellectual function, specific or global, are prominent, and psychiatric disorder may or may not coexist. Social and educational methods, correspondingly, are prominent in management.

The *physical disorders* discussed in Chapter 15 represent some of the questions of physical illness which recur in psychiatric work with adolescents.

Chapter 10

Problems of Feeling and Behaviour

INTRODUCTION

The problems grouped together in this chapter present in very different ways, yet have much in common. Like neurosis and personality problems in adult psychiatry, they range from the grossly atypical and disabling to the marginally normal; often the behaviour pattern or mood is strongly influenced by the situation, so that an adolescent who misbehaves or is miserable in one setting or with one group of people can be quite readily less disturbed, or even quite all right, in another. This does not mean that he or she is necessarily really all right, or 'putting it on', but that whatever the cause of the problem it is capable of being precipitated or maintained by particular circumstances and relationships and accordingly dealing with the latter (by advice, family therapy, or a change of school) may bring about considerable modification of mood or behaviour.

Often the behaviour pattern, for example school non-attendance, self-injury or delinquency, seems to have the qualities of an adopted strategy to deal with anxiety, sadness or a difficult situation, and while the latter will not be under the adolescent's control, the overt behaviour may seem so to some extent.

EMOTIONAL PROBLEMS AND DISORDERS

Emotional disorders, broadly defined, make up about two-fifths of the problems of psychiatrically disordered adolescents and a further one-fifth show both emotional and conduct problems (Leslie, 1974; Rutter *et al.*, 1976). These emotional disorders are not a clearly definable group. They include a variety of anxiety and depressive states of all degrees of severity, chronicity, and significance. Leaving aside the fact that any of the rather more circumscribed disorders in Chapters 11–15 may be accompanied by mood disorder, and often are, the clinician presented with an anxious or unhappy adolescent should have the following points in mind:

1. The mood disturbance may be a transient reaction to obvious stress, without pre-existing psychiatric disorder or long-term consequences; it may last hours, days, weeks, or months.

2. The mood disturbance may appear out of proportion to circumstances, although this is not an easy judgement to make since circumstances that seem unremarkable to the observer may be experienced differently, and not necessarily abnormally, by the adolescent and the clinician might miss a possible solution to the adolescent's problems which may respond to relatively straightforward advice or support, or by helping to modify circumstances. Among adolescents mood disturbances may be the relatively undifferentiated, apathy, sadness or fearfulness of younger children, or the anxiety, phobic, depressive or obsessional symptoms of adult-type disorders.

3. Mood disturbance may be transient or persisting, and may or may not be handicapping. It has long been believed that serious emotional upheaval is highly characteristic of adolescence (A. Freud, 1958; Gallagher and Harris, 1964; Mohr and Despres, 1958; Eissler, 1958; Geleerd, 1961; Lindemann, 1964), but this has been increasingly disputed (Bandura, 1964), and Rutter and his colleagues while confirming the relative frequency among 14–15-year-olds, of such feelings as misery, tearfulness, a wish to get away from everything, self-depreciation and ideas of reference, nevertheless showed that most adolescents do not experience marked emotional disturbance (Rutter *et al.*, 1976). As pointed out in Chapter 5, adolescents are referred to psychiatrists for a variety of family and social reasons; finding such symptoms as those above in an adolescent does not itself confirm that the boy or girl necessarily has an individual psychiatric disorder.

4. Whether mood problems are on a spectrum which ranges from normality through a variety of depressive reactions to a primarily endogenous, physiological depression is no clearer in children and adolescents than among adults (see page 79 and Chapter 13). Probably the range seen in clinical practice includes both similar presentations of fundamentally different conditions (for example social, individual, psychodynamic, physiological) and different presentations of similar conditions, with many different permutations of the 'levels' described on page 65. The clinician can assume that a proportion of the mood disorders that present in adolescence, including some that do not seem primarily depressive (see page 224) will respond to tricyclic antidepressants. For similar reasons mood disorders will sometimes

respond to minor tranquillizers such as diazepam, although for reasons given in Chapter 19 these should be prescribed with particular caution. Unfortunately the symptoms of most young people with major mood problems will not respond to medication, but a small group respond well and those that do will not always have shown the characteristics of adult-type depressive disorder.

5. Be prepared, therefore, for the nature of emotional problems to be complex. Eisenberg (1977) has pointed out that behavioural symptoms represent a final common pathway for the expression of multiple causes and, of course, these may include abnormalities reversible by medication, or any other relatively focussed therapy for that matter. I would take this further and suggest that a mood disorder, too, may be how a variety of quite different problems happen to present (see the 'Rubik cube' diagram on page 9) and a disturbed emotional state in an adolescent may be the expression, *the* cause, or *a* cause of whatever is the fundamental set of problems, or may be one manifestation of them, and again as discussed earlier (page 79) there are many reasons why sadness, or whatever changes underly sadness, may be expressed differently depending on the young person's maturity (see page 224 and Cytryn and McKnew, 1975).

6. As a diagnostic exercise which may be helpful in treatment always look for evidence of loss. Adolescence involves change, and change includes loss, and while most boys and girls cope with the move towards maturation and independence, some fear or are saddened by it; thus the sense of loss may be intrapsychic and largely unconscious, perhaps related to loss of a particular role, or the loss of aspects of childhood (see Malmquist, 1971); there may be a very obvious current loss, for example of a relative. Adolescents do not always show how fond they are of elder brothers, elderly relatives, even adult friends of the family; a particular person may occupy a particular place in the boy's or girl's view of the world, and if that person leaves home, leaves the area or dies this may matter more to the adolescent than people think; and indeed it may be convincingly denied at first, by adolescent and family. Past losses may be significant too; depression in adults may result from loss of a parent in childhood (Rutter, 1971b), and loss in adolescence may be particularly likely to be followed by depressive disorder later (Rutter, 1972c) But the effect on adolescents of loss of parents in earlier childhood, apart from obvious and normal distress and grief is uncertain.

There is fairly consistent evidence that parental loss by death or divorce is associated with depression. Prolonged separation of very young children from their parents produces a sequence of angry protest, depressive withdrawal, and recovery (Bowlby, 1973, 1980; Burlingham and Freud, 1943); and some retrospective studies have shown an association between adult depression and loss of a parent in childhood (Brown, 1966; Brown *et al.*, 1977). Among older children and adolescents depressive and related disorders (for example suicide attempts, psychosomatic symptoms) do appear to be more common among young people who have experienced parental loss (Caplan and Douglas, 1969; Seligman *et al.*, 1974).

Lowered self-esteem, which is a form of loss, is prominent in depressive and other mood disorders, and common among troubled adolescents. The approach taken in Chapter 4 has been that the move from dependence to independence is a challenge, and that most adolescents find ways of coping with it; not doing so is a double failure. There are those problems in relationship to parents, peers, and self that are not dealt with; and there is the failure to achieve what peers have achieved, for example independence, jobs, college places, friends of the same sex and the opposite sex. Another helpful model for lowered self-esteem derives from attachment theory (see page 108 and Figure 16). If a child has experienced highly perceptive, skilled parenting that responds in the right time and the right way, he or she may develop a very different self-image from the boy or girl who finds that in order to gain comfort and attention he or she must cry, scream, throw a tantrum or take an overdose of drugs. It is not simply that disturbed emotional behaviour may be learned in this way, though this may happen too; the self-valuation of a young person who has to go to such lengths to get what is wanted or needed is likely to be different from that of the child who is first amazed and later takes for granted that his or her parents seem to know what he or she really wants almost before he or she is aware of it himself/herself. Here, too, skilled parenting and good experiences are a matter of balance: parents who guess what the child wants or needs and are guided more by their own needs and fears than by their perception of the child will risk becoming overprotective and intrusive, and the child's self-esteem suffers in a different way: he or she may begin to have doubts about the significance of their special value, and begin to wonder if they are at risk in some way; what might there be to lose? Loss and other threats are those of imagination and fantasy as well as external reality (Hersov, 1977c).

7. Finally, in adolescence the clinician will come across a range of disorders in transition. Follow-up studies show that most children with emotional disorders improve, and become normal adults (Morris *et al.*, 1954; Robins 1966, 1979). Most children's problems are linked with their age, and those present before age seven have particularly little predictive value (Macfarlane *et al.*, 1954; Thomas and Chess, 1976). Two sets of symptoms if present at age seven, however, are likely still to be present in early adolescence: these are destructive, demanding, jealous behaviour; and sadness and shyness, the first characteristic of conduct disorder and the last associated with emotional disorder (Robins, 1979).

Rutter and his colleagues have shown that childhood disorders continuing into adolescence differ from those starting for the first time in adolescence (Rutter *et al.*, 1976; Graham and Rutter, 1977). In the Isle of Wight study

(Rutter *et al.*, 1970) just over half the psychiatric disorder found among young adolescents represented newly arising disorder, and just under half conditions persisting from earlier childhood, the latter contrasting with the findings of Warren (1965a, b) and Capes *et al.* (1971) who reported that most disorders among their adolescent patients had apparently begun in earlier years. Children with disorders persisting into adolescence tended to have more educational problems (particularly reading retardation) and more serious family problems, while difficulties arising for the first time in adolescence were not assoicated with educational problems, family factors were less prominent and less gross, and were more commonly found in girls (Rutter *et al.*, 1976). Thus the excess of boys over girls with psychiatric disorders in younger age groups diminishes in adolescence, the sex ratio then approaches equality, and by the time adulthood is reached more women than men are identified as having psychiatric problems.

The prognosis of these disorders does not seem to depend upon age of onset although in general the longer a problem or cluster of problems has persisted the longer it may take to go. Taking studies of adolescent disorders overall, most of them containing a majority of patients with diagnoses broadly in the categories discussed in this chapter (90% in Pichel's series 1975), the worst outcome tends to be for the psychotic disorders, schizoid personality disorders and obsessive–compulsive neuroses, the best for emotional disorders excluding obsessional states, with the outlook for conduct disorders in an intermediate position.

Perhaps the most important conclusion for the clinician about prognosis is that while transient emotional problems are frequent in adolescence, it cannot be assumed that emotional disorders will go away of their own accord, the boy or girl 'growing out of it'. The outlook for psychiatric disorder in adolescence is neither better nor worse than in any other age group (Masterson, 1967; Rutter *et al.*, 1976; Graham and Rutter, 1977).

PHOBIC DISORDERS, ANXIETY STATES, AND HYSTERIA

Anxiety states may present with the boy or girl complaining of his or her fears and subjective distress, or from parents' and teachers' concern about what the adolescent cannot do; the young person may be afraid of joining in games, be excessively shy or avoid separating from familiar people. While anxiety is common, many childhood fears quite normal, and some degree of anxiety a frequent accompaniment of every other disorder, an anxiety state as the primary problem is not particularly common among adolescents. Thus in Rosen's survey in the United States of 54,000 adolescents aged 10–19 discharged from 788 psychiatric clinics, anxiety as the main problem was diagnosed in 5.3% of boys and 6.1% of girls, and these included phobic states (Rosen *et al*, 1965).

Anxiety may arise in young people with no previous psychiatric problems, be precipitated by sudden loss or frightening events, be learned from chronically anxious parents (Eisenberg, 1958) or appear to be an expression of long-standing environmental stresses, temperamental vulnerability, or both (see Thomas *et al.*, 1968; Chess, 1973). A common theme in psychodynamic explorations of anxiety and consequent sympton-formation is that the symptoms represent an attempt to avoid or reduce anxiety generated by intrapsychic conflicts such as those summed up by Poznanski (1973) as representing fears of abandonment, fears of mutilation, and sexualized fears. Thomas *et al.* (1968), while acknowledging the presence of apparent intrapsychic conflict and psychodynamic defences in the children they studied, concluded that a more economical formulation could be made in terms of environmental influences, particularly patterns of parents' behaviour, interacting with temperamental vulnerability in some children (Thomas *et al.*, 1968).

Phobia refers to intense anxiety related to particular situations or objects. Among younger children common fears are of the dark, certain animals, insects, and going to school; in the Isle of Wight study there were no cases of handicapping social phobia or agoraphobia (Rutter, 1970) and these tend to make their first appearance in early adolescence (Hersov, 1977c) although according to Marks (1969) these disorders do appear in younger children, Phobia of school, and other reasons for avoiding it, are discussed on page189. Among younger children separation anxiety which is normal in infancy, is a prominent feature of a number of social handicaps, predominantly school refusal, but it does not invariably accompany school refusal in adolescents or even in younger children. Its relationship to school refusal is variable and unclear (Hersov, 1977; Gittelman, Klein and Klein, 1980; and page 188).

Hysteria is usually described in terms of an unconscious strategy adopted by a patient to cope with or avoid anxiety (the primary gain) and which is perpetuated by the secondary gains of interest, attention, and other responses on the part of parents, doctors, and others. Hysterical reactions such as convulsions or loss of sight, speech or movement occur in older children and adolescents; it is extremely difficult to distinguish the deliberate adoption of physical symptoms or disabilities from unconscious processes by which such conditions may arise; anxious and immature children can deceive themselves as well as others, and thoroughgoing self-deception, with a shifting of attention away from the chosen coping method is not so far removed from unconscious activity. Once a 'sick role' has been adopted, there is not merely secondary gain in the attention received, and indeed the attention does not always seem particularly enjoyable; it may also be very difficult indeed for the child to reverse the process without feeling or looking foolish. Minor hysterical or manipulative disorders are not uncommon in paediatric practice, and are sometimes relieved quite rapidly with confident assurance to child *and parents* that the problem will improve, particularly if (a) anxieties believed to be playing a part are treated without particularly relating them to the symptoms, (b) some modest help is given with the symptom, for example physiotherapy for problems in walking. That group of hysterical disorders that do not respond to such measures, however, may prove exceedingly difficult to treat It has been pointed out many times that hysteria is full of snags and pitfalls; it is difficult to define, there is controversy about its nature, and follow-up studies in adults (Slater, 1965) and children (Caplan, 1970; Rivinus *et al.*, 1975) have shown how often unusual symptoms presumed to be psychogenic turn out in due course to have an organic basis. Hysterical symptoms may also follow mild organic illnesses (Dubowitz and Hersov, 1976) and respond to cessation of physical investigation, physical rehabilitation (sometimes with operant behaviour therapy), and firm reassurance. A firm and confident approach to child and family is not always so easy to take by a psychiatrist if he or she is not completely certain of the diagnosis, which is not unusual in clinical work. On the one hand clinicians, and particularly psychiatrists, are often anxious about missing treatable and perhaps dangerous physical disorders; and the often repeated affirmation that it is just as bad, even dangerous, to miss psychiatric disorder seems a satisfying formula on paper but can ring hollow in clinical practice. The clinical psychiatrist has an extremely difficult task in being sure enough of the diagnosis to proceed not only with the confidence that the clinical relationship in general and much psychotherapeutic work in particular requires but with honesty too; and yet as a scientifically trained doctor he or she will more often than not entertain doubts about what is being treated. Are these to be shared with the child and family? The answer is yes, but explaining the clinical evidence to patients is a special skill in itself. A detailed theoretical discourse on the pros and cons of diagnosis and treatment is almost as out of place as deception. The clinician must take care not to be pressed by referring agents, colleagues or indeed by the chance outcome of mixed feelings into prematurely taking a particular approach. Highly anxious, perplexed and overprotective parents who want more investigations and second and third opinions may be right. But since so many heated feelings are getting in the way of everybody's sound judgement, the psychiatrist can appropriately offer to be the coordinator of further investigations; 'holding' the situation by seeing the adolescent and family, interpreting the results of investigations done so far and the advantages and disadvantages of further investigations that could be done, including the disabling effect of pressing on for weeks or months with more investigations.

The clinician should: (a) share his conclusions with child and family – it is always possible to do this in simple language, though it is not necessarily easy; (b) make clear what his own advice is, in the light of perhaps many people's views but *not* as a consensus view of the team; (c) explain what he is going to advise about such doubts as remain about physical disorder; for example, it may be clear that further tests will get in the way of treating the emotional problem and chronic nervousness and disability may be the greater risk, and should stop; or repeating a battery of physical investigations at, say, three or six monthly intervals may be appropriate; (d) avoid being pulled into acting as if psychology and physiology were in watertight compartments; of course there are mental and physical processes interacting in anyone with hysterical conversion symptoms, and it is hard or even impossible to say with certainty how much disorder is represented by each, and by their interaction; (e) finally, remember that no clinical decisions are certainties, but rest on balanced risks and probabilities, that psychiatric disorder and psychiatric treatment are themselves full of risks and that while sometimes mistakes will be made they usually happen because they cannot be foreseen.

Outbreaks of collapsing, overbreathing, and other distressing and alarming behaviour happen from time to time in groups of adolescents in schools or other communities or attending large meetings. The heightened tension caused by the 'attack' in one girl (it is far less common among boys), who may be psychiatrically disturbed, spreads by psychological contagion to less disturbed or normal young people (Moss and McEvedy, 1966, McEvedy et al., 1966; Benaim et al., 1973; Levine et al., 1974, Levine, 1977; Mohr and Bond, 1982). Most such outbreaks last only a few days and may affect up to one-third of the community involved. In the reports by Mohr and Bond (1982) the outbreak lasted for nearly two years, and the authors attributed this unusual chronicity to the large size of the community, a comprehensive school with 1,330 pupils, and because affected pupils (60 girls and 3 boys aged 12–15) used a variety of local general practitioners and hospital departments in the vicinity. A small core of eight girls with marked behaviour and family problems were repeatedly affected and may have acted as triggers for new cases. The authors found the incidence of faints during this period to be 335.1 attacks per 1,000 pupils and, interestingly, calculated the 'normal' rate in eight other co-educational comprehensive schools as 7.1 attacks/1.000 pupils. The management recommended is: (a) positive diagnosis without too long a delay; (b) identification and isolation of the 'trigger' adolescents and help with their problems; (c) attention to group tensions and emotions, which include reassurance and explanation to the adults involved, teachers, parents, and others; (d) coordination of the clinical resources involved (Hersov, 1977c; Mohr and Bond, 1982).

OBSESSIVE–COMPULSIVE DISORDERS

These disorders are relatively clearly defined in adult psychiatry; Schneider (1959) described compulsion as the individual being 'haunted by conscious contents although at the same time he judges them as senseless or at any rate senselessly insistent'. The 'conscious contents' take the form of recurring ruminations that the individual takes responsibility for (that is they are not attributed to outside agencies putting ideas into his head), and are described as *obsessions*; and the urge to ritualistic, repetitive behaviour, or *compulsions*; both are classically described as unwelcome and resisted (Lewis 1936; Despert, 1955;

Slater and Roth, 1969). In children and adolescents resistance is not so straightforwardly experienced as among many adults, and indeed Stern and Cobb (1978) have pointed out that in adults too resistance is not a universal component of obsessional behaviour, in that a patient may resist and resent repetition of the activity, but not the original idea. Certainly among children the reason why they must put out their clothes in a particular way, dress in a certain order, wash their hands with special thoroughness, check that they have said 'goodnight' to their parents (and been replied to) in the properly reasoning way, or carry out certain inner counting or statements before taking some action, may be experienced as most distressing and unwelcome but none the less necessary. The detailed questioning by which the adult psychiatrist hopes to show with crystal clarity if a man or woman's experience is delusional or obsessional runs into the sands with children. They are not sure; they are sure; they are easily led by the grown-up's questioning; they will not say, or they will not say everything. Obsessional doubt may affect the phenomenology itself.

Example 9
An intelligent sixth-former claims to know that his masturbating cannot possibly result in a stray sperm getting around the house and impregnating his sister; but then again he is not sure, and the strength of his feeling makes him feel grossly uncomfortable until all the doorknobs he touched and his own hands are thoroughly and repeatedly washed. Again, an obsessional girl suffers such internal pain at the feeling of being contaminated by germs that the conviction of being at real risk from germs and the psychic reality of feeling contaminated become blurred. She may understand that washing or rituals will not affect germs, and indeed the patient and clinician may be drawn into fascinating philosophical and scientific discussions of the possibility, which may last for hours. But she knows, unshakeably, that the feeling of contamination is insistent and painful and that the ritual provides relief, albeit fleeting.

Mildly obsessional behaviour is common, in children's traditional games (Opie and Opie, 1959) and indeed among professionals.

It is considered good luck if one meets a black cat and says 'black cat bring me luck' or if we stroke it three times from head to tail, and make a wish. But a black cat does not necessarily bring luck; much depends on the creature's behaviour ... if it crosses one's path from left to right, it is very bad luck. A Welsh girl says one must make the sign of the cross and turn completely round. A Shropshire girl says one must turn round three times. A Golspie boy says 'you must spit to avoid a terrible accident which is bound to happen'.
(Opie and Opie, 1959)

What is characteristic of such rituals is that they are part of play. In some children they are part of a general apprehensiveness and overconscientiousness, resulting, for example, in schoolwork which is regarded by teachers as excellent but which is the result of painstaking effort, re-checking, re-doing and some anxiety but some enjoyment and pride too. Alternatively, the work may never get done at all. The nature of the particular obsession or compulsion is less important than:

(a) the distress it causes the boy or girl;
(b) the individual social or educational handicap it causes;
(c) the effect on the child's family; it may become a source of serious conflict, result in over-indulgent helping with rituals (for example in order to get a child to school or to bed in a couple of hours instead of five or six, the whole family may join in the washing, organizing, door-knobs cleaning, etc.), or it may simply get in the way of ordinary family life, with the child and family learning to adapt to a marginally disabled style of life.

While repeated, ritualistic behaviour whose interruption causes distress is frequent, for example in autism, obsessional disorder in its own right is rather uncommon in younger children (Judd, 1965) and the small number found in the Isle of Wight Study (Rutter *et al.*, 1970) had symptoms of anxiety too. Adams (1973) reported that the 39 boys and 10 girls he studied tended to present at around the age of 10 or 11 but that they often had a history of several years' developing symptoms. They made up 1% of psychiatric clinic referrals. In nearly half the cases there had been a precipitating event, and in most cases other members of the family had experienced obsessive symptoms.

The origins of obsessional behaviour are uncertain. Family tendencies to obsessional behaviour are prominent, but the genetic contribution uncertain (see brief review in Thorley and Stern, 1979). Adams (1973) and others have suggested a relationship with ambitious, middle-class families with relatively strict requirements for behaviour, but the clear-cut disorder is relatively rare and the cases studied may be biased towards this group, particularly in the United States where his study took place. The clinical psychoanalytical explanation is that obsessional behaviour represents protective, quasi-magical efforts to deal consciously and by ritualistic behaviour with unconscious motivation that causes guilt and invites danger. In Example 9, mentioned above, the boy could be said to be guarding against incestuous wishes. As with so many psychodynamic explanations they are often general statements about human feelings and motivations that may be no less true of the patient in the clinic than of the individual walking cheerfully on his way outside. Something else selects, reinforces, and perpetuates the behaviour pattern: the boy in the example may have been more fearful about breaking unspoken family rules and 'being naughty' in general than about incestuous fantasies in particular.

In Example 9, the family members may have had mixed feelings about this too, so that 'being good' dealing with the obvious and maintaining a front ('getting him out of the house in the morning') may have tipped the balance towards encouraging rituals rather than confronting them and refusing to join in. Rising rage at the nuisance of the whole business would have challenged the family's self-image of being good and would have been swallowed, but not gone unnoticed, so that a vicious circle of rising tension and determined family effort at working away at the ritualistic behaviour in order to avoid rage would have become self-perpetuating. In turn, the boy himself would have learned to persist in his habits by learned avoidance (of anxiety and family conflict) a model for the development of obsessional symptoms suggested by Meyer and Chesser (1970), and which may be particularly potent in altered mood states (Rachman, 1971). Obsessional disorders in adolescence and their treatment have recently been reviewed and discussed by Bolton et al. (1983). Follow-up studies tend to show a good outcome for a single episode of minor obsessional symptoms, those with a short history and for some which are secondary to depressive disorder (Adams, 1973) which probably explains the helpfulness of the antidepressant drug clomipramine in obsessional adults who are also depressed (Marks et al., 1980). For many children and adolescents with marked and well-established obsessional symptoms, however, the outlook is not good, the relatively few studies of children show more than half experiencing long-persisting symptoms (Ross, 1964; Warren, 1965b). Bearing in mind the general notion of the 'good' hardworking, neat and tidy, reasonably inhibited child, and the frequency of mild obsessional symptoms, it is probable that it is obsessional adolescents with the problem in its particularly intractable form who are presented for treatment. What is well established, however, and allows a measure of reassurance in what otherwise can be a distressing, disabling, and chronic condition, is that it is rare for true obsessional disorder to deteriorate into a schizophrenic psychosis or serious depressive illness (Pollit, 1957; Goodwin et al., 1969; Elkins et al., 1980; Rapoport et al., 1981) although there can be quite serious and persisting impairments of social life and relationships (Hollingsworth et al., 1980).

Behavioural methods such as self-monitoring, thought-stopping, modelling, and response prevention may be helpful in some cases (see Hodgson and Rachman, 1972; Stern, 1978) but a number of special problems arise in the treatment of adolescents. Firstly, an adolescent's compliance in a response prevention programme may be ambivalent and variable. An adult may be expected to commit himself or herself fully, or decline. A boy or girl may have misgivings (and may express them in an appropriately childish, awkward way) and be as distressed by symptoms as by the treatment, wanting neither but wanting adult help none the less. He or she may make it clear that help is wanted, but cry and protest when treatment is pursued. Second, conduct disorder may be present too, and become particularly marked in treatment. Supervision and effective control of the treatment programme, and of the child's behaviour in general, may be very difficult for parents and (in residential units) nursing staff. Thirdly, and turning again to the formulation of the problem as one having both internal and family dynamic components, a behavioural treatment may work, but the parents find it impossible to be as consistent, firm and together in its application as is needed. In our own series (Bolton *et al.*, 1983) we began with the simple model of (a) applying effective behaviour therapy, (b) teaching it to the parents, and (c) dealing with the family or marital psychodynamics that got in the way of its being implemented. The approach undoubtedly meets the needs of some, but has major difficulties too, not least when obsessional symptoms simply disappear when the adolescent is away from home. In these and other cases the obsessional symptoms may be milder and a reasonably normal life livable if the boy or girl is found a place in an ordinary boarding school. Finally, although the 'pure' syndrome by definition lacks major symptoms of depression or anxiety, none the less family members characteristically felt disappointment, loss of self-esteem and were torn between independence of professional workers and dependence on them, and these feelings need help even if attending to them does not correct the disorder. In intractable obsessional disorder, as with other chronic conditions, the clinician has sometimes to abandon the search for a cure and instead help adolescent and family live as normally and fully as possible with their disabilities. However, we found response prevention helped many (Bolton *et al.*, 1983).

Suicide and attempted suicide

Like depressive symptoms, suicide and attempted suicide are practically unknown in young children (in whom neglect and self-neglect are increasingly hard to disentangle the earlier one goes), begin to appear in puberty, increase throughout adolescence, and reach the high levels associated with young adulthood in the late teens (Shaffer, 1974; Morgan *et al.*, 1975; Holding *et al.*, 1977; Wexler *et al.*, 1978; Lumsden Walker, 1980).

Shaffer (1974) in his study of children aged 10–14 in England and Wales during a seven year period, found that only 1 in 800,000 killed themselves, a low rate that appears not to have changed very much during this century (Mulcock, 1955) although suicide rates are notoriously difficult to be sure about because of the common tendency to avoid a verdict of suicide unless it is absolutely certain, particularly in young children and because of the uncertain effect on statistics of the acute medical services. With the exception of certain forms of cancer, accidents are a very prominent cause of death in adolescence, and the borderline between suicide, attempted suicide, risk-taking activity and casual self-neglect is not clear and deserves study. As far as completed suicide is concerned, 4,385 people were recorded as having killed themselves in England and Wales in 1978, of whom 108 were aged 10 to 19. No child under 10 years was recorded as having committed suicide. The male: female ratio for suicide has been 3:2 a proportion that has become less unequal in recent years (Office of Populations Censuses and Surveys, 1978). The pattern is broadly similar to that in the United States, where despite the vastly greater population only 1 child under 10 was recorded as having committed suicide during 1965 (Weiner, 1970b).

There is some evidence that the great increase in deliberate self-poisoning of recent years may have reached a peak (Holding *et al.*, 1977; Gibbens *et al.*, 1978) but the incidence of self-poisoning in adolescents, including younger adolescents, is continuing to increase (Hawton *et al.*, 1982a). In the studies by Hawton and his colleagues, 50 adolescents aged from 13–18 of whom 90% were girls were admitted to hospital after self-poisoning over an eight month period. Few had been under psychiatric care though one quarter had seen their family doctors in the previous week, a characteristic most marked for the older adolescents. About one-third of the girls and boys had recent or current physical ill-health such as asthma and juvenile arthritis, and two-thirds of the drugs employed were analgesics. Troubles with parents, friends and school or work were common difficulties preceding the overdoses. Family problems were prominent, and 14% of the whole group had been in the care of the social services, compared with 4% of 16-year-olds in general. In the majority of the cases described problems were transient, and referral to in-patient services was considered unnecessary, but 14% repeated self-poisoning in the succeeding year. The group for whom the outlook was particularly poor were those whose self-poisoning appeared to be part of a range of behavioural disturbance that included habitual drunkenness, stealing, and fighting (Hawton *et al.*, 1982b, c). The feelings expressed by the young people as a whole were that they felt lonely, unwanted or angry, and the self-poisoning had been to demonstrate their feelings or to try to alleviate them. One-third had wanted to die, a motive that clinicians in this study tended to underrate (Hawton *et al.*, 1982c). In Hawton's study, Leese's (1969) and Lumsden Walker's (1980) self-injury appeared to be part of a continuum of behavioural and family problems including poor communication with parents, absent parents (particulary fathers), a tendency for the overdose to be impulsive, and difficulties in fitting the children's problems into definite diagnostic categories.

The overwhelming method employed in attempted suicide is medication; Weiner (1970b) found that the methods used by adolescents who had completed suicide were different: firearms, explosives, hanging or strangulation being used, such methods being common in Shaffer's report too (1974), but with domestic gas being prominent (43%) a method which has been dramatically reduced since natural gas was introduced in Great Britain.

The treatment of adolescents who want to kill or seriously harm themselves is the treatment of emotional, conduct and family problems, but to this is added the alarming prospect of further and perhaps effective suicidal attempts.

It goes without saying that every threat of suicide should be taken seriously, although it is not possible to treat all young people who make such threats by confining and closely supervising them, even if this were sensible. My experience of disturbed adolescents is that while vague hints of what the boy or girl may do to himself or herself are common, adolescents whose feelings and attitudes are taken seriously by the clinician, tend on the whole not to issue empty threats. I am inclined to believe those boys and girls who say that although depressed and sometimes wishing they were dead, and even seeing suicide as an ultimate solution if life stays much the same, nevertheless say that they are not going to attempt suicide now, or in the near future. It is not a foolproof guide, and cannot be isolated from other clinical judgements, but it is one of several helpful indicators (Steinberg, 1979).

First, then, take any threat seriously, but also take seriously the other feelings the boy or girl is expressing, and hear about the circumstances, relationships, and grievances that are part of the young person's sadness, anger, and frustration. It is also important not to promise or hint at fairly rapid relief by medication, psychotherapy or simply by the contact with the psychiatrist. The adolescent will know that this impossible promise is well intentioned but more for the psychiatrist's comfort than his own; moreover it is not a promise that holds water in psychiatry. What is welcomed, and effective, is a determined offer to stick with the boy or girl and try to help. Unlike an offer of a cure, this is a promise that can be kept.

Secondly, the risk may be considered greater if attempts have been made before, and if means other than drugs have been used or are threatened. Access to the means and local and family tendencies to self-injury, should be noted too.

Thirdly, poor relationships, particularly social isolation, and problems associated with conduct disorder as much as symptoms of depression are risk factors. Of course these problems are common anyway, but an adolescent who threatens suicide, has done so before, and is aggressive, impulsive, and unhappy is at relatively high risk. Relationships with parents are important, but the type of relationship with therapists and other professionals is important too. A child with no successful relationships outside the clinical team or within it is particularly at risk.

Fourthly, in the history a story of loss, such as broken homes or parental death or divorce or the fear or threat of these, and recent serious problems with schoolwork or absence from school, particularly in bright, conscientious children, increase the level of risk.

Fifthly, in the mental state despair and a sense of hopelessness are high risk signs. There is a difference, in my view, between the adolescent who may have most of the characteristics already listed *but* can talk in a reasonably convincing way of the future, and how his or her future hopes are being frustrated, and the child with no sense of the future. Again, the latter is a dangerous sign. The minority of possibly suicidal adolescents who are also psychotic are at high risk too.

It is not possible simply to add up these risks to score whether suicide is likely or not, but with these areas in mind the psychiatrist must make a decision whether an attempt at suicide is likely before whatever help and supervision he is mobilizing has a chance to help. In this respect the role of the family as effective supervisors should not be ignored, even if they have found it difficult so far. The suicidal act or threat is a crisis, and the psychiatrist should do his best to involve the rest of the family in the offers of help being planned; the simple experience for the adolescent of sitting and talking about his worries with the rest of his family and the psychiatrist, and hearing the adults express their anxieties about the boy or girl and their wishes and plans to work together and help, honestly acknowledging any foreseen difficulties too, can be powerfully therapeutic. Part of the prognosis is, of course, how far a helpful therapeutic–supervisory alliance looks convincing. If the clinician is not convinced it is unlikely that the adolescent, who knows the family so much better, will be.

The effect of close supervision, whether by parents or by nurses on a ward, has to be weighed against the needs of treatment, particularly when an adolescent who has been recently suicidal now wants more freedom of movement. All clinicians know the unhappy youngster who has felt most secure when confined within a unit, and who as much dreads as hopes for the staff 'letting up' a little. If they do, will it mean to the adolescent that he is trusted or that they do not care? Probably both, in a fine balance that may tip either way. The relationships built up while the child has been contained are a guide.

In the final analysis, the clinician must decide whether or not he thinks the boy or girl will make a suicidal attempt: he cannot *know*, but he cannot fudge the issue. Either he must act as if the boy or girl will probably not attempt suicide, or as if he or she probably will. Either way he may be wrong, but it is not possible to supervise closely and yet not do so; in which context, vague advice to parents or nurses to 'keep an eye' on the boy or girl is unfair in the circumstances. If the doctor does not know or cannot decide if a possibly suicidal girl who may abscond should or should not be allowed to sit on the grass outside the unit, he should not expect a student nurse to make the decision. If the final decision is that the adolescent is indeed still suicidal, then close supervision at all times, and constant vigilance about access to the means, are essential.

Poisoning

Whatever the psychiatrist's predictions and precautions attempted suicide, self-injury, and overdoses will recur. One of the most difficult times is when an adolescent who has made a serious suicidal attempt and is being very closely supervised in hospital by nursing staff begins to show some modest improvement: characteristically the adolescent enters a period of many weeks when suicide is no longer consistently planned, but the boy or girl is still miserable, still ambivalent about whether or not life is worth while, still has suicidal ideation, and still has the general mood and family and other circumstances which led to the attempt in the first place. At such times it is clear that there is a risk of a further attempt, yet very close nursing supervision, causing as much irritation to the adolescent as a sense of being looked after, can begin to undermine therapeutic progress. There comes a time when the boy or girl will need to go for a walk, may dash away from the nursing staff, and go missing for 24 or 48 hours; and while away, whatever the clinical team has done so far, decide that because he or she has managed to get away this confirms the unwillingness or inability of the adult world to provide proper care. A suicidal attempt or suicide can follow.

The clinical team and the psychiatrist are not omnipotent or omniscient, and it is neither theoretically nor practically possible for any suicidal patient to be supervised in total safety until 'cured'; the former simply delays the latter, and in the long term prolongs the period the boy or girl is at risk. It is important for the suicidal threat or risk and the team's response to be an open matter between adolescent and staff, and talked about; the psychiatrist's responsibility is to make reasonable protective plans with senior nursing colleagues, and make them clear to all concerned, which includes recording them in the notes. It is not reasonable to expect a duty doctor and night nurse to make precise decisions about supervision ('I can't sleep if you keep looking in; I'm all right, really') which the clinicians who know the child best have left unclear. The clinical team should also be willing to search an adolescent and his or her room (and elsewhere) thoroughly in response to threats or suspicion that tablets or sharp instruments are being hoarded, and to have a well-established plan for emergency treatment, usually in conjunction with the local general hospital. Resuscitation equipment, needless to say, should be available, intact and working. Remember that salicylate overdose is particularly dangerous for the unwary because drowsiness and major metabolic changes may occur late, for example 24 hours later. Paracetamol can cause hepatic necrosis and this may occur soon after apparent recovery from the initial effects of the overdose. Oral methionine or I.V. acetylcysteine can prevent or reduce liver necrosis if given soon after the paracetamol overdose (within 10 hours) and may precipitate hepatic encephalopathy if given late.

Most psychiatric units (probably all outside general hospitals) cannot safely handle most overdoses. It goes without saying that vigilance and early diagnosis are vital; first-aid measures should be known about, up to date, and available; and the clinician responsible for the adolescent in the few hours following the overdose should collaborate with a general physician over monitoring and treating the boy or girl unless he is completely confident about the nature of the overdose and the psychiatric team's capacity to cope. In this connection, the more the team as a whole is used to dealing as a group with the fears and feelings about danger, death, and failure which are ever-present in adolescent psychiatric units, the more it will be freed to make rational judgements when emergencies arise. (For reviews of the treatment of poisoning, see Vale and Meredith, 1981; Vale et al., 1981; Valman, 1982. Note the number of the local centre of the National Poisons Information Service: 01 407 7600 in London, which also acts as the coordinating centre.)

SCHOOL NON-ATTENDANCE

School non-attendance is a common problem. It has increased from around 10% in 1967 in London secondary schools to 14% in 1978, reaching a 25% peak in the fifth (last compulsory) year class (Gray *et al.*, 1980). It can be assumed that for many late truants school absenteeism is a social, educational, and occupational matter, rather than indicative of individual disorder. Gray and her colleagues, in their recent study, could not support Tyerman's conclusion (1974) that truancy leads to work difficulties, other than through the consequences of low scholastic achievement. Probably the least affected young adults are those for whom school non-attendance was least determined by individual problems. However, for many young people presenting with school non-attendance the implications are more than educational and legal.

Hersov and Berg (1980) have defined *truancy* as unjustified absence from school without the parents' knowledge or approval. Some studies have shown an association with problems of conduct such as stealing, lying, destructiveness, excessive fighting, and delinquency, and there are often educational difficulties and family adversity. (Farrington, 1980). Persistent truancy in boys appears to predict personality and social problems in adult life (Robins and Ratcliffe, 1980). These associations are less well established in girls although they truant almost as much. It is to be expected that as with other problems of behaviour there are a wide variety of causes and consequences, and it is probable that among persistent truants, starting early, more problems will be found than among young people near the end of their schooling who find it a disappointment (Millham *et al.*, 1978b). The effects of unsatisfactory schooling and high levels of unemployment are likely to have variable effects on school leavers; some may choose to stay on at school, others to try to get a job before the jobs available are further reduced.

School refusal refers to a syndrome of fearful or angry unwillingness to go to school in a boy or girl who stays at home with parents' knowledge but disapproval. Some have additional emotional problems and some do not (Hersov and Berg, 1980). Resistance may be expressed in panic, anger or complaints of physical symptoms. *School phobia* is closely related to school refusal, and although the terms are quite often used interchangeably, it is best to restrict the term to those who seem fearful of the aspects of the school itself, for example its teachers, pupils, and buildings (Eysenck and Rachman, 1965) rather than fear of leaving home. Quite distinct phobias, for example of travelling, may also present as school refusal, while less commonly a more generalized disorder such as anxiety state or depressive illness may cause a range of social handicaps of which school refusal is one, and occasionally school refusal is reported as an early symptom of a psychotic illness (Berg *et al.*, 1974).

School refusal in adolescence is a different problem to that occurring in younger children, where the problems tend to be less severe, accompanied by fewer other emotional problems, and have a better outlook. In older children and adolescents the problem seems to have a more insidious onset, shows a persisting and excessive state of dependency between mother and child (Berg, 1980), is associated with other problems of emotional life and social adjustment, and is generally more severe (Eisenberg, 1958). A variety of studies have shown the persistence into adult life of problems in around one-third of school refusers, including major and minor phobic disorders and problems in college or work (Warren, 1965; Hodgman and Braiman, 1965; Berg, 1980).

The range of treatments used includes family therapy with special emphasis on asserting paternal authority (Skynner 1974, 1976a, b), graded reintroduction to school (Talbot, 1957), firmness and reassurance (Lewis and Lewis, 1973), antidepressants (Gittelman-Klein and Klein, 1973), behaviour therapy (Yule *et al.*, 1980), and residential treatment to ensure consistent management and help overcome anxiety about separation between parents and adolescent (Fleck, 1972; Hersov, 1977a). Overall, the younger the boy or girl the more acute the problem and the earlier it is tackled, the better the outlook.

Just as emotional problems and conduct problems overlap, so do problems of school refusal and truancy. Boys and girls and their families will be seen with the characteristics of both. For the more clear-cut cases of truancy, involving the law, the authority of school and reinforcing that of the parents is frequently effective. The parents of a child who will not go to school (or is not sent) can be prosecuted under section 40 of the Education Act 1974 which requires a child to attend school up to age 16; the authorized leaving date, incidentally, is at the end of term, not on the birthday; and Eisenberg (1958) among others stresses the importance in many cases of having the support of the education welfare services, and if necessary the courts, to allow a reasonable amount of pressure to be brought on the child. Pressure of this sort is not incompatible with either the principles of psychotherapy, behaviour therapy, common sense, or humanity: an anxious child of any age is likely to be made more fearful of a particular action by vague, anxiety-laden, and ambiguous advice to 'try' accompanied by obvious anxiety on the part of adults–a combination of firm determination and kindhearted interest and support is needed. Firmness is appropriate in both truancy and school refusal. In this context it is worth noting the relative effectiveness in truancy of using the pressure of the court, for example by repeated adjournments and injunctions to go to school (Berg *et al.*, 1978) and the preventative tactics of Rhodes Boyson (1974) who maintained close liaison with parents as soon as unexpected absence occurred, and rewarded children whose attendance records were good.

Given this very wide range of pathology (including the absence of pathology) implications and possible treatment, what guidelines can there be to help the adolescent referred for school non-attendance?

1. First, consider the referral. Why is the boy or girl being referred now? If he or she has just begun to absent himself/herself from school it is reasonable to accept school non-attendance as the primary problem; but if the adolescent has not been at school for a year or two, and is perhaps just coming up to school leaving age, the primary problems may be guilt and misgivings on the part of agencies who have unsuccessfully involved themselves with the young person's problems for too long without following through any action, legal,

administrative, or therapeutic. The problem may then need re-definition, for example as an upper-age adolescent with major educational and vocational disadvantage and the need for active help with both perhaps from special careers advisers, training centres, and youth opportunity projects. Sometimes a boy or girl in this position will find attendance at evening classes or a polytechnic more acceptable than school. Support and vocational counselling are important.

2. Second, is the boy or girl ill? Depression, rarely schizophrenia or very severe disorders of personality development (see Chapter 13) or clear-cut, severe phobic illness may be present. If so the disorder needs treatment in its own right and is not typically 'school refusal'. These are the only instances where a 'certificate' permitting time off school for treatment and perhaps home tuition may be appropriate.

3. Third, is the problem a clear-cut case of truancy? This is a rather difficult area. Adolescents who are neither ill nor typically school refusers may be quite clearly cheerfully misbehaving; clearly generally antisocial and sometimes quite unhappy and anxious behind a generally truculent manner; or withdrawn from school by parents for a variety of reasons (Berg *et al.*, 1978). I have seen psychiatrically normal young people kept at home by agoraphobic mothers who needed someone to do the shopping, by parents who objected strenuously to aspects of the only schools to which they had access, and a gypsy family who did not want their child to go to the local school because they were soon moving on. If there is no disorder evident in the child, either self-pepetuating or maintained by parental attitudes, the psychiatrist should be prepared to offer such immediate advice as he can, as would any other doctor, but should make it clear that the problem is one for the adolescent, parents, education department and the law to sort out together.

This will leave a mixed group of school-refusing children as defined on page 189 plus a number of truants who have some degree of emotional problems too: boys and girls who perhaps hang about on the fringe of a gang and who are willing to acquiesce in their parents' wish for help.

4. It is essential to engage the help of both parents. Family therapists will want to engage the help of the whole family. The aim of treatment must be explained to the boy or girl in the presence of both parents and with their support. It is essential to work with an identified member of the school's staff. If parental motivation and ability to get together in their child's interests and use help effectively is not in doubt, there may be no need to ask for the involvement of an education welfare officer (EWO), but usually it is extremely helpful to work with an EWO, or a social worker if the family situation seems particularly difficult and care proceedings may be called for. The ethical situation is a little difficult if the clinician thinks the help of an EWO or the social services department is needed but the parents refuse contact. If the psychiatrist thinks he and his clinical team can help sufficiently, they should proceed on that

basis. If they think it will be impossible, perhaps rendering chronic a condition that is known to get worse as time goes by, this fact and the reasons why the clinic cannot help should be explained to the parents and the referring agent.

5. With the goal of an early return to school clearly in view, the clinical team needs to clarify the difficulties threatening to prevent it. The adolescent may be moderately phobic or unhappy; resistant to parental pressure; playing one parent off against another; playing off parent against school; there may be organizational or attitudinal problems in the education department or school impeding a therapeutically guided return; the parents may not really be in agreement, or may be anxious or unable to cooperate.

6. A treatment plan which may include any combination of individual or family treatment is arranged; for example, a clinical psychologist may arrange desensitization in imagination to deal with separation anxiety or *in vivo* to deal with school phobia; he may enlist the help of an EWO in escorting the child to school, the parents in getting the child psychologically as well as physically ready for school, and the teacher to receive the child punctually and firmly take him or her to the first class. The psychologist or another team member may work with family on marital difficulties that get in the way of competent cooperation.

Persistence is important, so also is an early return to school, within days, if not the next day, of the treatment plan being agreed with parents and school.

7. Admission to hospital is appropriate if there are insuperable difficulties in getting parental cooperation (inability rather than resistance) or if the adolescent seems to have major fears or unhappiness or major problems in peer relationships. Unless the boy or girl is truly ill (page 191) the admission should be as brief as possible, and aimed at *either* an early return to day school with unit staff acting in *loco parentis* and then trying to share their skill and success with the parents, *or* arrangement of residential schooling. The latter may take a very long time to arrange, and preliminary enquiries and tentative applications are necessary as soon as the clinician thinks residential schooling is going to be needed. Occasionally a boy or girl will make reasonable headway but is clearly adversely affected and constantly undermined by irredeemably chaotic domestic circumstances. In such cases the possibility of a boarding school which makes its own holiday arrangements, a children's home for the boy or girl to regard as home in school holidays, or a therapeutic community, should be considered, rather than a prolonged hospital admission.

CONDUCT DISORDER AND DELINQUENCY

Conduct disorder is usually described in terms of persistently aggressive, destructive, defiant behaviour, sometimes including sexual misbehaviour, firesetting, and absconding. It is not a homogeneous group of problems but is not too difficult to differentiate from adolescents misbehaving because of current severe social stress, or as an apparent consequence of some other psychiatric disorder. It also tends to persist, tending to recur in many situations (but often with islands of activity or relationships where the boy or girl is 'as good as gold'). To this extent it is not easy to distinguish conduct disorder from an emerging pattern of personality development that may, in due course, be best considered as a personality disorder. The multi-axial classification scheme (Rutter *et al.*, 1975a) usefully sub-categorizes these problems into *mixed disorders of conduct and emotions*, where there is also considerable emotional disturbance, for example anxiety or depressive symptoms; *unsocialized disturbance of conduct* where problematic behaviour is very much part of the boy's or girl's own actions and reactions (for example solitary stealing, lying, teasing, tantrums); and *socialized disturbance of conduct* where misbehaviour recurs in a group of peers. Many younger children with conduct problems are also restless and overactive (see page 199) although by the time adolescence is reached overactivity is often replaced by apathy and inertia.

Conduct disorder is not synonymous with delinquency. The latter is a legal term, not a clinical one, and refers to law-breaking activity. Isolated acts of delinquency, like occasional misconduct, are common and normal; most adolescents taken to court do not have conduct disorders, and many are never re-convicted. Achieving the status of delinquent requires a series of events; the behaviour itself, the police being informed, getting caught, the action taken by police officers (which may depend on the demeanour of the adolescent and any preconceptions or knowledge the police have of the youngster and his or her family), and the outcome of a court appearance. Among the lower socioeconomic groups of adolescent boys, a quarter are convicted at least once as juveniles, and of these more than half are convicted at least once more, with a quarter becoming persistent offenders (Power *et al.*, 1972). It is members of the persistently offending group who may have much in common with adolescents with conduct disorder, but considerable caution must be exercised in relating socially disapproved and illegal behaviour to psychiatric disturbance (Taylor *et al.*, 1973; West, 1977). Delinquency is so closely tied to the official laws and unofficial rules and methods of a community, its incidence so dependent on how young people and neighbourhoods are supervised, looked after and provided for (Rutter, 1979), and psychiatric effectiveness in helping with delinquency so low (West, 1977) that the role of the clinical psychiatrist in delinquency is extremely limited. The psychiatrist should be able to contribute helpfully to research into the subject, and psychiatric and psychological skills may be useful in the management of residential and other programmes for delinquents, but delinquency is not a disorder and there is no treatment for it. The clinician's primary role here is to identify conduct and other disorders among delinquents, recommend management plans if he can, and offer some guidance about the likely future for the boy or girl (see also pages 194 and 196).

Having said this, the clinical psychiatrist in training should make sure he meets delinquents. Of course many young people in detention centres and borstal institutions are unhappy, unskilled, and without realistic hopes or plans; they often come from overcrowded socially deprived areas with high unemployment and from families with many problems, including psychiatric disorder and criminal convictions. Nevertheless many, particularly boys, seem to be basically normal young people, very different from those with conduct disorder among their own number and seen in clinics. Their need is for training in the widest sense: socially, educationally, and vocationally and with a reasonable expectation of adequate long-term rewards for their investment of trust and effort. It is the latter which is particularly difficult to provide and makes delinquency primarily a social rather than a psychiatric problem.

Conduct disorder is more common in boys than in girls (the ratio is at least 3:1), and the association with both educational difficulty in general and specific reading retardation in particular is striking. It does not seem that antisocial behaviour leads directly to academic failure, but possibly the reverse, or there may be underlying factors common to school and social difficulties. Despite the uncertainty underlying the relationships between the two, adolescents with conduct disorder need help with their educational and particularly their reading problems. With educational and vocational help as a focus, useful relationships may be built up, the boy or girl may begin to feel a sense of personal value and achievement, and at the very least another area of handicap is minimized.

The origins of conduct disorder are multiple, and several may be operating in the case of the individual boy or girl. Earlier childhood may have been characterized by unusual temperamental characteristics such as impulsiveness, aggressiveness, apparent lack of feeling for others, and relative unresponsiveness to praise and encouragement. They often come from large families where there is lack of supervision, inconsistent handling, extremes of discipline (none or excessive, perhaps alternating unpredictably), and marked marital and family discord. Many such families are grossly disorganized and live in neighbourhoods which are very deprived (see page 101). It is tempting to speculate that perhaps the human infant could be expected to develop into a conduct-disordered adolescent unless handled with that fine balance between permissiveness and limit-setting, affection and anger, protectiveness and the encouragement of independence, that competent families are able to achieve and the families described above cannot. It is important, also, to recognize that by the time the boy or girl is seen in the clinic, his or her habits, those of the family, and the responses of peers, teachers and other members of the community are thoroughly established in a way that can powerfully maintain the persistence of the repertoire of problem behaviour; interfering with such processes can be a daunting task. Many studies confirm that the outlook is not good for many, with conduct disorder in childhood leading to many problems in adult life, such as alcoholism, recurring problems with the law, repeated unemployment, poor interpersonal relationships and marital conflict, family problems and adult delinquency. Not all children with conduct problems have such a bleak outlook, but marginal problems in such categories are common and may be expected to lead to family and parenting problems, poor general achievement in poor neighbourhoods with poor schools and trouble with the children (see studies and reviews by Rutter and Madge, 1976; Rutter, 1979a; Robins, 1966, 1979).

From such follow-up studies a start has been made on predicting which children in adolescence are likely to show major conduct problems. Aggressive behaviour, poor peer relationships, underachievement for intellectual level, and failure to accept the teacher's authority, predict poor school attainment and antisocial behaviour including delinquency in later childhood and adolescence (Robins, 1979).

As with school non-attendance, an early task is to establish the authority with which the therapist can act; if the boy or girl is uninterested in help but the parents insistent, or if it seems that with time and patience their cooperation can be engaged and 'shaped up', it is worth proceeding. Alternatively, the boy or girl may be (or needs to be) the subject of a Care Order or of some other legal sanction before treatment can be contemplated: either the boy or girl wants some help (and ambivalence is often an acceptable basis on which to start, while unequivocal defiance is not), or the authority of parents, social worker or the law will be needed to guarantee a start being made.

It is important to make sure that the problem is not at least partly due to unrecognized psychiatric disorder. Is the child hyperkinetic, depressed, manic or does he or she have epilepsy? It is also important to make sure that the problem is not a transient one, or even a relatively long-standing one maintained in a previously normal child by current family, school or social circumstances that might be changeable. Diagnostic labelling is always imperfect, and individual children and families include many who are the exceptions to the statistical norms; it is worth at least setting out optimistically. What behaviour is expected of the child? How do the parents make this clear, and what are their sanctions? Are they consistently applied? More important, what are the rewards in the child's life? Are they consistent too? How do his teachers handle him? Is he in an appropriate school? Are the parents enjoying life? Adolescents with marginal problems can be tipped into giving up if adult life as practised by the parents seems to be a miserable, unrewarding drudge; this can be found in expensive private housing estates no less than in deprived inner city areas. Are naughty children receiving attention largely when being naughty, and ignored when behaving reasonably? Behavioural analysis of this type needs to be quite detailed, and may partially explain the successes of family therapy with otherwise intractable problems; it is not the occasional, or even the quite frequent, response to a child which influences it towards being disorderly or growing away from disorderliness. Nor is it the coarse aspects of behaviour. It is the finely graded social signals, sometimes represented as the outcome of competing and ambiguous statements and behaviour, operating relentlessly over the years, day in and day out, which gradually shape most children in one direction or another. These more subtle aspects of interpersonal behaviour, straddling behavioural and psychodynamic theory, require identification before it can be said whether or not they can be modified, and whether their modification will help the adolescent.

Often children with the more intractable behaviour problems arrive in residential institutions. What approach helps which children remains unknown. Some children, even with very difficult problems indeed, are helped by quite different institutions. All can claim surprising successes and surprising failures. Such settings – special residential schools, therapeutic communities, and community homes – are often very changeable too (see page 40). The best the clinician can do is to keep up to date with what those available to him are like, who they accept, and with whom they tend to have success. He must maintain a resource file, supplemented by visits to various children's homes, schools, and communities. Team members in training need to visit them, and their reports can be an invaluable source of information.

Yule (1978) has reviewed the use of behaviour modification techniques which include intensive training and supervision of parents applying them (Patterson· 1971, 1974) and the application of behavioural techniques in residential settings – the Achievement Place Project (Phillips, 1968; Wolf *et al.*, 1975a, b) which focuses on the training of boys in social skills. Both have achieved promising results, but require very specialized, sustained programmes; they can suffer in attempts at replication, and can be difficult to transfer to an ordinary clinical setting, in-patient or out-patient.

It is important, as already mentioned, to ensure that it is conduct disorder, not some other psychiatric or physical problem or a primarily social or family problem that is behind the adolescent's behaviour. If it is, the condition needs treating in its own right, whatever is done about the problematic behaviour. The clinical team, and the parents and teachers with whom they cooperate, should be clear about the behaviour that is being tackled, as should the adolescent. The way in which it is being dealt with should also be clear. If certain behaviour is to be tolerated while psychotherapy or counselling gets under way, this should be made explicit; it is possible to go in too heavily with a behavour programme at a time when a boy or girl needs time and space to build up self-esteem, and it is confusing for all concerned if it is not clear which behaviour is acceptable and which is not; if a period of tolerance is suggested it is important to make sure that normal expectations of reasonable behaviour are not abandoned. It needs to be made clear, to the family of an out-patient, or to the family and staff if the adolescent is an in-patient:

(a) What to do about unacceptable behaviour, such as threats or acts of aggression, with as a general rule a low threshold of tolerance for the behaviour of adolescents who clearly intend to test parents' and staff limits (see page 198). In in-patient units, group peer pressure to behave reasonably should be mobilized. This general approach is not to be confused with (b).

(b) Whether a formal behavioural approach is to be pursued, in addition. This may include time out, or operant training (for example via a token system). This requires expert supervision, for example by a psychologist.

(c) What other treatment is under way, and its relationship with (a) and (b). Thus it may be decided that a team member offering regular *counselling* may also act as disciplinarian if privileges are to be withdrawn for misbehaviour; or it may be concluded that a team member offering *psychotherapy* should not. There is no useful evidence about which of these roles can and cannot be combined; what matters is that the issue is aired, dilemmas and inconsistencies discussed, and a coherent, properly supervised management plan persued.

(d) Also the dual policy of *carefully supervising the whole management programme* (including sympathetic discussion about difficulties in implementing it consistently) and *charting progress* helps what may be a potentially difficult and initially unrewarding treatment policy to be pursued and persisted with. Small improvements should be spotted and worked upon, and the management plan adjusted accordingly with everyone involved and informed.

Finally, regardless of the place of individual, group or family counselling or therapy, it is important to pay attention to the boy's or girl's difficulties, fears, and misunderstandings about home, about school, and about the treatment programme itself.

Violence

The anger that spills into violence, like other moods, has too many possible causes and implications to set out a straightforward blueprint for handling it. The behavioural guidelines already given remain important: what exactly is the behaviour, in home or residential unit, that is causing concern? When does it occur, and in what circumstances does it stop? If an attempt is made to help in some systematic way, it is important to chart progress so that family, school or unit do not too readily assume that a further outburst represents a return to square one. Confrontation may be needed: if so, as already pointed out, it should occur at a lesser threshold than one which pushes people to the limit. If there is to be a confrontation over a defiant adolescent's behaviour, it should take place each time he is, say, unpleasantly and verbally abusive, not when he has hit someone with a chair. Family (or residential staff) should regard violent behaviour, its prevention and how to cope with it as a legitimate subject for discussion and training, led by the senior staff. It must not become a shameful subject which the most inexperienced staff try to handle alone, leaving their seniors to cope with higher clinical matters. Unless an adolescent is acutely psychotic or confused, *or being mishandled by adults or peers*, he or she must accept some responsibility, if not all, for his or her behaviour. It is neither therapeutic nor humane to accept that the adolescent 'can't help it'. He or she will have to be helped to do something about it, if a lifetime in and out of prison or mental hospital is to be avoided. In all cases an attempt should be made to involve parents (or the responsible social worker) in the plans for handling a violent adolescent in an in-patient unit, if only to affirm the authority to act which they are allowing the staff. The priority should be to stop anyone getting badly hurt, and misleading notions that 'letting off steam' by violence might be all right, or that stopping violence physically (or, *in extremis*, by drugs) is wrong, should be put firmly aside. Having said this, a little foresight is also needed; I would have no qualms about forcefully sedating an acutely enraged violent adolescent to stop more serious injury. But if a residential unit considers admitting a recurrently violent and possibly delinquent adolescent who is not mentally ill, the team should decide in advance its policy for dealing with dangerous behaviour: is sedation appropriate? Perhaps once, if it is the only way to bring an extreme emergency to a halt, but a delinquent young person near the normal end of the spectrum should not be repeatedly treated in this way: he or she should be invited to accept the help of the clinical team if some sort of therapeutic contract can be made, and this may well include suspension or discharge if he wants to knock staff or peers about, or says he or she cannot help it. It is not easy to decide whether a boy or girl should take his or her chances with the law and go his or her own way or alternatively comes into the category of one who should be contained and treated whether he likes it or not; but the dilemma of voluntary treatment, or containment and treatment (for example in a secure, highly staffed unit), is one to be faced.

Anger, even very noisy anger and the occasional window being broken is something a residential unit should be able to cope with without undue alarm. It is a step in the right direction from violence against people. A furious row that ends in the adolescent being held, with containment turning into a cuddle, is all right. In a residential unit the staff should be able to make crystal clear that they care about the boy or girl, yet can still feel angry with him or her, and moreover that violent behaviour is unacceptable. Calm, non-punitive containment is the ideal, though not easily achieved. Parents, too, may need help to see that firmness and hostility are not synonymous.

Such issues should be considered when a violent youngester is referred for admission because, it is said, he or she needs psychotherapy. The means for containing violence must be clear-cut; some therapeutic settings have a high capacity for containing violence, due to staff numbers, staff experience, and ethos of the community. But the most sophisticated psychotherapy stands no chance if the boy or girl cannot be contained. Physical security, special staff numbers and skills, or less often medication will be appropriate in different settings and for different sorts of problems, but the means for keeping the young person on the premises, and safely, should be clear, and thought through in advance.

Fire-setting

One of the most worrying forms of conduct disorder, and characteristically associated with other behaviour problems like fighting and disobedience, is firesetting. Family disruption is common in the child's background, boys far outnumber girls, and the general picture is that younger children tend to start fires alone and at home, and older children away from home and in groups (Lewis and Yarnall, 1951; Strachan, 1981; Stewart and Culver, 1982). The title of Strachan's paper, 'conspicuous firesetting in children', draws attention to the fact that not all childhood playing with fire is pathological; clandestine experiments are common, and it is likely that it includes reasonably responsible games with fire as well as risky experiments which go wrong. How this group compares with the young people who deliberately start serious fires and its relationship to poor adult supervision is not known. There are rather few detailed and systematic studies of the problem. All that can be said of fire-setting children who are referred to psychiatrists is that some stop doing so and some (about a quarter in Stewart and Culver's study) carry on, and that it was possible, but by no means certain, that the group who stopped came from more stable homes or were moved into more stable settings. However, there is no reliable way of predicting further fire-raising and the only advice must be to put right such emotional, family, and educational problems as one can, provide particularly close supervision for the most disturbed (some, for example, have been diagnosed as impulsive and hyperactive and psychotic; Kaufman *et al.*, 1961), and to give high priority to all aspects of fire prevention and fire alarm systems wherever people, disturbed or otherwise, are gathered together.

HYPERKINETIC DISORDERS

Hyperactivity is uncommon in adolescents although occasionally a younger, immature boy or girl will present with this problem. More often it becomes apparent in the earlier history of a young person who is now depressed, even withdrawn and apathetic, and has a long history of educational and social difficulties. It is very variably defined, which is presumably why it is regarded as common in the United States, but rare in Britain (Rutter *et al.*, 1970).

Hyperactivity (or *overactivity*) is a description rather than a diagnosis, and to some extent a point of view. Depressed or distracted parents may consider a lively child overactive, particularly if he or she becomes restless, demanding, and particularly exploratory in efforts to attract parental interest. A boy or girl may more appropriately be described as having a conduct disorder and perhaps be poorly and inconsistently trained and not given the guided stimulation that helps ordinary children direct their energies usefully and enjoyably; parental overindulgence can have the same effect. Almost invariably the overactivity varies from situation to situation. Anxiety states, depression, mania or autism may also cause motor overactivity but these diagnoses are usually obvious.

The *hyperkinetic syndrome* is a term which should be reserved for gross excitability and overactivity in most or all situations, accompanied by distractibility, a short attention span, impulsive and often dangerous behaviour (unexpected dashing across a busy road, for example), and major educational difficulties. Whether the latter are due to the child's poor attention and chaotic functioning, or like the behaviour disorder in some cases results from a primary neurological impairment, is not clear (see reviews by Cantwell, 1975, 1977).

While educational problems are prominent in hyperkinetic children, the relationship with intellectual level is not clear primarily because the syndrome is so variously defined. Thus Palkes and Stewart (1972) found mean IQs on the Wechsler Intelligence Scale for Children lower than for matched controls.

Some hyperkinetic children have clear evidence of brain damage, including temporal lobe epilepsy (Ounsted, 1955); some have evidence of 'minimal brain dysfunction', with abnormal EEGs (an increase in slow wave activity) in one-third to one-half of the children reported (Werry, 1979a) but most children diagnosed as hyperkinetic do not have evidence of cerebral dysfunction and most children with cerebral dysfunction do not show hyperactivity (Cantwell, 1977).

Treatment should begin with the approach as for any disorder of conduct: looking for emotional and educational problems to help, and offering whatever will help the young person's parents behave warmly and consistently towards the adolescent; parental or family counselling, family therapy, and sometimes marital work may be needed. One of the behavioural approaches, applied at home and if necessary at school, may be helpful. Drugs like methylphenidate are most likely to help when distractibility is prominent: attention problems can be confirmed by psychological testing if it is not clear clinically. For wildly overactive behaviour which stimulants fail to control, haloperidol or chlorpromazine may be useful, but benzodiazepines should be avoided. The drugs and their problems are discussed on page 328. White (1981) has pointed out that along with other measures they may help some impulsive, antisocial adolescents with a past history of hyperactivity and tricyclic antidepressants may be useful too.

THE MISUSE OF DRUGS AND OTHER CHEMICALS

Drug dependence in adolescents and its treatment is too wide a subject to be dealt with adequately here; Blumberg (1977) and Connell (1977) have provided helpful and comprehensive reviews. Drug misuse among children under 14 has been rare, and addiction in adolescents under 16 even rarer (Connell, 1977) and opiate dependence in particular may be becoming less common among adolescents in the United Kingdom (Rutter, 1979a). The misuse of alcohol, however, appears to be increasing in young people in Britain and the United States, with the possibility of a levelling out in the rate of increase in the United States since 1974 (Donnan and Haskey, 1977; Rutter, 1979a; Ritson, 1981).

Most young people learn to drink moderately; interestingly, Ritson (1981) considers that too much concern with alcoholism and its definition may distract us from the wider concern about the association of the sometimes casual abuse of alcohol with damage to jobs and family life, self-poisoning (Kreitman and Schreiber, 1979), road traffic offences, and criminal behaviour, rather than with alcoholism as a special disorder of certain vulnerable individuals. Ritson suggests that adults should think more carefully of the model they present, as drinkers of alcohol, to children; of education and information about its effects being provided in schools; of counselling for adolescents who begin to drink too early or too much. Is alcohol too cheap? Kendell (1979) has pointed out that between 1950 and 1976 the length of time a manual worker had to work to pay for a pint of beer fell by nearly half; meanwhile, young people have a lot to spend, it is not so easy for licensees to distinguish the under 18-year-olds from their seniors, and alcohol is very freely available (Kendell, 1979; Ritson, 1981).

The abuse by children and adolescents of solvents has become a recent cause for concern but in fact has been known for at least 20 years (see Tolan and Lingl, 1964; Press and Done, 1967; Skuse and Burrell, 1982). An extraordinarily wide range of substances are involved, including toluene, acetone, and naphtha (in 'Evostick' and model-making cement); benzene (rubber solutions); acetone and amylacetate (nail polish remover); carbon tetrachloride, trichloroethane and trichloroethylene (typing correction fluids and dry cleaning fluid); acetone (impact adhesives); benzene and naphthene compounds (petrol); fluorocarbon propellant gases (aerosols). These and other substances are sniffed from the bottle or tube or from a saturated handkerchief, inhaled from a polythene bag around the head or from an empty crisp packet, or sprayed from an aerosol directly into the nose or mouth. There is central nervous depression producing a sensation equivalent to alcohol intoxication, with excitement, blurred vision, visual distortion, dizziness, disorientation, occasionally memory loss for the episode, sometimes loss of consciousness and a variety of perceptions and experiences depending, like other drugs, upon the expectations of the user and the experiences and expectations of the group. These effects wear off quickly, but the chemical smell stays on the breath and a characteristic red ring may be seen around the mouth, 'glue sniffer's rash' sometimes accompanied by boils. These solvents are used as well as or instead of alcohol; users often prefer the latter if it is available and they can afford it (Burrell, 1982, personal communication; Camden and Islington Area Health Authority, 1981). There have been many reports of direct toxic effect. Sudden death due particularly to sniffing aerosol propellant gases and trichloroethane has been reported from the United States (Bass, 1970). There were under 100 such deaths in the period 1966–1969 during which time estimates suggested 1 to $1\frac{1}{2}$ million young people had 'sniffed' at least once. The evidence for brain damage appears to rest on few cases (Woodcock, 1976), but seizures and encephalopathy (King et al., 1981), polyneuropathy (Matsumura et al., 1972), liver disease (Litt et al., 1972), bone marrow disorders, chronic lung injury and renal failure have all been reported (Watson, 1977, 1980; O'Connor, 1979). Weight loss, anorexia, nausea and vomiting, acute bronchospasm, and cardiac arrhythmias have also been seen (Skuse and Burrell, 1982). The pattern of use, and the relation of this to the incidence of *direct* toxicity, is uncertain; thus there may be many adolescents abusing these substances casually and experimentally who are in less danger from this source than chronic users. Other dangers, for example suffocation, falling from heights or road accidents are more clear-cut. In the study by Skuse and Burrell (1982), of 45 adolescent solvent abusers (28 boys and 17 girls) most of the young people were found to have psychiatric problems largely classified as conduct or emotional (depressive) disorders, and delinquency was common among the chronic abusers, who were mostly boys. There was little evidence of physical dependence. Individual and family work was offered and half improved over about a year's follow-up and a good outcome correlated with high motivation for treatment. Masterton (1979) has stressed the need for community prevention by cooperation between general practitioners, schools, the police, and youth leaders.

Many drugs can cause toxic psychoses, including these solvents (Skuse and Burrell, 1982), and lysergic acid diethylamide (Sedman and Kenna, 1965) while paranoid psychotic states, usually transient, are associated with amphetamine use (Connell, 1958).

PROBLEMS OF PERSONALITY DEVELOPMENT

When does a persisting emotional or conduct problem become a personality disorder? I am reluctant to use the term in adolescents, whose personalities are still developing, but although this is justifiable clinically it admittedly evades an important question of psychopathology. As far as conduct disorders are concerned, we do know from the long-term studies (Robins, 1966; and page 194) that conduct-disordered children and adolescents include a proportion who in due course will be diagnosed as psychopaths and sociopaths. Of psychopathy it can be said: (a) that the term, like hysteria, is exceedingly difficult to define with any precision and yet it seems hard to do without it; (b) that it carries connotations of impulsive, irresponsible, immature behaviour with a need for immediate rather than postponed gratification; (c) that a lack of empathy with other people's feelings is characteristically included in the description of psychopathic individuals, and selfishness predominates; (d) that there is no mental disorder or retardation that would alone account for the disordered behaviour and relationships; (e) that the troublesome behaviour may be either primarily aggressive or primarily inadequate. All these qualities are found in normal infants, and one way of describing the various forms of psychopathy would be as infantile behaviour occurring in an adult in the absence of mental illness or mental retardation. As the years go by, some adolescents seem to be developing in this direction.

Sexual questions and problems

Another maturational task with occasional clinical implications is that of sexual choice. Parents, teachers, or occasionally the adolescent himself or herself may wonder if he or she is growing up homosexually, or in a deviant way. The adolescent may fret about masturbation and need the information that it is a universal, normal, and desirable aspect of sexual development. Choice of sexual behaviour is apt to be a hot topic, with the paternalistic and the libertarians taking sides. Younger adolescents tend to be a more conservative group than those 10–15 years their senior, and challenging and provocative ambitions, sexual or otherwise, tend to be the exception rather than the rule, though very difficult when they arise. If sexual behaviour is legal and harmless and not driven by emotional problems (for example promiscuity because of loneliness or disinhibition, or as a way of showing off or achieving notoriety), and if it does not risk seriously hurting other people's feelings or pregnancy, I would not make a big thing of it; like so much else in the way of adolescent experimental behaviour, the social skills of tact, discretion, and regard for others' feelings (peers and parents) can make all the difference between what is normal, sensible, playful, experimental behaviour and what is exhibitionistic, hurtful, and destructive. Questions about choice of sexual behaviour and relationships are only difficult for the clinician because he may be drawn unwittingly into issues that are not medical, and yet feels an adult obligation to guide a boy or girl into what is wise, which is not a new dilemma.

Example 10

A 16-year-old girl, among her other worries, has a lesbian relationship with a 13-year-old girl at school. Parents and teachers find both children ambivalent, that is both are worried about their relationships, somewhat embarrassed by it, and not sure whether they want to be homosexual or not. It is not a big problem for the younger girl who, with relatively little, non-intrusive advice from parents and teachers is readily 'released' into taking up friendships of both sexes, although still primarily other girls, and is encouraged into having a few more years in which to make up her mind what sort of young woman she wishes to be. In her case the issue was less a sexual one that a premature, intense, rather prolonged involvement with one friend to the exclusion of others.

The older girl, however, has a more preoccupying and troubling problem. Torn between wanting to have sexual relationships with women, and the shame she feels about being homosexual, she wants to have a surgical operation to turn her into a man. She has many problems in her family, and is also profoundly depressed, and sees suicide as the only alternative to being offered an operation which is often unsatisfactory. The first question is whether her ambition is an illness; her conviction that only the operation would resolve her muddled feelings is near-delusional. The second question is how much what she says represents what she really wants. It is a difficult philosophical and ethical dilemma, to differentiate free, personal choice from an ambition coloured by muddled and unhelpful experiences in a boy's or girl's life so far and family background. It is decided that (a) she has a depressive disorder, for which she readily accepts antidepressant medication, and (b) she and her parents should be helped to talk about *how* she is going to make her own mind up about having an operation and why becoming lesbian is regarded as shameful. Some things she is unwilling to discuss with her parents, and vice versa, so the co-workers seeing the girl and parents together hold separate sessions for them too. As her depression changes from illness into normal worry and unhappiness, she sees the operation as a premature and inappropriate way of dealing with her problems. She does not want to be a man; she wants to be a happy lesbian; and she is not even sure about that. The focus of the problem (it has now ceased to be disorder) is now clearer; first, she has mixed feelings about her sexual interests and feelings, which means she is bisexual, not homosexual; second, the only hurry is the rush to resolve painful family conflicts, and the fear of never being able to assert her own individuality without causing damage to a vulnerable family (and marriage) emerges as the sharpest issue. She is helped to see that she has no special responsibility to hold her parents' marriage together, that while marital matters are painful her parents are stronger than she thought, that in any case she is now quite right to contemplate independence and the pain of separation on both sides is one of those things to be born, and that learning to bear it will help avoiding a precipitate rush into independence.

The process of finding out what other people really think helps her get her sexual guilt into perspective too, and she feels free to think more clearly about her sexuality. The dilemma she is left with is a social as much as a personal issue: homosexuality is stigmatized and growing up to be homosexual will be a challenge. But she remains uncertain about he sexual feelings, and how much the choice of a homosexual orientation represented for her a depressive choice approaching martyrdom. By this time she is 17, accepts individual psychotherapy to help her with her own autonomy as the focus, and is put in touch with an independent sexual counselling service, unconnected with clinics, for her to use when she wants. Should she grow from a muddled, bisexual adolescent into a troubled homosexual young woman, she should be put in touch with a responsible self-help organization; information about any sort of self-help organization, which is really helpful as opposed to indocrinating, should be kept in an up-to-date resource file. This applies to any problem and not just sexual troubles.

It is most important for the clinician to keep his head over any matter for which there is fashionable pressure in one direction or another, particularly in connection with 'permissiveness', and clinical discussion can readily be drawn towards the moral and political convictions of members of the team, something which can cause great anxiety and inhibition among people who have become quite relaxed about such topics as sex and death. The clinician's duty is to his or her patient, and helping the young person work out what he or she wants; a crusading zeal towards one of the 'liberation movements' on the part of the professional working with adolescents is as inappropriate as a preoccupation with keeping the peace; these rebellious *versus* conservative instincts are for the most part the crises of early middle age rather than childhood.

Green (1977) has helpfully reviewed problems of psychosexual development in younger children, and points out that while atypical gender role behaviour in boyhood correlates positively with atypical sexual behaviour in adults, what happens to adolescent experimentation with sexual role and preference is less clear. It does seem that most early adolescent homosexual genital experience does not endure as a homosexual style of life. On the other hand the outcome of fetishistic cross-dressing in adolescence is not known.

The overall picture at present is that while gender identity and gender role are learned and become apparent in early childhood (Stoller, 1968, 1975; Money and Erhardt, 1972), sexual orientation, which is more a development of adolescence, is less well documented and understood, particularly in boys (Green, 1975; Jones, 1981).

The sexual abuse of children and adolescents is an area full of uncertainty and contradictory findings. The incidence of reported rape, incest, and other sexual experience between adults and children is rising, but whether the incidence or the rate of reporting is rising, the contribution some children may make to seduction, the effect of different sorts of sexual experience, and the effect of the response of other adults to the fact of the experience, are all open to much speculation (Mrazek, 1980, Pomeroy *et al.*, 1981). Among the children and adolescents who come to psychiatric attention, family and social disruption is common, the young people tend to be unhappy in general if not always about the sexual experiences, and premature self-reliance and pseudo-maturity are common in some (the 'street wise' child) and helplessness, passivity, and compliance common in others. Muddled feelings and behaviour about sex, aggression, and affection are common and staff looking after such children in residential settings need support and advice about how to respond to a child who needs adult affection and physical contact but who is also (or seems) sexually seductive. This problem is not difficult if it is brought into the open and made the subject of staff teaching and consultation.

NOTES ON MANAGEMENT

The very disparate group discussed in this chapter represent a large proportion of adolescents seen by psychiatrists. The problems presented are widespread and a proportion can be grossly handicapping, and through example, neglect or in other ways lead to similar problems in other family members, contemporaries, and future generations. Through suicide, accidents, and homicide this category of problems causes more deaths than, for example, anorexia nervosa or depressive illness. Nonetheless every sub-category, including attempted suicide, delinquency, and drug abuse, includes a substantial number of adolescents with no discernible psychiatric disorder, and differentiating which boys and girls need psychiatric help is difficult, philosophically, diagnostically, or by looking at the outcome of psychiatric intervention.

In this broad group more than any other, the approach taken by the clinician must be an adaptable one. His special priority is to identify psychiatric or neuropsychiatric disorder, and particularly disorder for which treatment exists. In parallel he must help to mobilize those other things which the conduct disordered or emotionally disturbed child must have whether clinical treatment is relevant or not. These include proper care and upbringing, with its balance of affection, interest, stimulation, responsiveness, and limit setting, against a reasonable material background; the most suitable education for that boy or girl, including attention to special difficulties; the opportunities of a normal social life, including hobbies and fun; and a job, if not a career. It is difficult and sometimes impossible to provide such things and sustain them, but such normal expectations for the boy or girl, including the expectations of reasonable behaviour and the law, are usually at least as good a guide to management as an understanding of individual and family psychodynamics. Often the clinician must use his medical authority to say precisely this, that whatever treatment is hypothetically indicated, proper caring, schooling and upbringing must have priority, first because they are essential anyway and cannot be replaced by psychiatry, and second because treatment is relatively impotent without this sort of foundation. It is no less than an exercise in the psychiatric equivalent of public health, with the physician pressing for proper nutrition, clean water and good drains rather than antibiotics, vitamin pills, and isolation hospitals. One way of doing this is by the normal means of professional and public education; but in the individual case of each child the responsible adults (parents, social workers, teachers, education officers) must be identified, reminded of their responsibilities if necessary, encouraged in them, and helped to work together on these common-sense tasks. Often it will be said that all this has been tried; equally often it must be simply tried again, with more attention to detail, including the detail of modest areas of progress, and with some means built in (which may be consultative or psychotherapeutic) of coping with the irrational feelings of helplessness and anger that naughty adolescents provoke in adults.

Chapter 11

Anorexia Nervosa, Obesity, and other Disorders of Eating

ANOREXIA NERVOSA

Phthisis, the old term for tuberculosis, means wasting, becoming emaciated, and long before anything was known about the tubercle bacillus phthisis was attributed to 'Grief, Fear, Cares, too much Thinking, and other such-like Passions of the Mind' (Morton, 1689). One form of phthisis was known variously as latent tubercle, nervous consumption, apepsia hysterica, anorexia hysterica, or anorexia nervosa, and was described as the latter by Gull in a lecture given in Oxford in 1868 (Gull, 1874). The descriptions he gave would be familiar to clinicians today.

In adolescence, it is usually anxious parents who bring their child's problems to the attention of the doctor.

The immediate and striking clinical feature is usually emaciation. The anorectic is not just a thinnish person, small boned but fully formed; she is skeletal in appearance and with a marked absence of subcutaneous fat. She may weigh as little as four to five stones (56–70 lb; 25–32 kg) . . . she may wear clothes of a kind which effectively mask much of her bodily appearance but her face is likely to look gaunt, though it may rarely by puffy if she has recently overeaten. Swelling of the ankles if present is a more chronic feature and is almost always an indicator of severe starvation associated with low protein levels and severe electrolyte disturbance in the tissues. These latter disturbances are features of current, chronic and often secretive vomiting and/or excessive purging. The anorectic's extremities are usually cold and often red or blue in colour. Chilblains are not uncommon. The pulse rate is slow (but eating can produce tachycardia) and the hands and feet cold. There may be a growth of fine downy hair over the face and back (Crisp 1980).

Crisps's most valuable account of this condition, which he summarizes as 'a

207

distorted biological solution to an existential problem for an adolescent and her (or occasionally his) family' begins with historical evidence for the frequency of fasting and for that matter overeating as an historical tradition whether in the Carnival (which literally means farewell to flesh) or in self-starvation being used as an act of anger, protest, or revenge.

The key feature of anorexia nervosa is not primarily a revulsion for food but a fear or revulsion of size and weight, and the overriding goal of the anorexic patient appears to be to gain control over her weight and reduce it at all costs. There is also amenorrhoea and anxiety about developing physically and sexually.

Incidence

Anorexia nervosa occurs primarily in young women and older adolescent girls, the average age of onset being around 17–18 years, but as is well known it occurs in boys and young men too (Falstein et al., 1956; Hay and Leonard, 1979) the female : male ratio being about 10 : 1, and several cases have been reported in prepubertal children (Lesser et al., 1960; Blitzer et al., 1961; Warren, 1968; Minuchin et al., 1980). Among adolescents, the condition appears related to membership of higher socioeconomic groups, and although it is known throughout the world, including the Muslim world and Eastern Europe (Crisp, 1980) it is particularly widely reported in European, Australasian, and North American cultures, and seems related to social circumstances where the availability of food is not a cultural problem. It appears to be increasing in Britain, especially in the southern part of the country, and is more common in private schools than in the state educational system. Thus Crisp found severe anorexia nervosa in 1 in 200 girls (1 in 100 among those aged 16–18 in independent schools compared with 1 in 300 in the state system) (Crisp et al., 1976; Crisp, 1980). Crisp considered that the condition was likely to be even more common than this because of the stringent limits set on the inclusion of cases.

Course

The beginning of anorexia nervosa is characterized by a feeling of being fat and an urge to reduce it; the girl or boy then begins selectively to avoid carbohydrates, although protein may be eaten readily and this, plus gorging followed by secret vomiting, may mislead other family members into believing that a full diet is being taken. The patient regards control of times and content of meals as important and accordingly becomes interested in the household's cooking and meal-planning arrangements, and characteristically is in a good and even euphoric mood while her plans run smoothly, becoming very angry and anxious if there is any attempt at interference. Rapid weight loss and the cessation of menstruation occurs early. Anorexia, since it means loss of appetite is a misleading term; patients are often hungry and indeed preoccupied with food, which adds to the fear of loss of control. In general, weight continues to fall but there may be periods of plateau. Vomiting may be accompanied by massive self-purgation and the metabolic consequences, including the loss of potassium, can lead to cardiac arrhythmia or arrest. Acute gastric dilation, epilepsy and, ultimately, gross emaciation may result, and the metabolic imbalance may be complicated by large quantities of water if the patient uses this as a means of producing a transient weight gain to deflect suspicious clinicians. About 5 or 6 people in 100 with the condition die of suicide or severe inanition. The disorder may last for years, and in the chronic disorder the young woman seems able to maintain her body weight at a level (around 35–38 kg) a few kilograms below that at which menstruation usually begins (46–47 kg). According to Crisp (1980), while the statistics of outcome without treatment are hard to establish, probably 40% recover to some extent after a few years but with persisting social and psychological problems. Amenorrhoea persists until normal weight is regained, and may even then be delayed by several months. Wakeling *et al.* (1977) have suggested prescribing clomiphene to cut short a long delay.

Aetiology

There are many different views on the cause of anorexia nervosa but since the disorder has so many individual psychological, family, social, and physical consequences, all interacting with each other, it is difficult to discover in which system the vicious spirals start. Minuchin's and his colleagues systems model (1980) of family function (page 120) could be accurate yet this still allows for some adolescents' problems to begin in the family, some with individual vulnerability, and both aspects of the system are not incompatible with the various psychological, social, and physiological mechanisms that have been postulated.

Bruch (1974, 1978) sees the disorder largely in individual psychological terms, as an attempt to gain personal effectiveness and autonomy through the control of weight, coupled with disturbed perception of body feelings (such as hunger) and body image (size and shape), both of which are consistent with the findings that anorexic patients perceive themselves as fatter than they are (Slade and Russell, 1973) and misinterpret hunger pains (Silverstone and Russell, 1967). A number of studies have suggested a primary disorder of hypothalamic functioning. Once normal weight is regained by a successfully treated anorexic patient not all of the physiological abnormalities are corrected, which suggests that they may not necessarily be secondary to self-starvation or weight loss, although it remains possible that the latter could selectively damage some hypothalamic functions and not others. This aspect of the physiology of anorexia nervosa has been helpfully reviewed by Russell (1977a). The explanatory model used by Minuchin and his colleagues has already been mentioned: they suggest that anorexia nervosa (and conditions like asthma and disbetes mellitus too) may be considered primarily or secondarily psychosomatic. In the former, a physiological abnormality is already present; in the latter emotional conflicts are expressed somatically. In either case four patterns of family organization were noticed, which in combination (but not alone) were able to cause or expose psychosomatic vulnerability. These were: *enmeshment* (intense mutual involvement with poor boundaries and unclear individuality and individual roles); *overprotectiveness*, with 'nurturing and protective responses constantly elicited and supplied'; *rigidity*, with heavy family commitment to avoiding change, including the changes in the whole family which are part of one member negotiating adolescence; and *lack of conflict resolution*: possible conflicts are avoided by physical and verbal detours, issues diffused, and disagreement treated as threatening.

Crisp, while reminding us that like other disorders anorexia nervosa both blends with normal variation and can present in atypical forms (some of which may be depressive; see page 213) sees phobia of normal weight as central (Crisp, 1974) and rooted in anxiety about being carried forward with biological maturity, and hence may be seen as a state of psychobiological regression. This may be the 'final common path': an imperative desire not merely to stop the clock, but to turn it back to achieve a safety margin. The physiological vulnerabilities and the psychological processes which make growing up frightening may presumably vary considerably; Crisp describes them in terms of the social maturational crisis that precedes the phobic illness. The crisis is no longer a psychic reality by the time the disorder is established because it has achieved its purpose of reversing the pubertal process. The anorexic adolescent is no longer anxious or distressed about anything except adult efforts to make her proceed with growth once more. Part of the clinical presentation is a relatively good mood; this, and the restless overactivity that results from starvation, helps perpetuate the *status quo*. The clinician's task is to bring about the very changes that the anorexic adolescent has invested time, effort, energy, and a formidable range of social skills into avoiding.

Management

Most treatment systems have in common a firm and structured programme of weight gain which assumes that psychological problems cannot be tackled until weight loss has been corrected, and a good deal of sympathy and support in everything except the wish to avoid this (Russell, 1977b; Kalucy, 1978; Dally *et al.*, 1979; Dally, 1981). Most treatment programmes emphasize the importance of involving parents or family; recent studies have suggested that family therapy may be remarkably effective, at least in some cases (Selvini-Palazzoli, M, 1974; Minuchin *et al.*, 1980) although the nature of the type of problems treated and the outcome make comparison with other approaches, so far, difficult.

At Bethlem our strategy can be broadly outlined as follows:

1. *Establishing the diagnosis*, following Crisp's (1980) advice to make the diagnosis in terms of overt physical and behavioural characteristics, in terms of the patient's central fear (of weight gain), and in terms of a formulation of the individual and family psychodynamics which uniquely lead this person to behave in this way. To this we add physical assessment, particularly of current height, weight, nutritional state, and in particular hydration and electrolyte balance.

2. *Out-patient family therapy* if it is physically safe to do so, which depends as much on the feasibility of close out-patient supervision as on the patient's state and family willingness to cooperate. A strategy currently being studied is the use of family therapy backed up by admission to a hospital unit if necessary and at the family therapist's request.

3. *Admission*, with family therapy if possible, if out-patient work is impracticable. Regardless of the possible family dynamics in the aetiology of the condition, it is assumed that if the boy or girl is to be safely discharged in due course both parents, and if at all possible the whole family, should be involved in the treatment programme. As discussed on page 275 clarification of authority to treat is crucial. In a boy or girl of 16 or over, the agreement must be his/her own and a contract made with the clinical team. Crisp (1980) has discussed how the patient's cooperation can usually be gained but affirms that, rarely, compulsory detention and treatment under the Mental Health Act 1959 may be needed, for example if the patient is in serious physical danger and unaware of the seriousness of his/her condition, or if he or she is suicidal. Crisp stresses also how this can only help temporarily; voluntary participation in treatment is the necessary goal at the earliest opportunity.

   For a boy or girl under 16 parental authority to treat is sufficient; but it must be adequately expressed, and backed up by parental action. From time to time the situation arises where parents agree to hospital treatment when the child is *in extremis* and allow themselves to be manipulated by the adolescent into abandoning treatment as soon as the danger is past. Repeated attempts at treatment, sometimes in a series of different clinics and units, become the pattern, with the boy's or girl's problems becoming perpetuated. The adolescent and parents should be confronted firmly but with understanding if this pattern is beginning, and the facts made clear that the disorder has a morbidity and mortality rate, and is usually effectively treated if clinical team and parents work together consistently. If an adolescent under 16 is at serious physical risk, because treatment is undermined by parental ambivalence or opposition, seeking a Care Order may be more appropriate than invoking the Mental Health Act. It may seem a drastic move to contemplate, but the boy's or girl's life, health and development is threatened, and the matter can be decided in open court, with proper legal processes observed.

4. *On admission*, a normal (50th percentile) weight gain chart is constructed for

the young person's age, height and build and he or she is put to bed. All nurses not familiar with anorexic adolescents' ploys of manipulating their weight (heavy objects in pockets; drinking vast quantities of water, then vomiting; exercising; hiding food) are taught (a) what to look out for, and (b) what manipulative diversionary behaviour to be prepared for. The boy or girl is allowed some choice of food, and meets the dietician to discuss the options, but the calorific value of the diet and its nutritional balance is not negotiable. The patient is reassured that the staff's control of his or her weight includes making sure that he or she does not become overweight and that he or she is wrong in the belief that he or she is overweight already. On the contrary, the authority of the doctors and nurses in matters to do with what constitutes a normal, healthy weight chart is not for discussion. Meals are closely supervised, an experienced nurse sitting with the boy or girl and persuading him or her to eat all he or she is given. Massive meals are not given; it may be physically impossible for a chronic anorexic patient to eat large amounts at a time because the stomach and small bowel may be wasted and underfunctioning. The expected rate of weight gain is usually somewhat less than that planned for adult patients because a return to a normal developmental trajectory rather than a single 'target weight' is the aim. Usually a 3,000 calorie diet with the aim of achieving a weight gain of about $1\frac{1}{2}$ kg a week is prescribed, and as weight gain proceeds along a prearranged curve towards the norm, prearranged (and agreed) privileges are allowed, for example being allowed out of his or her room, and joining in activities. Two further points: first, the object of the exercise is to return the adolescent to normal health. Of course honesty and consistency are required but if for unforeseen reasons plans (for example calorie intake) have to be modified the clinician explains this firmly to the adolescent, and does not negotiate about it. Second, adolescents are naturally active and energetic, and many anorexic adolescents are bright, ambitious young people. Once the danger period is passed, there is no objection to their being normally active, joining in the fun and games and hobbies expected of healthy young people *but* they must eat enough to take part in such activities while maintaining normal growth.

5. *Transfer of authority*. Throughout admission, parental authority has been used to back up medical authority, and medical authority has been used to diagnose an unhealthy, unacceptable state and prescribe treatment (c.f. discussion on page 277). Also throughout admission, regular meetings with the whole family if possible or at least child and parents have been held too, to explain treatment, discuss progress and begin to plan for the time when the parents will take over the adolescent's feeding. They will have many mixed feelings of anxiety, guilt, a sense of failure, ambivalence about accepting professional help, distress about sanctioning the firm line that has been taken. When the boy or girl is physically out of danger and at a normal weight discharge begins to be discussed. The clinical team member seeing the family

reminds them of the serious social and educational handicap of a relapsing state and repeated admissions to hospital, and explains that the next step is for the adolescent and family to be able to maintain the normal rate of weight gain *without* nursing pressure and persuasion and the use of operant methods. As progress is made, in individual and family change as well as in weight maintenance, the adolescent's new capacity is tested by weekends at home and, all going well, the family are asked to decide in a responsible way (that is not taking chances about relapses) when the discharge date should be. During this process it is decided whether individual psychotherapy should be offered too, in addition to family therapy.

Medication is not usually needed. High levels of excitement and anxiety should be managed by a firm, supportive, confident approach by staff; but if this is insufficient chlorpromazine, initially in small doses, may be prescribed. However, it may produce spurious weight gains and should be avoided if possible. Depression, too, is best helped by social and psychological means, but if severe and not amenable to such approaches, tricyclic antidepressants may help.

With so many possible dynamic formulations of the adolescent's individual feelings and the family's interaction the nature of the psychotherapeutic work cannot be summarized here. Some common themes, however, can be stated. In the adolescent common feelings are of repulsion towards bodily growth; fear of loss of control; fear of loss of identity and autonomy; fear of sexuality and sexual relationships; and adulthood not seeming an attractive prospect. I do not believe psychodynamic interpretations of such feelings and fantasies are helpful, but (as discussed on page 289) the therapist can use these insights to inform and modify the types of conversations he has with the patient. In the family, fears of asserting parental control, fears of the consequences of the child growing up including changes in the family's balance, fears of the emergence of the adolescent's sexuality and its effect on siblings and parents are common. Fear of change in general is characteristic; in child and family there often seems to be a heartfelt wish for things to somehow be 'better' while staying the same.

Outcome

Anorexia nervosa is a disorder which includes both the most severe and intractable and the marginally normal. The statistics of outcome of treatment depend on the severity of the problems in the individual case, and in that clinic. Experience is important; a skilled and experienced clinical team is in a better position to manage the many diversions involved in this condition. About 40% of severely ill anorectic patients will make at least a partial recovery after six years. Overall, two-thirds can be expected to be much better but, though few die, dietary, emotional, and social problems become chronic and recurrent in many.

BULIMIA NERVOSA

Self-induced vomiting, as well as being common in anorexia nervosa, has recently been described as a syndrome in its own right (Russell, 1979; Fairburn, 1980; Pyle *et al.*, 1981; Fairburn and Cooper, 1982). It is characterized by a powerful and intractable urge to overeat accompanied by a morbid fear of becoming fat, a dilemma coped with by resort to vomiting and the abuse of purgatives. Fairburn and Cooper (1982) through their survey conducted in a women's magazine concluded that the condition is not uncommon, is accompanied by significant psychiatric morbidity, and appears to be largely unknown to doctors. About one woman in five in the survey was aged between 15 and 19, and none was younger. Whatever their age, at the time of the survey, most had begun binge-eating in their late teens, with vomiting tending to occur a mean of one year later. Menstrual problems, including irregularity and amenorrhoea, were common. Its relationship with anorexia nervosa is uncertain and its prevalence unknown at present. Like all psychiatric disorders it has had its place in normal behaviour too, as in the Roman *vomitorium* where in the excessive amounts of ingested food were ejected, and in the supposed habit of city aldermen attending banquets who could relieve themselves by stimulating the auricular branch of the vagal nerve for the same purpose (the 'alderman's nerve').

OBESITY

Self-esteem and attracting the admiration of parents and peers are important and the fat child is often a figure of fun. Obesity has sometimes been admired, representing fertility, abundance, and success while the Spartans examined children monthly and made the overweight take exercise. The current fashion at least in the West is to see slimness as the ideal for children, particularly in the upper socioeconomic classes (Howard *et al.*, 1971; Stunkard *et al.*, 1972), and some studies have demonstrated that both adults and children tend to consider disabled children as more likeable than obese children and the latter as having themselves to blame for their physical state (see Goodman *et al.*, 1963; Maddos *et al.*, 1968; Chisholm, 1978). According to Canning and Mayer (1966, 1967) and Bray (1976) obese young people and adults are sometimes discriminated against educationally and in finding employment, while it has also been shown that obese adolescent girls show attitudes similar to those of racial minorities (Monello and Mayer, 1963), tending to be passive, isolated, and easily hurt.

Chisholm (1978) describes a range of possible causes of obesity, including disturbance of perception and body image, overeating as a means of gratification and anxiety reduction, and much of it is also influenced by genetic inheritance (British Medical Journal, 1975) and family patterns of feeding. It is important to determine why obesity is a problem and who perceives it to be so, if a boy or girl is referred as overweight, especially since from the point of view of general health there is little evidence that any but the most extreme obesity is a serious matter (see Brook, 1980). Often the focus of work will be: (a) to make sure that no serious psychiatric or physical disorder is the cause of obesity or the wish to slim; and (b) how decisions are reached by adolescent and family (in this case concerning slimness) and acted upon. Such factors apart, diet of about 1,200 calories is prescribed to return the weight to normal. It is important not to add to the young person's problems by undermining self-esteem and confidence when weight loss proves hard to achieve (Bruch, 1971, 1974; Chisholm, 1978). For a particular boy or girl individual, group or family work may emerge as the most helpful setting in which to get the balance right between firm expectations and support.

PICA

Pica, which is the Latin for magpie, is the ingestion of inedible objects. It is found particularly among children of low intelligence, but may occur at any intellectual level. Some blind children tend to identify and familiarize themselves with objects by mouthing them. Occasionally pica leads to intoxication, particularly with lead, and hairballs in the stomach. Pica requires supervision, discouragement, and help with alternative sources of stimulation (see Bicknell, 1975).

A NOTE ON THE 'TOTAL ALLERGY SYNDROME'

Recently quite considerable newspaper and television attention has been given to a condition occurring in young women who have become supposedly allergic to an extraordinarily wide range of materials, including food and water but also plastic, paper, and ordinary everyday materials, and as a result have become extremely emaciated, grossly handicapped or both. The condition causes considerable distress and anxiety and like many allergies defies treatment. However, doubt has been expressed about its truly allergic nature, and with its severly disabling effect and the possibility of psychological contagion in mind, it is worth noting suggestions that at least some forms may be psychogenic, and that the syndrome could be adopted as a variant of anorexia nervosa (Lum, 1982; Crisp, 1982, personal communication), possibly accompanied by recurrent hyperventilation.

Chapter 12

Enuresis, Encopresis, and Tics

ENURESIS

Bladder control is acquired as normal development proceeds; at age 7, about 20% of boys and 15% of girls wet their beds at night at least occasionally, and by age 14 the respective figures are about 3% and 2%. (Rutter *et al.*, 1970, 1973). In adolescence, therefore, dry nights are the normal expectation, and the persistence or reappearance of wet sheets is a cause of considerable distress and social disability.

Aetiology

The cause of enuresis in any boy's or girl's case is likely to be the outcome of a balance between three processes: the maturation of the physiology of bladder control; the effect of training; and the effects of the young person's emotional state, which may be mildly, normally and temporarily disturbed or represent a persisting emotional problem (see review by Werry, 1979b).

The following factors are associated with enuresis: a strong genetic component (higher incidence in relatives and greater concordance in monozygotic than dizygotic twins); upbringing in an institution or a large family: socioeconomic classes 4 and 5; male preponderance, and a tendency for the intellectual level to be below average; a history of stressful events in early childhood; a relatively small bladder capacity; the presence of urinary tract infection, particularly in girls; and for a minority, the presence of psychiatric disorder, with stronger association between enuresis and emotional or behavioural disturbance in girls than in boys.

Bed-wetting may present as a persisting or recurrent problem in an adolescent who has never been dry at night (primary enuresis) or as a new problem (secondary enuresis); some children, especially those from chaotic families and

216

with relatively low intelligence and poor social skills wet by day, and if so usually wet by night as well. In such cases the general social problems will be evident. In young people who do not have these general disadvantages, particularly when bed-wetting presents and recurs or persists in an adolescent who has previously been dry at night, there is a tendency to assume that there is emotional stress or an emotional disorder behind it. However, the disadvantages of delving into an individual or family's psychopathology to seek the supposed cause are considerable.

It is reasonable to assume that: (a) different people have different physiological susceptibilities and that minor, normal stresses (intrapsychic or external) may interfere with acquired developmental skills; and (b) in many cases both the bed-wetting and the emotional disorder that goes with it may be as readily helped by reinforcing bladder training as by embarking on some form of psychotherapy.

Treatment methods

There is no evidence for psychotherapy being helpful in enuresis (see Werry and Cohrssen, 1965) although if there is definite evidence for emotional disturbance coexisting with enuresis (and not apparently caused by it) it should be considered. In such cases my own view is that attention to the young person's self-esteem, autonomy, and mood is likely to be more helpful than working on supposed psychodynamic interpretations of the nocturnal activity.

Many drugs have been tried. Pituitary snuff for its anti-diuretic effect, amphetamine for lightening sleep, and the tricyclic antidepressants (see also page 334). The latter seem helpful but only for the period during which they are given. The beneficial effect seems due neither to sleep lightening nor antidepressant action, but to local and central bladder control mechanisms.

Imipramine, amitriptyline and nortriptyline are equally useful (Blackwell and Currah, 1973). Shaffer recommends a single dose of either 35 mg or 50 mg imipramine in mid-afternoon or evening for older children (those weighing over 30 kg), avoiding higher dose levels which may actually reduce the drug's effectiveness (Maxwell and Seldrup, 1971). This will reduce wetting frequency in 85% of bed-wetters and suppress it completely in 30%, the maximal effect occurring within a week of starting treatment, that is before any anticipated antidepressant effect (see Shaffer et al., 1968; Shaffer, 1977a). It is important that parents and adolescents know of the effectiveness of the drug, particularly if it is given for a brief period to cover a social occasion such as a holiday; in which context it is worth noting that many enuretic children drop the habit when sleeping in unfamiliar surroundings.

Conditioning by bell-and-pad ('buzzer method') in which the passage of urine on to a pad completes a circuit and sounds an alarm, is an extremely effective cure for bed-wetting in 60 to 100% of cases (Kolvin et al., 1972). Various permutations have been put forward as to how it works, the consensus appearing to be that waking becomes a conditioned response to the bladder being in that state at which urine is about to be passed. Often, however, a boy or girl will be presented with the story of the bell-and-pad having failed. One history of three months' apparent failure of this method turned out, in fact, to have been an example of incompletely explained (and understood) instructions, somewhat casual and intermittent efforts with the equipment, battery failure and too quiet a 'buzz' to wake the child on most occasions; careful history-taking revealed that the treatment had actually been carried out as intended, at best, on seven or eight nights spread over three months. This is not atypical, and in addition parents and child may have mixed motives about bothering to use the method.

Other methods, including fluid restriction at night, and waking during the night to go to the lavatory, generally seem ineffective, but Shaffer (1977a) points out that an alternative possibility is that they are effective methods which therefore do not result in clinical referral, psychiatrists seeing the minority in whom such methods fail.

Treatment plan

1. *In assessment*, ensure that there are no symptoms or signs of urinary infection or neurological abnormality, and obtain as detailed a story as possible of the conditions under which bed-wetting has occurred or improved, including attempts at treatment. At the same time a picture of the organization and capacities of the household will emerge; poverty, overcrowding, shared beds and bedrooms, lack of laundering and drying facilities, and angry, punitive or mocking attitudes from other members of the family, or the subject being a great source of embarrassment (perhaps because of its history in a parent), all raise tension and on general principles may be assumed to undermine bladder control.
2. *Start a progress chart*, preferably one that will be completed for a period before treatment begins.
3. *Explain the nature of the disorder*. It is widely believed to be evidence of weakness, nervousness or being neurotic and is a source of shame. A careful balance has to be achieved between explaining the facts (that is that its relationship with psychiatric disorder is in most cases tenuous) while not being falsely reassuring; the adolescent's shame and distress and the family's reaction are facts too.
4. Use *medication* (imipramine) if temporary relief is an urgent need but teach the use of the bell-and-pad and explain the need for using it properly and persisting.
5. Use failure to use the equipment properly as a focus for family work, involving those members of the family who are involved in the problem and its treatment, normally the adolescent affected and his or her parents.

ENCOPRESIS

Encopresis, or faecal soiling is unusual in adolescence, and the few cases I have seen in this age group were boys whose problems had proved intractable in earlier childhood. The term is best regarded as a generally descriptive one, and means lack of bowel control in the absence of physical abnormality or disease. Bellman's study (1966) of nearly 9,000 Swedish children showed a steady decline of encopresis with age. Age 8 years the prevalence was 2.3% in boys and 0.7% in girls and it reached practically zero at 16. In the Isle of Wight (Rutter *et al.*, 1970) the equivalent figures for children aged 10–12 were 1.3% and 0.3%. Nearly all children are continent of faeces by age 4; most authorities set the age limit after which faecal incontinence is considered abnormal at 2 years. All studies confirm the higher rate for boys at all ages (Berg and Jones, 1964; Bellman 1966) and there is a significant association with enuresis (Stein and Susser, 1967; Rutter *et al.*, 1970).

The evidence for an association with psychiatric disorder, developmental problems, intellectual and educational difficulties, and other problematic behaviour is unclear. Probably encopretic children have more of a variety of family and individual problems, but the nature of the evidence so far is that it is not possible to say how far this is secondary to the encopresis itself. (See reviews by Hersov, 1977b and Werry, 1979b).

Part of the uncertainty in the literature is due to the varying definition of the disorder. It has been used to describe constipation with overflow (which can be an effect of tricyclic antidepressants or due to a painful anal fissure), defaecating in inappropriate places due to lack of training or in order to make a point, usually interpreted as anger; or as a result of anxiety-laden, coercive toilet training which breaks down under stress (Anthony, 1957).

A blocked bowel can lead to overflow of liquid faeces, whatever the cause. Physical examination will reveal this, and a microenema, containing sodium alkylsulphoacetate (Micralax) followed by regular bowel training and the prescription of mild laxatives (Senokot) and a stool softener such as lactulose (Duphalac) is suggested by Hersov (1977b); together with the involvement of parents in the retraining programme. Operant methods, that is systematic rewards for depositing faeces in the right place, help. In immature adolescents of low intelligence from chaotic, multiple-deprived backgrounds, this close attention to very basic toileting can result in overdependence on the detailed care involved, and may perpetuate the problem. It is important to provide in parallel with bowel retraining other forms of interest, care, and attention.

TICS

Tics are quick, sudden, repetitive, apparently purposeless coordinated movements of small groups of muscles, usually of the face, head and neck, and occurring in descending order of frequency from head to feet (Wilder and Silberman, 1927; Corbett *et al.*, 1969; Corbett, 1971) in a motor pattern. Corbett (1977b) describes the movement as very similar to that seen in the startle reflex, a flexion reflex which appears in infants at four or five months in response to sudden loud noises. Tics usually begin in younger children; it is unusual for them to appear for the first time in adolescence or adult life. Usually they are transient, recovering without treatment, frequencies of the order of 5–10% at about age six to seven being reported (Pringle *et al.*, 1967), with most studies giving a male : female ratio of about 3 : 1.

Tics may persist and if they become progressively more complex and accompanied by vocal tics, that is apparently purposeless, involuntary utterances – the syndrom is known as Tourette's (or Gilles de la Tourette's) syndrome, which he reported in 1885. The content of the utterances may be barks, grunts or throat-clearing noises, and in some cases swearing (coprolalia). These are sometimes accompanied by obscene gestures (copropraxia). Persistent tics and Tourette's syndrome differ largely in the vocal accompaniment of the latter, its tendency to persist into adult life, and the frequency with which it is associated with emotional disturbance. Other aetiological and clinical character-istics are similar (Corbett, 1977b).

Tics sometimes arise out of overactivity syndromes (Eisenberg *et al.*, 1959) which possibly indicates a common temperamental vulnerability in some cases of both disorders. The status of tics as a primarily neurological disorder remains uncertain. Evidence of minimal brain dysfunction has been reported, including non-specific EEG abnormalities (Field *et al.*, 1966; Lucas *et al.*, 1967) but such findings are common among children seen in psychiatric clinics (Werry, 1979a). Involuntary movements and vocalizations occurred after the epidemic of encephalitis lethargica early in this century, and it has been suggested that disorder of neurotransmission particularly in the basal ganglia plays a part, possibly due to excess dopaminergic activity, which haloperidol (see below) may block (Shapiro *et al.*, 1978) but overall the neurological evidence remains inconclusive (Tibbets, 1981).

The evidence of a family history of tics is conflicting. Corbett *et al.* (1969) found a high incidence of parental psychiatric disturbance, particularly affective illness among mothers, rather than a family history of tics, and in this study a high incidence of emotional and conduct problems, not dissimilar to those of other children attending the hospital, was found. The main differences were an excess of gratification habits, speech disorders, encopresis, obsessional be-haviour, and hypochondrias among the children with tics; and more misbe-haviour, aggression, and depression among the others, consistent with the possibility of tics being an alternative or supplementary mode of emotional expression.

The nature of tics gives the syndrome qualities associated with delays in biological maturation: its similarity to the startle response; its frequency as a transient phenomenon in childhood; its greater frequency in boys and its association with speech disorder, encopresis and immature habits like thumb sucking.

In the child's history both long-standing family stress and, less often, acute distress apparently acting as a precipitant are found. As in so many disorders, the general formulation of individual biological vulnerability that results in a particular style of responding to family and individual arousal or distress, and then becoming perpetuated by the anxiety and other responses (for example attention) it generates, is a compelling one. It may not be the whole truth nor a sufficient explanation, but in our present state of knowledge it is reasonable to try to treat the problem physiologically, behaviourally, and psychologically.

First, the family should try to disregard the tics as far as they can. In so far as they have difficulty this may be a focus for work with family or parents. Has the child always tended to be a focus of close attention and anxiety for some reason? Why? Not infrequently there is anxiety that he may be like a relative who was disturbed in some way, and tics, like fits and other forms of dyscontrol, are often associated fearfully with emerging madness. If one or other parent feels that the other is making too much fuss, how is he or she to resolve this difference in the child's interests?

The evidence for psychotherapy being helpful is conflicting. The rule should be to respond to the adolescent's or family's need and problems by advice, reassurance, counselling or psychotherapy, but there are no grounds for believing tics to be directly responsive to this treatment. If psychotherapy results in less tension and more attention to aspects of life other than tics, and helps child and family cope with this severe social handicap, it is worth while for this reason.

Massed practice, the deliberate, voluntary repetition of the behaviour has been successful in some cases (Yates, 1958; Clarke, 1966). Operant conditioning and aversion techniques have also been tried.

Drug treatment has helped, but controlled studies are few; Werry (1979b) considers only that by Connell et al. (1967) adequate in this respect, and they found haloperidol significantly reduced tic frequency compared with diazepam and placebo. Haloperidol should be prescribed initially at 0.5 mg TDS, slowly increasing if necessary to achieve maximum benefit without troublesome side-effects (see page 333). Ophenadrine (Disipal) 50 mg TDS may be needed. Children and adolescents with tics seem particularly vulnerable to developing motor restlessness; this does not respond to antiparkinsonian drugs, and a small dose of Amytal (30 mg TDS) is worth trying if the haloperidol is significantly helping the tics (Corbett, 1977b).

The overall strategy is to try a combination of individual and family guidance and support (which may or may not become individual or family psychotherapy); various behavioural approaches, especially massed practice, with careful attention to (a) how the tic starts (thus Corbett (1977b) has observed that the eyeblink tic may act as a trigger to more complex tics) and (b) charting and working on small areas of improvement; and using haloperidol.

When improvement takes place it tends to be in late adolescence, the best outlook in the study by Corbett *et al.* (1969) being where age of onset was between six and eight years. Presentation in adolescence (or before age six) and the presence of multiple, severe tics, tend to persist into adult life. Nevertheless, in this series, followed up by Corbett and his colleagues 1–18 years after the first attendance, 40% had completely recovered, over 50% had improved, 6% were unchanged, and none had deteriorated.

Other follow-up studies have found comparable results, with at least half much improved if not tic-free. Most tics had lasted five or six years, and persisted when there was associated mental retardation, epilepsy, severe home difficulty or when parents had persistent tics too (Zausmer, 1954; Torup 1962). The syndrome can be most disabling when it persists, and understandably causes anxiety and depression, but there is no evidence for deterioration into more serious mental illness, which has occasionally been reported in the earlier literature, possibly through misunderstanding or misdiagnosis.

Chapter 13

Depressive Disorders, Affective and Schizophrenic Psychoses and Major Disorders of Personality Development

DEPRESSIVE DISORDERS

When a clinician describes an adolescent as 'depressed' he may mean any one of a number of quite different conditions. He may mean that the boy or girl is ordinarily and appropriately unhappy because of current or recent circumstances, perhaps following a loss. He may mean that the sadness is understandable but nevertheless out of proportion, a notion which has something to do with our ideas of the natural limits of sadness in length and depth and something to do with what we can expect of normal social coping mechanisms: thus a child may be diagnosed as having a depressive reaction to stress which is hardly pathological but with which parents and teachers cannot cope without help. Moving further along the spectrum towards true disorder, an adolescent may be described as depressed in a way explicable in terms of psychodynamic or family functioning; the boy or girl is maintained in a depressive state by self-reproach (Freud, 1917), by internalized anger (Abraham, 1927), by lost self-esteem (Bibring, 1953), by feelings of helplessness and the inability ever to be able to acquire a feeling of being loved and comforted (Sandler and Joffe, 1965), or by a combination of a sense of loss, a sense of lost autonomy and a sense that things cannot change for the better (Beck, 1967). In terms of family and social interaction, depression may be maintained by a failure to elicit support from others, with the result that the young person becomes increasingly unhappy and by his/her move from relatively mature to more immature attempts at care-eliciting behaviour becomes harder to respond to and more readily rejected

223

(Liberman and Raskin, 1971; Coyne, 1976 and page 108). The demonstration by Paykel *et al.* (1969) of an accumulation of life events, particularly involving different sorts of loss, in the months preceding depression in adults is of interest in the light of Coleman's notion (1980) that to maintain normal functioning and development adolescents seek to space out their life events.

These hypotheses tend to imply that depression is part of the normal human repertoire, like inflammation, and can be evoked if the necessary conditions prevail. Thus a clinician may also feel able to describe disturbed adolescents in terms of 'masked' or 'atypical' depression (Glaser, 1967), with the assumption that because of their circumstances or presumed personal or family psychodynamic state they *ought* to be depressed, even though their behaviour is, for example, that of school refusal, drug abuse or other misbehaviour.

Finally, there are many hypotheses of neurochemical and other neurophysiological dysfunction involving body water and electrolyte distribution, endocrine activity, and central neurotransmission (see review by Bhanji, 1979), consistent with the genetic influences in certain types of depression (Robins and Guze, 1972) and the undoubted value of drugs like antidepressants and lithium in certain cases. This is the depressive disorder generally regarded as 'psychotic' or 'endogenous' depression.

To add to the complexity, it is generally assumed that the absence of typical adult-type depressive symptoms in young children and their appearance in adolescence is connected with the maturational process, but whether this represents psychodynamic, social or neurochemical development, or an interaction between all three, is not known. In attempting to formulate why a particular boy or girl is (or ought to be) depressed, the clinician will usually find himself operating two conceptual sliding scales:

1. How far the disorder is understandable in psychosocial terms of stress and loss both as external realities and as inner feelings; and how far a predisposition to the neurochemical state that underlies some depressive states is involved.

2. How far the boy or girl has developed psychosocially and physiologically. Have they conceivably developed the social relationships, personal psychology, and neurochemical state to make a formulation in the above terms tenable?

The clinician cannot know the answers to these questions, but they can help to inform the clinical process of trial and error.

The 'depressive equivalents' described by Glaser (1967), Toolan (1962), and others have been summarized by Weiner (1970b) as: persistent, intolerable boredom interrupted by periods of restlessness; an exaggerated approach to, or withdrawal from, parents and friends, sometimes expressed as promiscuous sexual behaviour; fatigue, bodily preoccupation, and physical symptoms; problems in concentrating, for example on schoolwork (see page 253); and antisocial, sometimes delinquent behaviour, as preceded some of the suicides in young adolescents reported by Shaffer (1974). The risk of suicide should be judged by an adolescent's ideas and feelings, not by trying to diagnose whether or not the depressed state he or she suffers from constitutes an endogenous illness (see also page 186). The same applies to the above symptoms of 'masked' depression; there is no evidence that, in so far as they indicate a depressive state, it is primarily a depressive disorder or an affective illness.

The main value in trying to identify the 'endogenous', physiologically based depressive state is because of the frequent effectiveness of drugs in such cases. Depressive states which are relatively mild, or understandable in psychodynamic or psychosocial terms *and* responsive to psychodynamic or psychosocial methods, require management along the lines described in Chapter 10. Where symptoms are severe, particularly if they include adult-type depressive characteristics like weight loss, sleep disturbance, suicidal ideas and guilt, where they make little sense in psychodynamic terms, and where there is little apparent response to psychological or social measures, it is reasonable to try medication. This advice needs three qualifications: first, the presumed presence of a physiological component to the depressive state does not rule out the psychosocial component, nor vice versa; second, a careful clinical judgement has to be made about the psychological impact of using medication, and the by no means certain advantages weighed against the possible undermining of adolescent and family learning to cope with painful feelings in a constructive way that enhances emotional growth. The clinician cannot know for certain whether a painful therapeutic experience (painful for the therapist, too, sometimes) is necessary or not, any more than he can know for sure if medication will help. What is important is to allow room for both aspects of the formulation, and both sorts of help. Third, here and in the section which follows, I have assumed that one particular group of depressive disorders, those that are physically based and often respond to physical treatment, deserve identification as affective illness, psychotic or 'endogenous' depression, or manic depression; there is good evidence for their physical basis, but no definite biochemical basis for distinguishing each from the other. I have therefore included under the general heading of affective illness all these disorders, but their association with the term psychotic illustrates the imprecision of the term; here it refers to a supposed aetiology rather than to a particular mental state, but it is important to remember that the nature of the physical component remains obscure.

AFFECTIVE ILLNESS

The characteristics of adult-type psychotic depression are a persistent sense of sadness and despair – usually believed to be worse on waking – disturbed sleep, ideas of inadequacy, unworthiness, persecution and guilt which may become delusional, hypochondriacal ideas or delusions, ideas or plans about suicide, and sometimes auditory and visual hallucinations with a depressive content.

Tearfulness is common, there is loss of appetite and weight, and either apathy, motor retardation and withdrawal (even into stupor), or agitation and restlessness. Often there is a family history of depressive disorder. In addition, some patients have periods of manic excitement (hypomania if relatively milder) in which there is euphoria accompanied by swiftly alternating bonhomie and irritability, grandiose ideas, pressure of thought, speech and activity, flight of ideas with joking and the making of puns, and social and sexual disinhibition. The thought processes are often quite coherent if the clinician can keep up, the jumps from topic to topic seeming to be the impulse of the moment, an amusing diversion or association, rather than representing chaotic conceptualization as in the patient with schizophrenia. Anger and aggressive behaviour and bouts of profound depression, too, are never far away, often fleeting, yet quite dangerous when they occur.

Schizoaffective psychosis is the term applied by some clinicians to illnesses with the characteristics of schizophrenia (see page 229) but with a strong manic or depressive component, often with a history of affective illness in the family, and a tendency to return to a reasonably intact personality between episodes of illness, instead of the decline of process schizophrenia, where there is a steady deterioration in thinking, motivation, and social skills. The nature of this disorder and its variants has preoccupied many clinical workers, and the history of the description of these and similar schizophrenic variants is reviewed by Hamilton (1976) in his revision of Fish's well established work.

Adolescents present with adult-type manic, depressive, and schizoaffective illnesses, and some studies suggest that adolescents presenting with apparently acute schizophrenic illnesses may occasionally be suffering from manic-depressive illness, or at any rate a disorder which in due course is controlled by lithium carbonate (see page 336; and Horowitz, 1977). Frommer has been prominent in recognizing the existence of adult-type or atypical but drug-responsive depressive disorder in children and adolescents (Frommer, 1968), and a number of studies have confirmed the infrequent though unequivocal appearance of adult-type manic-depressive illness in adolescents of all ages (Wertham, 1929; Barrett, 1931; Campbell, 1952; Sands, 1956; Anthony and Scott, 1960; Perris, 1968; Winokur et al., 1969; Berg et al., 1974; Youngerman and Canino, 1978). The clinical stereotype of the manic-depressive boy or girl is outlined on page 337, and in these young people lithium for the acute manic illness and for preventing recurrences of mania or depression, and tricyclic antidepressant drugs for periods of depression should be given (see page 334 and 335). Cambell (1952) described cyclothymic symptoms in a minority of the young people he reported before the emergence of a severe illness, and also described a characteristic premorbid personality in several others, consisting of tension and sensitivity with a tendency to extraversion, anxiety for group approval and fears about the future; the earlier frank mood disorder occurred the stronger was the family history of affective illness. Strain and responsibility in adolescence seemed a prominent precipitant of the illness, and he noted that the cyclothymic children had special problems in adjusting to family life with a manic-depressive parent. In adults, Brodie and Leff have reported environmental stresses preceding the first admissions to hospital of depressive and manic-depressive patients, and suggested that further episodes seemed more randomly determined (1971). Apart from Campbell's account the relationships between environmental stresses and acute psychotic illness among adolescents have not been reported, but as a general rule family and school tensions and disruption should be dealt with as far as possible, because they may play a part in precipitating the acute illness, because proper control of the disorder (lithium) requires meticulous dosage and attention to side-effects, and because the boy or girl will have experienced considerable upheaval in any case. Mania in particular comes close to one of the lay images of madness, and the young person who has been behaving in what is usually a most uncharacteristic manner in a wild, disinhibited and foolish-seeming way can have great difficulty in re-establishing relationships and esteem among all but their closest friends; the prevention of further attacks is a very high priority, but every effort should be made to help adolescent, family, and school live and cope with further attacks, and the possibility of further attacks. If, in addition, there is an individual or family problem that may be helped by individual or family psychotherapy, it is reasonable to embark on this. A focus for work that I have found helpful is to try to establish in a few key people – parents, selected friends, and *long-term* clinical workers, that degree of trust that will enable someone to persuade the manic adolescent to accept help when he or she is beginning to feel 'high', has decided that everyone else is being a wet blanket, and stops taking medication. After a painful, acute illness, which may be exceedingly hard to control the young person will often be able to recall finally accepting that help was needed because a familiar person was around to say so; but even so the situation with an acutely manic adolescent can be decidedly brittle.

The outlook for both manic and depressive illnesses is variable. With lithium and antidepressant treatment respectively, the evidence is that lithium is effective in reducing recurrences of mania, and depressive recurrences seem less severe; correspondingly, tricyclic antidepressants (in lower doses) reduce relapses of depression (see review by Bhanji, 1979). Murphy *et al.* (1974) followed up 37 patients with depressive illness: 6 were ill throughout, 9 remained well, and the rest, just over half, had 1–9 recurrences lasting from two weeks to a year. Angst *et al.* (1973) followed up 1.000 patients with depressive and manic-depressive illnesses; the vast majority had further episodes, and each episode lasted about the same time for each patient. Recurrences numbered 7–9 for manic-depressive illness and 4–6 for depressive illness over some 20 years. However, the median age of onset of this large group was 43 for manic-depressive illness and 30 years for depressive illness, and the natural history of the disorder beginning in adolescence is not well documented. Most authorities are not specific on the question of how long lithium prophylaxis should continue. Several severe episodes which proved hard to treat would justify prescribing lithium for many years if a close eye were kept on dose, side-effects and renal and thyroid functions. On the other hand many years on a toxic drug would not be justified following a single episode in an adolescent; I would give an adolescent lithium after an unequivocal manic episode and supervise him or her on the drug throughout his or her education. If he or she remained well throughout that period, after discussion of the pros and cons of stopping medication with the adolescent (and parents, if still involved) a supervised period off medication would seem reasonable. By then, one would hope, research into the prognosis of manic-depressive illness in adolescence would have made more headway. Some studies indicate that bipolar (manic and depressive) affective illness with an onset early in adolescence has a particularly poor prognosis, with frequent episodes of illness and a high incidence of suicide (Welner et al., 1979). Certainly a large proportion of bipolar illness in adults appears to have begun in adolescence (Loranger and Levine, 1978), characteristically beginning with depression foreshadowing a first episode of mania.

In addition to the many adolescents who present with depression, those who are thought to be atypically depressed, and the very few with unequivocal manic-depressive symptoms, there remains a group of young people with episodic disorders which are not apparently related to external circumstances, and not particularly affective in symptomatology, some of whom respond to lithium treatment. The majority of accounts that report this describe recurrent behaviour problems, sometimes in mentally retarded young people, sometimes in autistic children, and occasionally in seriously aggressive young people who have simply failed to respond to all other treatments (Annell, 1969a, b; Dostal and Zvolsky, 1970; Sheard, 1975; Lena et al., 1977; Youngerman and Canino, 1978; Kymissis et al., 1979), while Stein et al. (1982) have described the prescription of lithium reducing mood swings in an anorexic girl and enabling dietary treatment which had so far failed to proceed; these authors point out the connection that some authorities have suggested between anorexia nervosa and affective disorder (Cantwell et al., 1977). It is worth considering the use of lithium in adolescents with serious episodic problems whose recurrence, after scrupulous history-taking, seems to arise primarily from within rather than from without, particularly if there is a family history of affective illness, and particularly if the clinical phenomenology gives a strong impression of fluctuations in arousal – tension, excitement, or withdrawal and apathy – even if finer distinctions about mood cannot be made. The use of lithium in such cases should always be treated like the experiment it is, with careful charting of the progress of symptoms and behaviour it is hoped to change. If the illness is not too severe, it is worth considering using a crossover trial of lithium and placebo, with parental knowledge and approval, rather than embarking on a long period of using a toxic drug unnecessarily. Probably there will be few conduct-disordered young people who will be helped by lithium, but the outlook for some versions of the later group of disorders is so bad that it is worth bearing the use of lithium in mind (Steinberg, 1980).

From time to time the question of prescribing antidepressant or mood-stabilizing drugs while an adolescent is receiving individual or family psychotherapy will arise. I do not believe the two approaches are necessarily incompatible. There should be no 'rule of thumb' about this; of course, the use of drugs can change the whole appearance of a problem, and thoroughly undermine a psychotherapist's efforts to help a child or family take responsibility for their feelings and behaviour. Equally, medication can completely relieve symptoms and disability in weeks with less in the way of side-effects than a year or two of psychotherapy produces. Antidepressive drugs help some adolescents with dramatic speed, and completely fail with many others, even when the symptoms are characteristically physiological in type. It is important for the clinician not to be drawn into an ideological battle with others (or even within himself) about whether drugs or psychotherapy are naturally right; both are most unnatural. Rather, treatment should be prescribed according to a diagnostic formulation that makes sense, and it may include psychodynamic factors, physiological factors, neither, or both. If there does seem to be a physiological component, and if troublesome and protracted symptoms make medication justified, the fact of its prescription and all that it means to patient and therapist should be a legitimate focus for some of the work; its use should not be denied.

SCHIZOPHRENIC ILLNESSES

Adolescent psychiatrists will know the young patient with the unequivocal, characteristic signs of schizophrenic illness; but also the boy or girl who defies diagnosis, who in his or her mental state is neither deluded nor thought disordered, has good interpersonal rapport, but whose behaviour is guided more by unrealistrc attitudes and fantasies than by the exigencies of real life or the expectations of other people, sometimes to disastrous effect. Often we do not know what will become of them; not enough is known to predict which adolescent will become ill, who will get by in an eccentric and perhaps disadvantaged way, and who will in due course acquire the unsatisfactory label of 'simple schizophrenia' because of an insidious and inexorable social decline, perhaps into vagrancy.

As with depression (page 223), the clinician working with adolescents is up against the dual problem of the variability of schizophrenic and schizophrenic-like disorders, and the effect of maturation. Perhaps the most important single characteristic of a schizophrenic psychosis is the delusion: a belief held with absolute conviction as a self-evident truth, usually of great personal significance, not shared by other people with the same social and cultural background, fantastic or unlikely in nature, and amenable neither to reason nor by the evidence of experience (Mullen, 1979). Immature adolescents, and many boys and girls seen by adolescent psychiatrists are immature, are often not so dogmatic; they are not sure, and their version of their perceptions and experience is coloured by childlike fears and fantasies, changes from time to time and can be variably modified depending on the person with whom they are talking. Obsessional ruminating can include very bizarre content, be acted upon, and be of considerable importance to the individual (see Hamilton, 1976). Bizarreness alone does not constitute a delusion, and in any case what is abnormal is not the belief itself but the value attached to it. Thus an obsessional, hand-washing adolescent will not *know* that there is dangerous contamination on his hands, but he may think there could be, and explain that while he can understand other people's incredulity about his precautions, he himself is not prepared to take the risk. Can the psychiatrist guarantee that it is impossible for him to come to harm from something picked up on his hands? The honest scientist cannot guarantee this, but only talk about its extreme unlikelihood (if he is so off his guard as to be drawn into this sort of discussion with an obsessional adolescent) and the conversation ends with talking about risks the psychiatrist is willing to take but the patient is not. Like the paranoid idea, which also characteristically contains a grain of truth, the obsessional idea can also have qualities of such special importance to the individual that, particularly in the young person with doubts and mixed feelings, it seems to have the potential for becoming delusional. Usually it does not (see page 183).

When schizophrenia was first described as *dementia praecox* by Kraepelin (1899) he regarded it as a disorder appearing typically in adolescence or young adulthood, a view shared by E. Bleuler (1911). Over the years, however, it became clearer that different types of schizophrenic illness develop at different times of life, for example paranoid psychosis in middle life, while Post (1966) showed that paranoid psychoses indistinguishable from schizophrenia can develop after the age of 60. Nevertheless, many forms of schizophrenia make their first appearance in adolescence (Weiner, 1958). The study of schizophrenia has been dogged by efforts to define the syndrome tightly alternating with variants of the disorder, or personality anomalies with an uncertain relationship with the disorder, creeping in (see review by Murray, 1979). The closest we have come to a widely accepted definition of schizophrenia, though with by no means all the problems of classification resolved, is by using Schneider's (1959) first rank symptoms of schizophenia, and the findings of the International Pilot Study of Schizophrenia (World Health Organization, 1973) which showed how wide a degree of agreement could be reached in the diagnosis of schizophrenia in a wide range of cultures.

The first rank symptoms of Schneider are:

1. Hearing his own thoughts spoken aloud.
2. Hallucinatory voices speaking about the patient in the third person, or as a running commentary.

3. Feelings of influence on body functions which are known by the patient to originate from outside agencies, and other passivity experiences.
4. Thought withdrawal or insertion by outside agencies and the communication of his own thoughts to others.
5. Delusional perception, that is to say the attribution of special significance, usually self-reference, to a normal perception.

The WHO pilot study showed that the most useful discriminatory symptoms were delusions of control by outside agencies; thought insertion, broadcast or withdrawal; auditory hallucinations in the third person, and non-affectively based auditory hallucinations addressing the patient. In the absence of organic (including toxic) disorder, no probability of cultural beliefs (for example religious or magical beliefs) mimicking the symptoms, and the patient is believed, the diagnosis of a schizophrenic illness is definite. There is an additional quality to the expressed feelings and behaviour of the patient with schizophrenia which is known to every clinician and hard to put into words: it is largely to do with feelings of passivity. The schizophrenic patient does not seem to feel in control of himself or of his own destiny; whatever the doubts about his delusional conviction, or whether or not he is really experiencing hallucinations, there is a definite sense of things affecting him from *without*; even if he has bad internal experiences (and some patients will agree on close questioning that their hallucinations are indeed in the 'mind's ear', so to speak, rather than heard outside in the room) there is, in many forms of schizophrenic illness, a certainty that the origin of the experiences is external and current.

These are the core symptoms of 'nuclear' schizophrenia. In addition there is often considerable distress in the form of high arousal, anxiety, or sadness. Lack of affect is often described, but is more apparent in the remote, shallow and sometimes flippant manner of the hebephrenic type of schizophrenia, where silliness, mannerisms, and irresponsibility are particularly marked. In paranoid forms of schizophrenia, more common in more mature personalities, hallucinations are less evident and systematic, stable delusions, that is conveying a particular message of persecution or specialness more prominent. It is usually to require the symptoms to be present in a state of clear consciousness; but in some acute schizophrenic episodes, particularly in adolescents, there is an apparent slight clouding of consciousness and perplexity, the oneroid state or oneirophrenia described by Meyer-Gross and by Meduna and McCulloch (see Hamilton, 1976). Another concept is of residual schizophrenia, a state of emotional blunting and lost social skills which persists after an acute illness has passed.

The general principle recommended is to diagnose schizophrenia in adolescents when the clinical presentation includes some of the above features, but particularly some of the Scheiderian first rank symptoms; whatever the aetiology of this condition, it does seem to represent a disorder which is found with reasonably high consistency in many different cultural settings, and regarded in them all as abnormal. In addition, adolescents with schizophrenic illnesses tend to show a number of characteristic patterns of behaviour such as high levels of anxiety, incoherent speech, grimacing or stereotyped movements, intense preoccupation with inner thoughts with a corresponding distancing from other people (for example by avoiding eye contact or maintaining minimal facial expression), poor emotional control with socially inappropriate outbursts of rage, poor social judgement, and a seriously declining social and academic performance (Sands, 1956; Spivack and Spotts, 1967; Weiner, 1970a).

In clinical assessment, one of the more difficult tasks is to remember that there is a great deal more to the boy or girl than a set of symptoms and signs. The clinician can all too easily share the boy's or girl's preoccupation with strange and troubling experiences and have too solemn a conversation about them. If it is at all possible to engage the adolescent on a lighter topic or on some realistic concern, for example about friends and schooling, this will not only help the young person remember that he or she is still part of the human race, but also the topic may be a more manageable focus for helping with fears and sadness, rather than trying to cope with delusions about wickedness, world destruction, and the devil. In schizophrenia, as in manic-depressive illness, I believe it important to affirm the much maligned sick role; frightened young persons having terrifying and perplexing experiences should be told by adults looking after them that they are not well, and that the care and medication they are being given is designed to help them feel better. This is perfectly consistent with setting limits on wild or mad behaviour and expecting the adolescent to begin to take some responsibility for what they do; one would (after all) do the same with a confused, delirious adult. Talk also about real issues; what is going on here and now; how it feels to have become ill in this way, to be brought into hospital, to be trying to talk to a stranger about experiences that must be hard to put into words, and the pain and difficulty of finding himself or herself away from home and among strangers it is impossible at first to trust. Assume that the adolescent will be worried about the worries of his or her family; explain that the staff know that he or she is naturally worried, and will be helping him or her. At least some discussion about what seems wrong, what sort of investigations will be needed, what sort of treatment given, and how to help with parents' worries should be undertaken by doctor, nurse, and social worker with adolescent and parents. In a confusing and frightening situation it helps for the boy or girl to see everyone talking together, rather than to have a series of fragmentary interviews in a succession of rooms. We can only guess what the experience of acute schizophrenia must be like; possibly many times worse than being lost on a foreign railway station in the early hours with one's train about to leave from an unknown platform. Acute schizophrenia is very interesting, but for the boy or girl and parents concentrate on the muddle and fright and explain carefully and clearly what is going on, and why.

If I am certain of the diagnosis I tell adolescent and parents that the disorder is one of the schizophrenic illnesses, adding that there are many different types with many different sorts of outcome, an impression they might not get if they look the term up in a book. If admission to hospital is needed, as it usually is, explain why; that the boy or girl is not well, will be helped by medication, and will need a professional eye kept on progress and medicines. If one of the reasons is strange and upsetting behaviour such as stripping off in the street, explain that whatever the boy or girl thinks about it other people will think what the adolescent does is strange, and in due course he or she would be glad that someone took a firm hand and insisted on a period of relative privacy until he or she was behaving in a way that did not seem so crazy; this can, and of course must, be put kindly, and is an appropriate approach to take. The same applies to an explanation of the use of compulsory admission to hospital; that as an adult who cares about what happens to the boy or girl you want to do all you can to stop him or her hurting himself or herself, and that, for the moment, you know best. Do not worry if you think you are talking like the psychiatrist in an old antipsychiatry film; your concern and responsibility is the patient and family, not cinema audiences and radical theoreticians.

Causes

The nature and cause of the schizophrenic illnesses are not known. There is now no doubt about the genetic predisposition; the stronger the genetic relationship between people with schizophrenia and others, the higher the risk. Thus children of parents both of whom have had schizophrenia have a 25% chance of developing it themselves, a 12% chance if one parent is affected, 2.5% for second degree relatives, and so on down to the 1–2% risk of the ordinary population (see Kety et al., 1968; Heston and Denny, 1968; Rosenthal et al., 1971; Murray, 1979). These studies, of course, include careful research into the progress of relatives brought up in completely different environments. What is transmitted, and the link between genetic influences and whatever develops physiologically or biochemically in the individual remains unknown (Shields and Gottesman, 1973).

Some recent long-term studies of special interest and importance have been attempts to identify high risk factors other than genetic ones. Children at high risk appear to be characterized by an unusual autonomic reaction to stress (marked reaction, rapid recovery, and slow habituation), disturbed cognitive associations, an excess of perinatal complications and early and stressful separation experiences (see Garmezy 1974a,b; Mednick et al., 1974; Schulsinger and Mednick, 1975), a picture consistent with the possibility that adult patients with schizophrenia are over-aroused and hypersensitive to their environment (Venables, 1968, 1978). The strongest predictor of later breakdown with schizophrenia (diagnosed by Schneider's first rank symptoms) in children at risk appears to be abnormal autonomic reactivity as measured by skin conductance response – a short recovery and high amplitude (Venables, 1980), early physiological characteristics which appear to persist (Mednick *et al.*, 1978). Schizophrenia also seems more likely to develop in socially isolated, oversensitive, odd children, although there are no more specific premorbid characteristics (Sands, 1956; Symonds and Herman, 1957; Masterson, 1967; Warren, 1965a, b; Offord and Cross, 1969).

A number of well-known theories have been put forward to suggest environmental causes of schizophrenia, although in recent years there has been more acceptance of the model of genetic predisposition and external influence interacting to cause schizophrenic disabilities. These include the double-bind or contradictory message (Bateson *et al.*, 1956); marital schism and distress with parental irrationality and reality distortion (Lidz, 1958); confusion and mystification as a means of control of the patient by the family (Laing, 1960); pseudo-mutuality (Wynne *et al.*, 1958) and other abnormal and misleading communication patterns. The studies by Wynne and Singer (see Wynne and Singer, 1963; Wynne 1968) suggested vagueness, irrelevance, lack of closure and other verbal communication defects as characterizing the parents of schizophrenic patients but not neurotics, but a particularly careful replication of this work found only that the fathers of schizophrenic patients talked more than the fathers of neurotic patients (see review by Hirsch and Leff, 1975). There is, however, good evidence for the precipitation of schizophrenic episodes by social factors (Brown and Birley, 1968; Birley and Brown, 1970), and the vulnerability of schizophrenic patients to overinvolvement with a critical relative (Brown *et al.*, 1962; Brown *et al.*, 1972), influences which can be dealt with by giving appropriate advice to families, and against which phenothiazine medication has a protective effect (Brown *et al.*, 1972).

However, the evidence for specific precursors of schizophrenia, including autonomic and attentional anomalies, remains inconclusive (see review by Steinberg, 1983).

Outcome

The best outlook is for patients (adults or adolescents) with acute onset, marked affective symptoms, the presence of confusion in the acute illness, clear-cut precipitating factors, a normal EEG, a family history of affective disorder, above average intelligence, a friendly and outgoing premorbid personality, and relatively late onset (in studies of children, onset after the age of 10 years) (Pollack, 1960; Annesley, 1961; Vaillant, 1962, 1964; Stephens *et al.*, 1967; King and Pittman, 1971).

A bad outcome tends to be associated with a strong family history of schizophrenic disorder (McCabe *et al.*, 1971), an insidious onset, low intelligence, an abnormal EEG and early onset – in children, before the age of 10.

Positive symptoms like hallucinations and delusions give little guidance on prognosis (Jansson, 1968; Strauss and Carpenter, 1972); symptoms such as lack of affect and disturbed interpersonal relationships are associated with poorer outcome.

Differential diagnosis

The biggest problems are the schizophrenic-like disorders discussed in the last section of this chapter (page 238). If there is no firm evidence of a schizophrenic illness as described above then it is less definite that medication will help, and the outlook is as for other personality disorders, that is uncertain. However, it is reasonable to use medication such as the phenothiazines or haloperidol, particularly if the adolescent is highly aroused and anxiety is distressing or disabling. As with clear-cut schizophrenia, dealing with the various social and educational handicaps and family problems remains important. Probably the more understandable the disorder, that is the more it can be formulated in psychodynamic or sociodynamic terms, the more likely a diagnosis other than schizophrenia will be made, and the more likely will psychotherapy be attempted. The relationship of 'understandability' to diagnosis, treatment and outcome, however, remains unclear.

The second question is that of the schizoaffective psychoses. If the clinical features of mania (page 226) are present, and they do not readily subside with phenothiazine medication, lithium should be tried. The more characteristically manic the illness, particularly if there have been relatively circumscribed episodes before, and if there is a strong family history of affective illness, the more should prophylactic lithium be seriously considered. The contribution of depression is a matter of clinical judgement. Acutely schizophrenic adolescents are particularly likely to be depressed too, and phenothiazines and haloperidol can cause depressive symptoms. Persisting sadness as a primary problem is hard to distinguish from the low mood which may accompany the illness or medication, and a trial of tricyclic antidepressants in addition to antipsychotic medication is worth while in such circumstances; antidepressant drugs should be prescribed with particularly careful supervision, and initially in low doses, because they can worsen the schizophrenic state, or precipitate mania if the disorder was primarily an affective one.

Intoxication with various drugs can cause psychosis and mimic schizophrenia (see below) and some organic conditions can do the same (see page 258). All adolescents with an affective or schizophrenic disorder should have a thorough physical examination and investigations for neurological disorder, however typical their symptoms.

Management

1. Of course diagnosis is important, but the priority for management is to treat the handicaps. Treatment should be guided by the diagnostic formulation: educational and social handicaps should be helped by educational and social measures; family problems by family work (which is not necessarily family therapy). Family therapy cannot be expected to cure schizophrenia, but work

with parents or, with care, with the family in order to reduce criticism, anxiety and intrusiveness or muddling communications, may be helpful.

2. Chlorpromazine, building up from small doses (50 mg TDS) to adult levels, guided by avoiding oversedation and troubling side-effects, is the most useful drug where there is overactivity and high levels of arousal; haloperidol is a good alternative, and trifluoperazine or pimozide the better drug when there is apathy or inertia. Depot preparations are more reliable and often regarded as more convenient by patients for long-term treatment. Drug therapy is discussed in more detail on page 324. Remember that new learning is always important in psychiatric treatment as part of the recovery process, education is important for all children, and it is in this context that tranquillizers such as the phenothiazines can interfere with the learning process (Eisenberg and Connors, 1971, McAndrew et al., 1972).

3. Some form of regular, individual work with the boy or girl is important; whether it is called psychotherapy rather depends on the work being undertaken and what the clinician chooses to call it. The schizophrenic adolescent needs: (a) support in a frightening illness with an uncertain outcome; (b) reminding that in some ways he or she is not well and needs to learn to trust the people looking after him or her, but he or she has his strengths and responsibilities too, like anyone else with an illness; (c) explanation about the management being undertaken, for example group work, what the drugs are for, their side-effects, how his or her parents are being given encouragement and kept informed; (d) advice about how to cope with peer relationships and how to use various therapeutic and educational sessions; (e) friendly, non-critical feedback about bizarre statements and behaviour, for example 'I didn't understand that; could you put it another way?' as a response to a chaotic, thought-disordered statement; (f) acknowledgement of the difficulty of putting muddling and bizarre experiences into words, and (g) affirmation that the psychiatrist cannot read the boy's or girl's mind and that the adolescent will want to keep some troubling thoughts private to himself or herself.

4. Normal behaviour should be expected, though not made into a great issue. Thus it is not too much to expect a newly admitted adolescent with an acute schizophrenic illness to take part in a disco, but he should be invited along even if he only sits there for a time with a nurse. Broken windows or other people's property should be paid for, and crazy behaviour kindly but firmly stopped. His or her opinions should be sought, along with that of the other boys and girls, on ward or school matters, and the unit school should be attended except in the most florid stages of illness.

5. Assuming that the boy or girl is in hospital, plans for discharge should be made from the start. How will the rest of the family cope? What help do they all need together? If, as in some chronic illnesses or persisting handicaps, where after consultation with adolescent and family it seems that the young

person will do better away from home (for example in a therapeutic community or Rudolf Steiner home), how can they be helped to make a decision, cope with separation, and retain close contact during holidays? What sort of school, work, or training should the adolescent be returned to if he or she does return home? What preparation is needed?

6. Another aspect of treatment in hospital is that it is best if the adolescent is among young people with other and less severe disorders too, and indeed can benefit from being in social skills and activity groups with them (Steinberg *et al.*, 1978).

7. Unless the psychotic illness is a transient one, long-term problems can be anticipated. For the foreseeable future, which in practical terms means the next two or three years, there may be continuing handicap, medication and its side-effects to be monitored, anxieties about schooling, social life, independence and work, and occasional relapses of illness. Before discharge from the hospital unit, as stable plans as possible should be made about supervising and supporting the adolescent, helping the family, consultation with teachers or residential workers and, later, career advisers and employers. These plans cannot be made in advance, but plans can and should be made about who will be responsible for maintaining contact and monitoring progress. The fact that an adolescent may need readmission a couple of years after he or she has outgrown a children's and adolescent's service, for example, should not be allowed to take everyone by surprise. Rather, at the appropriate time a thoughful handover of care to an adult psychiatric team with the knowledge and agreement of the family doctor, and the transfer of social work from the clinical team's worker to a local authority social worker or community psychiatric nurse should be planned.

8. Finally, progress should be carefully monitored. Symptoms, disabilities, varying responses to medication, deteriorating abilities and areas of improvement should be recognized and treatment plans changed accordingly. It is difficult to keep the impetus up over the years, but persistence and attention to detail should be the aim (see also Steinberg, 1983).

PSYCHOTIC STATES WITH A PHYSICAL CAUSE

Physical illness causing psychotic and other abnormal mental states are discussed in Chapter 15.

Intoxication by drugs or other chemical substances should always be considered in the differential diagnosis of psychotic states, and particularly in acute disorders urine and blood samples should be taken as early as possible; it is best if this is a routine arrangement in hospital units made between psychiatrist, nursing staff, and the clinical laboratory so that the right specimen in the right container is got to the laboratory at the right time; there may not be a further opportunity.

Of the drugs that are misused, lysergic acid diethylamide (LSD) and similar substances are the best known for mimicking schizophrenic illness. There is pyrexia, dilatation of the pupils, visual hyperaesthesia, illusions and occasionally hallucinations, accompanied by any extreme of mood change. The individual's personality, expectations of the drug and the circumstances under which it is taken will colour the experience. The effects of the drug (and its duration in the body) are transient, but lasting personality changes, including persisting psychotic disorder, have been described (Sedman and Kenna, 1965; Hatrick and Dewhurst, 1970) including depressive disorders. Flashbacks are brief re-experiences of aspects of the LSD 'trip', characteristically experienced as feelings of paranoia and unreality accompanied by paraesthesia. They may last minutes or hours and occur up to 18 months after the drug was used. Their nature has not been fully explained (Dusek and Girdano, 1980). The latter authors also review the conflicting evidence that LSD could cause chromosomal damage.

In the psychotic states described by Connell (1958) in people taking amphetamine in the range 50–325 mg daily, ideas of reference and delusions of persecution were prominent. These drug psychoses subside in weeks or months, and prolongation suggests either a schizophrenic illness or continuing use of the stimulant drug. Amphetamine is usually completely excreted in two days, but may be detected in the urine for up to 10 days. It is excreted quickly in an acid urine so urine tests may only be briefly positive in a disturbed, anorexic, acidotic patient.

Solvent abuse (page 200) and alcoholic intoxication (Cutting, 1978) can produce acute psychotic states accompanied by mood changes, delusional ideas and confusion. Psychotic reactions to cannabis (grass, weed, hash, hay, hemp, bhang, ganja, charas, etc.) have been reported (Kolansky and Moore, 1971; Spencer, 1971) but the evidence is inconclusive (Rathod, 1975). Considering its widespread use it is probable that such psychotic reactions as have occurred may have been in unusually vulnerable individuals (Dusek and Girdano, 1980). Cocaine, much favoured by Sigmund Freud although he eventually acknowledged its dangers, can cause euphoric, excited, hyperactive states followed by depression, which have been described as psychotic (Post, 1975).

So wide a range of prescribed psychotropic drugs may cause abnormal mental states including psychotic symptoms that this possibility should be considered in all acute psychotic disorders. Anticonvulsants like primidone, phenytoin, carbamazepine and sulthiame may do the same (Stores, 1975).

SCHIZOID PERSONALITY AND THE 'BORDERLINE STATE'

There are a very large number of permutations of terminology and definitions used to describe unusual and often disabling personality characteristics which do not fit into the more clearly defined psychiatric disorders. Although the following categories can be defined in such a way as to exclude others, they are also used interchangeably sufficiently often to cause considerable muddle; for example: schizoid personality; Asperger's syndrome; atypical autism; latent schizophrenia; pseudoneurotic schizophrenia; pseudopsychopathic schizophrenia; borderline state; psychotic character; schizotypal personality disorder.

The concept of *schizoid personality* has a respectable tradition in British psychiatry, beginning with Kraepelin's description of young people who were shy, quiet, unable to make friends and predisposed to schizophrenia; Kretschmer's account of schizoid people as unsociable, oversensitive, cold, stubborn and pedantic; and Bleuler's use of the word to mean shut-in, suspicious, sensitive and 'pursuers of vague purposes' (see reviews by Nannarello, 1953; Wolff and Chick, 1980). Some patients with schizophrenic illnesses had been, in childhood and adolescence, socially, emotionally, and behaviourally odd in such ways (Rutter, 1972c; Garmezy, 1974a, b), and some have claimed schizoid behaviour patterns in adolescence as an important predictor of adult schizophrenic illness (Demerath, 1943; Kohn and Clausen, 1955; Bower et al., 1960), but the careful, long-term follow-up studies of O'Neal and Robins (1958) and Robins (1966) showed no such association, and on the contrary conduct problems (truancy, running away, and incorrigibility) were more evident in the personalities of children who later became schizophrenic, which compares interestingly with the findings by Symonds and Herman (1957) and Masterson (1967) that psychopathic rather than schizoid characteristics predominated in the presentation of schizophrenic adolescents. Wolff and Chick (1980) conclude that the schizoid personality type exists among children as an enduring characteristic and presents problems of its own, but its relationship with adult schizophrenia is unknown; they also consider it the same as the syndrome described by Asperger, with the differences that girls too can be affected, and schizophrenia may develop in later life.

Weiner (1970a) points out that it is the uncertain cases where diagnosis is most important; the acute, florid illness is the most easily identified and has the better prognosis, while the insidious form of the disorder is most readily confused with personality oddities. He suggests three guidelines. First, the longer equivocally schizophrenic symptoms persist, despite successful efforts to alleviate situational problems, the more likely is the disorder genuinely schizophrenic; second, the more normative the adolescent's preoccupation (school, family, sex), the less likely is schizophrenia, other things being equal, a diagnostic point made earlier by Warren (1949); third, the more the process of thinking (as opposed to its content) is disturbed, and the less the adolescent's ability to distance himself from abnormal aspects of his thinking or behaviour (Easson, 1968), the more likely is schizophrenic disorder. This last point is probably the most helpful of the three: the adolescent who, however bizarrely troubled, sees his or her experiences in perspective, as a problem for patient and therapist to work on, 'feels' less psychotic; there is a feeling of a shared task, rapport is better, and this view of the problem comes close to that elusive concept 'insight'. The adolescent who is as muddled about the therapist, the clinical relationship, the clinic, and the world as he or she is about the problems, and who seems overwhelmed by it all more or less equally, will seem closer to having a schizophrenic illness. However, children and adolescents have difficulty anyway in standing outside their own emotional and intellectual problems and being objective about them; and the impaired ego functioning that would give the boy or girl the above perception of themselves and the world comes close to another concept: *the borderline state.*

Weiner, in his excellent and comprehensive book, does not mention the borderline state, which is unusual for an American work; the term is more determinedly avoided by the British (except where psychodynamically oriented psychotherapy is practised) (Macaskill and Macaskill, 1981). These authors suggest that psychotherapists favour the term because it describes primitive defence mechanisms which fall short of frank psychotic states, that is it is an aetiological rather than a descriptive term because such phenomena are more readily evoked in the unstructured relationships of psychotherapy and because psychotherapists, particularly in America, may more often see *in psychotherapy* people with rapidly resolving, transient psychotic states.

A composite picture of the borderline personality from the American literature is as follows: *presentation* is characteristically with complaints of misbehaviour (antisocial behaviour, drug abuse, running away, promiscuity) or with troublesome boredom, restlessness, and educational difficulty. There may be poor impulse control, suicidal threats or attempts. *On examination* there may be depression, withdrawal and a sense of futility, or enraged hostility. The clinician will have a sense of an individual with a poorly integrated sense of self and others; transient psychotic states occur. There are major problems of autonomy, attributed to maternal discouragement of childhood independence, leaving the child trapped between safe passivity and frightening, inept self-assertion. This identity diffusion is general, persisting, and distressing; it is not a relatively minor ambivalence about a particular person or circumstance. Defences centre upon splitting, that is people and things are perceived as wholly good or wholly bad and in opposition to each other (see page 84). Reality testing is maintained, as judged by: (a) absence of hallucinations and delusions; (b) there is reasonable capacity to empathize with the therapist's comments on unusual aspects of what the patient says or does; and (c) comments on defence mechanisms – that is cautious interpretations – are to some extent acceptable. A *history* of painful separation is often present, but may not be prominent, and there is evidence of prolonged dependence and passivity and defects in ego development, for example poor impulse control, poor tolerance of frustration and problems in social relationships. The *parents* are often described as having borderline personalities themselves: they cannot parent competently, and 'perceive their children as parents, peers or objects and are unable to respond to their child's real needs' (Masterson, 1973). Mothers are demanding, dominating, controlling, and intrusive towards the child, often alternate between being punitive and permissive, and are maintained at a distance from (and by) passive, inadequate fathers. The most striking family communication pattern is an unnoticed or unresponded-to appeal by the child for care (see Grinker *et al.*, 1968; Mahler, 1971; Kernberg, 1975, 1976; Masterson, 1972, 1973; Schwartzberg, 1979).

Treatment is inevitably uncertain in a condition that almost certainly includes a number of quite different individual and family patterns of adaptation and behaviour; what is described above has a certain consistency, but it is largely understandable as a developmental abnormality in emotional life stated in terms of ego psychology, and this could well represent the final common path of a number of quite different psychopathological factors. Thus one adolescent's problem may be largely derived from a traumatic separation as Masterson (1973) suggests, another due to highly disturbed parenting, and another due primarily to constitutional vulnerability. Thus the genetic studies of Rosenthal, Kety and their colleagues (see page 233) do suggest that there may be a spectrum of schizophrenic disorder which is variably expressed (see Rosenthal, 1975), and some young people with this vulnerability in some family circumstances may present with 'borderline' problems and be diagnosed as such. Nevertheless, although borderline patients are vulnerable to psychotic states, there is fairly wide agreement that the borderline disorders are clinically distinct from schizophrenic illnesses (Knight, 1954; Masterson, 1973). Whether they are aetiologically distinct remains to be seen; certainly the diagnosis once made, appears to hold up over the years (Aarkrog, 1981).

The family problems in these adolescents' cases are considerable, and the adolescent's capacity for an independent life a central issue. Shapiro and his colleagues (Zinner and Shapiro, 1975; Shapiro, 1978) recommend concurrent individual and family therapy. Long-term individual psychotherapy is the priority for the boy or girl who can use it, and long-term stability of healthy relationships, for example in a therapeutic community, may be needed if the adolescent cannot use individual psychotherapy, or cannot use it yet. Psychotherapy and therapeutic communities vary too much for a particular type to be recommended; I would emphasize the relationship, or the setting, which is most likely to help that young person develop autonomy and a sense of self-esteem and which will persist with him or her through alternating periods of withdrawal, anger, anxiety, and rejection. Stability over a reasonably long time is needed, and (in a residential setting) staff sufficiently experienced to perceive and cope with the adolescent categorizing them all into 'good' and 'bad'. The object of individual psychotherapy and the therapeutic milieu is to be supportive, responsive, encouraging, and reality-focused, limit-setting and to patiently and persistently help the adolescent accept and take responsibility for his or her own feelings and ideas, and to see that neither the adolescent nor the therapeutic team is good or bad but human and ordinary. If this balance can be maintained over a long period, the young person may develop emotional maturity. At the same time he or she will often need help with basic social skills, sometimes even self-care, and may have great difficulty with art, games, and play. Interest and success in these areas should be helped and encouraged. I would not avoid medication if the young person is constantly highly aroused or anxious, or profoundly depressed, and if as time goes by psychotherapy does not help with these moods.

Work with the family is always important, with the aim of helping individuation and, if necessary, separation, but individual psychotherapy should continue in parallel with whatever family work or family therapy is undertaken. There are two possible strategies: one of the family co-workers can also see the adolescent regularly as individual therapist, and join the boy or girl in the family sessions; or individual and family workers can be kept separate. The indication for short-term or long-term separation, for example by admission to hospital or to a special community is persisting disability and distress which, despite help and effort, the family cannot respond to. Often the adolescent continues to feel intensely responsible for other family members, and is helped by being made to understand that they are being looked after by the clinical team, by work continuing with the parents once the child has left home, reaffirmed from time to time (for example in holidays) by family meetings.

Masterson (1980), perceiving the psychopathological flaw in the borderline state as not only a fear of abandonment by the mother as the penalty for attempting to achieve individuality, but loss of self too, made disturbed self-image, problems in self-assertion, and lack of autonomy the main foci of his therapeutic programme. This entailed a period of separation from the family in a highly staffed residential unit where limits were firmly set, school, social and occupational skills taught, and this firmly reality-orientated setting provided a framework for individual psychotherapy. Parents were seen separately for a time, joint interviews following later, and the expectation was that after a prolonged admission the patient would live away from home. In a four year follow-up of 31 patients just over half had maintained the improvement achieved by discharge and were judged to be minimally (16%) or mildly (42%) impaired. The patients regarded on admission as being closer to neurosis than psychosis in symptomatology did best, this judgement based particularly on their capacity to acknowledge their symptoms as problems, an ability that seemed to correlate with higher tolerance of anxiety. Persistence with treatment after discharge was also associated with a better outcome.

Asperger's syndrome, which Wolff and her colleagues (page 243) associates with the schizoid personality, was described (Asperger, 1944), as 'autistic psychopathy of childhood', characterized by grossly impaired social relationships marked by a lack of empathy with other people, solitariness, non-conformity, extreme sensitivity and egocentrism, narrow and idiosyncratic tastes and preoccupations (for example unusual hobbies whose pleasures others find hard to appreciate), poor coordination and visuo-spatial perception, and usually normal intelligence. Most patients regarded as showing the features of

Asperger's syndrome are boys, and schizophrenia does not develop. In the study by Wolff and Chick (1980), they considered the group of children they studied as resembling schizoid personality and borderline states as described in the adult psychiatric literature, with the distinction (from Asperger's syndrome) that they found girls who were also affected, and (from Asperger's syndrome and the borderline state) schizophrenia could develop.

The relationship between these three broad groups of personality problem, and of autistic psychopathy with autism, remains unclear. Like depression, anomalies in the sense of self in relation to others may represent a pattern of feeling and behaviour which may be expressed as the resultant of a wide range of possible constitutional, experiential, and circumstantial influences.

Chapter 14

Autism, Mental Retardation, and Learning Disabilities

CHRONIC INCAPACITY IN ADOLESCENTS

Birds and beasts after a certain time banish their offspring, disown their acquaintance and seem to have no knowledge of objects which lately engrossed the attention of their minds and occupied the industry and labour of their bodies. This change in different animals takes place at different distances of time from the birth, but the time always corresponds with the ability of the young animal to maintain itself – never anticipates it . . .

In the natural and instinctive feelings of man as contradistinguished from those which have been modified by reason, something of the same kind can be observed. The mutual relation of protection and dependence produced by power and weakness is of this description. A helpless infant excites much stronger sympathy in the mother than a child that can shift for itself. Hence that partiality, accompanied by blindness to defects which most parents entertain towards children whose natural deficiency, whether bodily or mental, throws them on their care long after the season of infancy.

Brougham and Vaux, 1845
Quoted in Ounsted et al., 1966.

A recurring theme in some parents of adolescents with long-standing disabilities is their anger and grief. They are usually most solicitous towards their child, and are frequently described as overprotective, although the mixed and sometimes muddled and misleading advice they have been given over the years by clinicians and others makes their characteristic suspicion of professional opinion understandable. Nevertheless they find themselves dependent on the people they cannot completely trust. The lack of confidence has another facet; it is not only to do with conflicting advice about diagnosis, prognosis, handling, schooling, the effects of treatment, and the generally parsimonious provision of residential help when they cannot cope at home. It is also to do with the quite common failure of professional workers to face, and help with, the parents' feelings of profound disappointment, despair, anger, anxiety, and shame about the less than perfect child (Bentovim, 1972a,b) and the less often recognized sense of unassuagable chronic grief they experience because of the loss of self-esteem (and sometimes mutual esteem), the loss of the ideal child they hoped for up to (or sometimes after) they asked 'Is it all right?' and their loss of a normal life (see also Olshansky, 1963; Gath, 1972).

The younger the child, the more this can sometimes be coped with; the child may improve; parents may believe that various developments such as having other, normal children will make things all right; research may produce new forms of help (often many 'second opinions' will be sought) and administrative developments new facilities; they themselves may 'learn to adjust'. Facilities for young children, too, are quite often relatively bright and new and with an optimistic atmosphere, with emphasis on the feelings of the family. The parents are also younger, and the boy or girl usually relatively more amenable, than he or she will be 10 or 15 years later when adolescence is reached, by which time various hopes will be unfulfilled, the parents are in middle age and experiencing other losses (for example of parents and health). Their other children, too, may not be unscathed, the boy's or girl's lack of ability or wish to lead an independent life is becoming an ever-clearer reality, a series of doctors, social workers, education departments and others have failed to help enough, and the future holds no place for the boy or girl than, perhaps, the adult mental handicap hospital.

This may be the picture in the families of mentally retarded or autistic children and some with long-standing disorders like epilepsy, schizophrenic illness, and the more severe disorders of personality development. In adolescence, when the boy or girl needs to challenge his parents' care in order to experiment with being independent (a finely tuned piece of serious play – see page 89) things can go badly awry.

This is a bleak picture, and is by no means universal, but it is not uncommon in adolescent psychiatry where an attempt is made to help families and adolescents with these long-term intractable problems. The clinical workers, after a honeymoon period in which, if at all reasonable and competent, they may feel themselves to be the only professional people who have really begun to meet that family's needs for some 10–12 years, will sooner or later have to face the parents' rage. Without this happening, useful work cannot be done and this requires seeing this long, painful and stormy period through without abandoning the family and while maintaining reality about what the things are that cannot happen and will not be done (for example, a 'cure'; the 'ideal' placement). Most clinical workers who take on this therapeutic task find that in much of the work they are doing they are dealing more than anything with unresolved grief.

AUTISM IN ADOLESCENCE

The literature of adolescent psychiatry gives the impression that autism is a disorder of infancy. It certainly begins almost invariably before the age of $2\frac{1}{2}$ years, but is a lifelong handicap; as many adolescents as younger children have autism.

An important development in recent years has been the clear distinction that has been made between autistic and schizophrenic disorders: the two groups of conditions are quite different (Kolvin, 1971a,b; Kolvin *et al.*, 1971; Rutter, 1968, 1970, 1972a). Childhood schizophrenia resembles adult schizophrenia in epidemiology, genetics, and in clinical phenomenology, and is extremely rare before the age of seven or eight years. Children with autism have no greater genetic connections with schizophrenia than has the normal population, and its clinical signs are quite different. Moreover, while most patients with schizophrenic illnesses are of normal intellectual level, most autistic children (three-quarters) have intellectual levels in the retarded range (Rutter and Lockyer, 1967).

Some children have the most characteristic features of autism which include the features of Kanner's early descriptions (1943, 1949) which he summed up with the epithet, 'extreme aloneness and insistence on sameness'. They respond abnormally to sounds, have poor comprehension of gesture and speech, lack imaginative or cooperative play, and their speech is markedly delayed and abnormal, including echolalia, pronoun reversal, neologisms, immature 'telegrammatic' syntax, and concreteness of expression. Their eye to eye gaze is poor and they have weak or unusual attachments to their parents, but rigid, stereotyped attachments to certain objects and rituals, and show great arousal anxiety and rage if these are interrupted. They are sometimes overactive. The children's parents often think they are deaf, or cannot see properly, and report how they are not cuddly; unlike ordinary children, they do not lift their faces and arms towards approaching parents. About 2 children in 10,000 show this typical clinical picture, and the same number again have a similar but less typical condition (Lotter, 1966, 1967) The male:female ratio is about 3:1.

About half autistic children, especially those with higher levels of intelligence, gain reasonable ability in language by the time adolescence is reached, but a monotonous delivery lacking emotional expression and inflexion, and obsessive questioning about current preoccupations is characteristic although this may improve by late adolescence, during which period what had been rigid routines may develop into obsessional symptoms. Some autistic children develop epileptic fits during adolescence, and this is particularly associated with low IQ (Rutter, 1977b).

The cause of autism is almost certainly a biologically based cognitive deficit affecting the understanding and use of language, although the precise disorder is unknown. Various EEG studies indicate a higher than average rate of non-specific EEG abnormalities (for example Creake and Pampiglione, 1969) while Hauser *et al.* (1975) showed an association of autism with left temporal lobe enlargement. The only observations on the characteristics of autistic children's parents that have stood the test of replication is that they tend to be middle class, but this association may be due to factors affecting referral and diagnosis (Wing, 1980).

About 60% of autistic children remain very disabled and cannot lead an independent life; about 16% make a reasonable social adjustment and are able to work, the best outlook being predicted by high IQ, the earlier attainment of useful speech, good, appropriate schooling and a home free from disruption and social disadvantage.

The following tasks should be fulfilled when treating autism in adolescents:

1. Continue those efforts to support, inform and guide the family and be available to help if feelings such as those outlined at the beginning of the chapter are intruding in any way.

2. Continue to manage behavioural problems such as tantrums and destructiveness, which may become rather more prominent in later adolescence as the boy or girl tries to assert his or her independence belatedly and inappropriately. Physical size and normal sexual development may cause new parental anxieties. Sometimes drug treatment is considered for the first time, for example to maintain a child in a school or special community that has so far coped reasonably well, and where it is important to try to avoid interruption of painfully acquired stability. The phenothiazines or haloperidol are the most useful drugs, and larger doses than usual may be needed, inadequate doses causing only irritability (Corbett, 1976). Epilepsy may occur for the first time in adolescence, and need anticonvulsants; these drugs should only be used for treating overactive or aggressive behaviour if it is clearly associated with seizures. Similarly antidepressants are only useful if depressive illness is present (for example Campbell *et al.*, 1975), although lithium (page 335) may help some autistic children if there is a strong cyclical quality to periods of behaviour disturbance which cannot be explained in other ways (Campbell *et al.*, 1972; Corbett, 1976).

3. Corbett (1976) has helpfully discussed the problems of sexual behaviour in autistic adolescents, which generally amount to sexual inappropriateness (for example masturbating in public), or seeking physical affection in a childish way but which may appear sexually precocious to others and be misunderstood. This behaviour like other inappropriate social behaviour requires firm management by the parents, who need reassurance that this will not cause emotional disorder if the adolescent is handled kindly, firmly, consistently, and without undue anxiety. Most autistic girls learn to cope with menstruation by themselves. If periods are painful or irregular low oestrogen dose contraceptives may help, and by rendering the menstrual cycle predictable help with self-care.

4. Predictability, consistency, and patient perseverance with everything that helps – behaviour management, family counselling, the most helpful schooling, the most appropriate residential care if this is necessary, are all important. Autistic children and adolescents have great trouble coping with change, and with all but the simplest explanations too. Changes may be needed, for example, a change of school in adolescence, or a move away from home, and this can cause great pain, distress and disruption, which sometimes leads to yet further changes if home or residential setting cannot cope. Helping the parents help the adolescent (Howlin *et al.*, 1978), a supportive and consultative role with schools and children's homes, may all help minimize changes and the effects of change. It is important constantly to remind the boy or girl (and parents too) of what they can do, enjoy, and achieve together.

5. Autistic children can enjoy themselves, and are particularly fond of music and rhythmic movement, although they have difficulty in learning and copying skilled movement, areas in which music therapists and physiotherapists can help.

6. When residential care, all the time or some of the time, is needed it is important to maintain such parental contact as is helpful, providing a sense of continuity even if the boy or girl is away from home. Suitable day and residential centres are few and far between and there is a need for much more specialized training of all staff, including teachers, care staff, speech therapists, and music therapists. (Wing and Wing, 1976).

MENTAL RETARDATION IN ADOLESCENCE

It will be clear that mental retardation and autism are quite separate problems, but many of the points made above apply here too, particularly the importance of helping adolescent and parents cope with chronic disappointment and worry, and with social handicaps which may become more troublesome in adolescence. As with autistic children, if the child cannot manage or be managed at home, there may be considerable and often justifiable concern at the resources available in the mental handicap establishments. In this context parents of mentally retarded or autistic children have a common fear which emerges particularly as the boy or girl reaches adolescence and they themselves middle-age: 'who will look after him when we've gone?'

Some definitions

Mental retardation and *mental subnormality* are the terms commonly used to describe intellectual deficit and its consequences; Rutter (1971a) has suggested using the term *intellectual retardation* for the psychometric concept of low intellectual level, and *mental handicap* for social, psychiatric or physical handicaps associated with it.

Intellectual retardation in this sense is a social and administrative and therefore largely arbitrary concept (Corbett, 1977) and refers to performance on standardized tests (such as the Wechsler Intelligence Scale for Children; WISC) at least two standard deviations below the mean. With a mean of 100 and a standard deviation of 15 intellectual retardation applies to that 2.5% of children who have an IQ of 70 or below.

The categories in axis three of the multi-axial classification scheme (see page 153) include:

Normal variation IQ 71 or more, including superior intelligence
Mild mental retardation IQ 50–70
Moderate mental retardation IQ 35–49
Severe mental retardation IQ 20–34
Profound mental retardation IQ under 20.

Brain disorder and psychiatric disorder are both separate concepts from that of intellectual retardation. The majority of intellectually retarded children and adolescents have neither, and retardation is the result of an interplay between genetic and environmental factors, which at its simplest amounts to inheritance setting the upper limit and environmental factors such as stimulation and type of education determining the actual level achieved. Environmental factors include less clearly defined physical factors too. The lower socioeconomic classes get less antenatal care, experience more obstetric problems and have more children of low birth weight, which may be associated with 'minimal brain damage' (Knobloch and Pasamanick, 1962).

Brain disorders are more likely to be found at the lower levels of IQ. Thus nearly all children with severe intellectual retardation have organic brain disorder. There are many causes: *genetic*, for example tuberous sclerosis, phenylketonuria; *chromosomal*, for example Down's syndrome; *prenatal environmental causes*, for example infection with rubella or syphilis, rhesus incompatibility, maternal alcoholism or diseases like toxaemia complicating pregnancy; *brain injury*, for example in premature birth or hypoxia; *injury in early infancy*, status epilepticus, encephalitis, meningitis, lead poisoning, head injury. (See Kirman, 1977, and Taylor, 1979, for fuller accounts of the medical aspects of mental retardation.)

Psychiatric disorder and *behavioural disturbance* both occur more frequently in intellectually retarded children than in the general population although the types of disorder are much the same as among children in the average intellectual range (Rutter *et al.*, 1970).

Educational subnormality (ESN) is another administrative term, referring to mildly retarded young people who cannot make progress in schools for the average range.

Psychiatric disorders

The psychiatric disorders seen in mentally retarded children and adolescents are very much the same as those occurring in young people of normal intelligence, and for the most part appear due to similar influences such as problems in personal relationships and emotional life rather than low intellectual level as such, or brain disorder (Philips, 1967; Philips and Williams, 1975). In the latter study the authors found a higher incidence of psychotic disorders the causes of which were unclear. The term psychosis is often rather loosely applied to chronic or recurrent chaotic, bizarre behaviour accompanied by high degrees of distress; it is usually present from early childhood, and sometimes has autistic features. Occasionally mildly retarded adolescents under severe stress who have so far been psychiatrically well present with acute, bizarre, chaotic behaviour accompanied by near-delusional or frankly delusional fears and paranoid ideas. Occasionally this is the beginning of a severe mental illness, but as often it has the qualities of an acute psychotic reaction, resolving fairly quickly with relatively smaller doses of tranquillizing medication than usual. A possible explanation of such disorders is that the boy or girl has experienced severe distress with which he or she cannot cope, lacking the intellectual, emotional and interpersonal resources and the verbal and social skills to make sense of the experience to himself or herself or to others. An anxiety state or depressive disorder, or painful domestic circumstances may be the nearest thing to a cause that can be identified, and it may be possible to prevent recurrences by family work, reappraisal of educational and training provision for the boy or girl, and by counselling or support. These episodes are not well documented, and their nature and implications require study.

Problems of independence

Less dramatic but painful feelings surround the issue of the mentally retarded adolescent's capacity for future independence. Most mentally retarded people tend to be compliant and submissive rather than pressing for their rights, but always in their parents and often if vaguely, in the young man or woman there are questions to be faced about living independently, having friends including friends of the opposite sex, sexual relationships, marriage, finding work, and having children. These issues can cause considerable anxiety, so much so that they may not be raised; the clinician who believes that they are behind sad or worried feelings or even more acute reactions should explore them. It is a matter of fine judgement how and when to deal with them with the family as a whole. Communication problems may justify a little rehearsal first about how best to put things; explaining to a young man or woman about his or her job, marriage, and friendship prospects, or whether he or she will be able to have children and look after them, can be quite daunting. It is often true that the level of social functioning a mildly mentally retarded adolescent will be able to achieve eventually is in fact uncertain, and it is not dodging the issue gently to reflect back questions about how the young person is going to achieve this thing or that, what difficulties he or she has had so far, and how he or she is going to use further training, educational and social opportunities; on the contrary, this is more realistic than issuing optimistic or pessimistic predictions, and more honest than resorting to heavily qualified expressions of hope that may well be misunderstood.

Job prospects are not always appalling; some mildly mentally retarded young people slip happily into reasonable work 'helping someone' or in some local authority work; it is important to arrange for someone to keep an eye on their self-presentation and timekeeping, to make sure that they do not miss continuing training opportunities, and that they are not exploited. Nevertheless there can be major disappointments and much hurt pride, and particularly for the more severely retarded day care and sometimes residential care will be needed. With regard to the latter, the strain on well intentioned families can be severe, and sensitive work is needed to be sure how far to encourage a family to try to cope, and how far to recommend residential care for everyone's sake. The provision of services is very variable and sometimes very poor; Wing (1971) has helpfully reviewed some questions about the provision of these services.

There are many approaches to independence training for mentally retarded young people, involving both individual and parents; it is worth remembering how even quite simple skills like the mechanics of shopping, basic housekeeping, using a phone, or travelling on a bus can be difficult, confusing and frightening, and can be systematically taught (Matson, 1981). Group work can be helpful in assisting in the transition from a training setting to the community and the advice given to group leaders, for example to be active, responsive, and to provide structure (Slivkin and Bernstein, 1970) is not dissimilar to the approach taken by many who take adolescent groups in general (see page 298).

The mentally retarded adolescent's sex role perception and preference can be muddled and this can be exacerbated by institutional life (Biller and Borstelmann, 1965). Sexual education, learning about opportunities and about what is or is not socially acceptable, is needed, often missing, and can be difficult (Kempton, 1972; Craft and Craft, 1980, 1981). The possibilities of marriage, childbearing, birth control, and parenting also cause disquiet. The studies on marital success and parental competence, as might be expected, include extremely variable results from good to disastrous, and depend upon intellectual level, family size, personality and age of the marital partners, and outside support needed and given (Shaw and Wright, 1960; Rosen, 1972; Scally, 1973; Mattinson, 1975; Craft and Craft, 1979). Many of these are studies of adults, but they help inform the expectations and advice of the clinician working with mentally retarded young people and their families.

Self-mutilation

Repetitive, stereotyped self-injurious behaviour is an infrequent but persistent and, rarely, quite dangerous pattern of behaviour seen among mentally retarded children and adolescents. Corbett has estimated severe self-injury of this type being present in around 1 in 10,000 of the total mentally handicapped population, and it can result in irreversible mutilation, blindness or brain injury as a result of head-banging, eye-punching and gouging and biting of the extremities. Rarely there is an associated biochemical abnormality, as in the Lesch–Nyhan syndrome but the cause is generally obscure, with such factors as self-stimulating behaviour which is to some extent reinforced by adults' efforts to intervene probably being significant influences in many cases. Medication, restraint, and neurosurgical procedures have been disappointing (Corbett, 1975), time out procedures are occasionally helpful (Corte *et al.*, 1971), and an active programme to stimulate and encourage other activities is always important. If all else fails, and the self-injurious behaviour becomes life-threatening or likely to lead to brain damage, blindness, etc., aversion techniques using mild electric shock should be considered, with great care taken to obtain full parental consent, to avoid any possibility of abuse or misuse of the technique, and to help with the inevitably mixed feelings of staff. (See reviews by Corbett 1975; Corbett and Campbell, 1981.) Like other therapeutic and ethical dilemmas presented by young people, the clinician must weigh the risks of acting against the risks of not acting, rather than hope to prophesy a definite outcome; involve all concerned as fully as possible in discussions about the pros and cons of the treatment, although if the parents cannot finally make up their minds (as opposed to disagreeing) it is up to the clinician to make a definite recommendation; if parents agree, staff anxieties and misgivings must be faced helpfully, but in the final analysis it is the senior staff prescribing and carrying out the treatment who should make the decision to proceed; it cannot be debated endlessly. Written consent must be obtained and the whole procedure kept as 'open' as possible, within the obvious limits of the patient's and family's confidentiality and privacy. Finally, every step from discussion to results must be documented meticulously. There are many lesser ethical problems in child and adolescent psychiatry which require an equivalent approach.

READING DIFFICULTIES AND SPEECH DELAY

The understanding, acquisition, and use of language is fundamental to mental life, social functioning, and creativity; much of teaching and psychotherapy is about the use of words. Reading difficulties and problems in the development of speech are common, disabling, and persistent. These two areas of development and disorder cannot be reviewed adequately here (for full accounts see Rutter and Yule, 1977; Rutter, 1977c; Howlin, 1980; Frith, 1980). Two aspects will be briefly considered: educational failure in adolescence; and elective mutism.

Educational failure

'Succeeding' at school requires getting there in the first place, getting by without attention being drawn to social and academic performance, and then 'getting on' at a standard which meets the expectations of pupil, parents, and teachers. All three aspects depend upon the aspirations and competence of adolescent, parents, and school, and while the first two have long been taken for granted, recent evidence has confirmed the variations in schools that bring about different behaviour and academic performance in equivalent intakes of children (Rutter *et al.*, 1979). Epidemiological evidence, of course, does not tell us about the individual case, although it shows us what to look for.

School non-attendance (page 188) in adolescence may turn out to be a more serious matter in terms of outlook than school non-attendance in the younger child. In the wide spectrum of disorder there will be some boys and girls, particularly truants, whose educational and social performance when in school, and therefore their relationships with teachers, is problematic (Farrington, 1980), while others, particularly school refusers, include many who claim to like school and whose educational performance is satisfactory when they are there. Dislike of school and acting upon it, for example by not attending or not taking work seriously is, as expected, more a characteristic of the adolescent, although what happens to younger children who do not like school but cannot get out of it needs further study (Mitchell and Shepherd, 1967).

Poor educational performance and delinquent behaviour often coexist, possibly because similar family and temperamental characteristics predispose to both, and poor attainment in reading or in general can lead to that low self-esteem which in some young people leads to discouragement in schoolwork and gravitation to gangs, groups, and sometimes individual 'clowning' behaviour which provide an alternative source of status and support, and sometimes a very powerful one at that (see review in Rutter and Madge, 1977).

The frequency of *reading difficulties* and their association with behavioural and psychiatric problems in both clinic studies and the general population has been frequently noted (Rutter *et al.*, 1970; Rutter, 1974). It is important to distinguish between general backwardness and specific retardation, the latter representing a group, more often boys (sex ratio 4:1), where reading, speech, and language impairment form a special cluster of disability less related to intellectual level, other neurological or developmental disability or social disadvantage, while general backwardness is related to these four other sets of problems (Yule, 1974; Rutter and Yule, 1977). The difference, if any, between the concept of specific reading retardation and dyslexia remains obscure and controversial (see Rutter and Yule, 1977).

Educational failure may present as a problem in its own right, or may emerge when the history is taken. It is unusual for an adolescent's problems to have no repercussions in some aspect of school life. The first step is to be clear about the nature of the problem, which is partly a matter of careful history-taking and getting detailed school reports, and partly a matter of psychological testing. In these respects it is important not to overestimate the accuracy and validity of detailed and neatly written educational and psychological reports – they may be more subjective than they seem. A psychologist or teacher on the clinical team should review past reports and talk to the child's teachers, and his or her own objective and interpretive conclusions about these, and of the boy or girl, will provide a more complete and useful picture. It should then be clear in which areas, generally or specifically, the adolescent is having trouble. This cannot be isolated from the question of the ambitions of adolescent, family (or individual parents), and school.

There may be considerable investment, emotional and sometimes financial, in a boy or girl staying at a particular school, and great anxiety about changing to an alternative; as we have seen, schools vary considerably, and not only in the private sector. There will be similar anxieties about reappraising ambitions, a shift from higher to lesser standard examinations, for example. Parental expectations may be too high or too low, so may be those of the school. It is extremely difficult to set guidelines on how to balance competing hopes because they are tied to cultural attitudes which are matters for the community rather than the clinic: professional workers in secure jobs should not too readily dismiss the anxiety of parents and child to succeed academically as indicative of neurotic attitudes or wrong values. It is important to check that the boy or girl is having a reasonably well balanced life, with friends and play complementing academic work. There may be too little of the latter or the former. It can be particularly difficult for a rebellious teenager to assert that he or she *does* like school if stuck with an anti-school peer group and if the parents are ambivalent anyway. My own inclination is to start with the ambitions of the parents and expect them to underwrite and press for a necessary minimum standard (which is not the same as a low standard) of expectation of their child and of the school, in terms of attendance, behaviour, and educational performance. Higher ambitions or additional aims should, finally, be those of the boy or girl. Family discussions can then be on a basis of respecting the aspirations of the adolescent while affirming the parents' concern and responsibilities too.

Educational failure is not always a matter of motivation, although, in general, problems presenting for the first time in adolescence are rather less likely to be due to previously unrecognized general or specific cognitive problems. Having established that poor performance is a fact rather than an opinion, and its precise nature, it is important to get as full a picture as possible of changes over the years, which include developmental milestones and general mood and social functioning as well as specifically academic achievement, remembering that intellectual development is uneven and troughs and peaks are to be expected, including IQ changes of as much as 20 points (see Rutter and Madge, 1977; Rutter, 1977d). Attention to detail is important; minor emotional or social problems, bullying, friendships and losses, relationships with teachers, changes in teaching methods, deflection into alternative absorbing pursuits, may trigger off a vicious circle of failure and labelling as failure which shape what could have been a minor educational hiccup into a problem. Rarely, a serious psychiatric or neurological disorder is the cause: see page 258. Finally, a most important rule in any problem presenting as 'failure' is to remind child, parents, and perhaps teachers too of areas of progress and success.

Elective mutism

Mutism – inability to speak – can arise in serious psychiatric disorder (for example some schizophrenic or depressive states) or neurological abnormality (for example deafness). Elective mutism refers to children who are silent in certain situations when speech is expected, for example at school, or with any but a very small group of close friends, and was first described by Tramer in 1934. It usually develops in early childhood after several years of normal speech development, occurs equally in boys and girls (unlike developmental disorders of language), and on the occasions that the child does speak comprehension and expression are usually normal. However, Rutter (1977c) points out that the psychiatric literature has tended to overemphasize the purely emotional and motivational nature of the problem, and that in a minority of cases there may be a language handicap or speech defect (see Rutter, 1977c; Smayling, 1959; and Wright, 1968). For these, speech therapy will be needed, and sometimes there is a history of abandoned speech therapy (perhaps after a period of success) which needs to be enquired into and taken up again.

For the majority of children, the problem is an emotional one, and the nature of the condition, with intrusive adults trying to cajole a fearful and sometimes irritable boy or girl into saying something can raise anger and tension all round and make matters worse. In the few cases I have seen in adolescents the usually effective treatments have already been tried, for example desensitization to deal with social fears, or systematic encouragement by operant training such as social reinforcement (see Straughan et al., 1965; Reid et al., 1967). The eventual outlook is usually good, but the going tough meanwhile. In intractable cases, a decision must be made whether to press on firmly and systematically with behaviour therapy explicitly focused on the speech problem, or to let this retreat into the background.

If no treatment has worked, my preference would be to try the latter: (a) make relationships with other children and within the family the focus of work, using family work, groups and social skills training, explaining to the child that these things and education too must be helped even though they are not yet ready to join in and talk sufficiently; reminding the boy or girl, as always, of the many things he or she can do; and (b) those working with the family, school or nursing staff (if the child is admitted for a time) should consult regularly with an experienced behaviour therapist to learn how, with patience and tact, to shape the child into gradually widening the circle of those he or she will talk to. Allow plenty of time, for example reviewing progress every year.

Chapter 15

Physical Problems

UNCERTAIN NEUROLOGICAL SIGNS

A number of apparent deviations from the physical norm are common in children and adolescents; as development proceeds it can be quite difficult to be sure what statistical normative data apply to the boy or girl in the clinic. Thus pubertal changes occur at different times in different children (page 69), developmental abilities like bladder control are acquired with similar variation (page 216), and some biochemical normal values such as blood haematocrit and serum alkaline phosphatase vary with maturity, sex, and growth velocity (see Daniel, 1977).

'Soft' neurological signs are so called because they are minor, hard to interpret reliably, age-related and therefore changeable, or uncertainly related to development and possible pathology. They include clumsiness, difficulty in producing rapid alternating movements (dysdiadochokinesis), involuntary choreic or athetoid movements and inability to identify or reproduce shapes outlined on the child's palm (see Rutter *et al.*, 1970; Shaffer, 1978). They vary with age and IQ, occur in children with no other problems at all, and when age and IQ are taken into account these signs do not discriminate between children with problems and others. An association between such things and psychiatric disturbance in adolescence has been noted (Hertzig and Birch, 1966, 1968) but these studies did not exclude patients with neurological disease, and included patients on drugs and counted hyperkinetic behaviour as a soft sign. Quitkin *et al.*, 1976, reported an association between delayed development, learning problems at school, and the later emergence of certain forms of schizophrenia and personality disorder both associated with 'soft' neurological signs.

Electroencephalographic examination can cause similar difficulties. Many brain-damaged and disturbed children have normal EEGs and many children whose emotional, behavioural, cognitive, and neurological state appears perfectly normal have EEGs reported as abnormal. Except when there is a specific abnormality (for example, diffuse, severe, slow wave abnormality in encephalopathy, or focal discharges) a deviant EEG can only be evaluated with the other clinical evidence. It is then at its most useful as part of the monitoring of progress and response to treatment over time. For example, Satterfield (1973) found that more hyperactive children improved with methylphenidate treatment if they had 'soft' signs and EEG abnormality (see also page 337).

Electroencephalographic findings change with arousal, medication, mood, circumstance as well as age, and a single recording may not tell us more than, for example, a single blood-pressure measurement. If brain dysfunction is thought to be related to clinical abnormality, psychiatrist and clinical neurophysiologist should collaborate in planning what sort of serial investigations might answer which sort of question (see review by Harris, 1977).

BRAIN INJURY AND PSYCHIATRIC DISORDER

Leaving aside obvious, severe neurological disease, the diagnosis of brain damage usually rests upon an uncertain history (for example of head injury at birth or in an accident), the sort of neurological signs described below, or when psychological testing supports the possibility of brain disorder by confirming and measuring defects in memory and learning. Studies of the relationship between brain injury and psychiatric disorder are complicated by the well-established associations between low IQ, educational difficulties, physical handicap, and obstetric problems, and the association of the latter and educational problems with social disadvantage. Such factors were taken into account in the Isle of Wight study (Rutter *et al.*, 1970) which demonstrated a real association between epilepsy or unequivocal brain damage and emotional or behavioural problems. The incidence of disorder was highest when there was neurological disorder of this sort, there was a significantly lower incidence of psychiatric disorder among children with non-cerebral physical disorder, and the latter had more psychiatric problems than the general child (10–11-year-old) population.

Overall, brain injury appears to increase the risk of subsequent psychiatric disorder. It does so in complex ways which include family, social, and educational effects as much as neuropsychiatric impairment. It is correspondingly modifiable by educational and psychosocial means, at least in principle, and the age at which injury occurs can be significant for future risk, for example psychiatric abnormalities in adults are more common when temporal lobe epilepsy begins in childhood (Taylor and Falconer, 1968). Although the locus of damage has relatively specific cognitive effects, it does not seem related to particular emotional or behavioural conditions in childhood with the possible exception the association of between temporal lobe epilepsy and some conduct problems. How this may be compared with Lishman's findings in adults that psychiatric disorder is more common after left hemisphere or frontal injury is not known. (See reviews by Shaffer, 1977b; Werry, 1979a.)

ORGANIC CAUSES OF PSYCHIATRIC DISORDER

As discussed on page 138, the psychiatrist should be vigilant for evidence of psychiatric symptoms being caused by physical illness, and particularly when disorder seems to arise from within. Adolescents with recent onset of a psychotic illness (affective or apparently schizophrenic) should be particularly carefully investigated, and a consistently declining educational performance should be treated with a particularly high level of suspicion, for example when psychiatric disorder follows viral infection (Steinberg *et al.*, 1972).

Corbett and his colleagues (1977) have described two adolescent boys both of whom had prolonged behaviour problems in a setting of grossly disturbed family psychopathology before the appearance of neurological disorder and, in due course, dementia and in one case, death. Both were suffering from neurodegenerative diseases, with metachromatic leucodystrophy confirmed in one child's case and probable in the other. Both cases were characterized by the absence of neurological signs for a long period, uncertain and sometimes conflicting physical investigations, and florid psychiatric symptoms, including first rank signs of schizophrenia. There have been several other accounts of physical disorder first presenting with psychiatric symptoms, for example Caplan described 28 children diagnosed as hysterical nearly half of whom were shown in due course to have organic disorders related to the presenting symptom (Caplan, 1970), while Rivinus *et al.* (1975) reported 12 children and adolescents with psychiatric symptoms (psychosis in two cases) who were found to have neurological disorders.

The range of possible neurological disorders is unlimited, but four rare disorders in particular may first present in later childhood or adolescence:

Hepatolenticular degeneration (Wilson's disease)
Huntington's chorea
Metachromatic leucodystrophy
Addison–Schilder's disease

In *Wilson's disease*, which is an abnormality of copper metabolism, almost certainly inherited as an autosomal recessive disorder, there is liver and neurological disease possibly related to the deposition of unbound copper in the liver, basal ganglia, and elsewhere. According to Bearn (1972) 40% of cases first present with liver dysfunction (which is particularly the case in children); 40% with neurological disorder such as rigidity, tremor, athetosis, dystonia, lack of facial expression, a flapping tremor at the wrists and occasionally fits; and 20%

with psychiatric disorder, including school phobia and behaviour problems (Scheinberg *et al.*, 1968; Walker, 1969). Depressive, hypomanic, and schizophrenic clinical pictures have been reported (see review by Lishman, 1978). Remission and fluctuation in the disorder may occur, with death occurring in a few years, with the worse prognosis the younger the age of onset. The most important signs on investigation are the Kayser–Fleischer ring, a brown coloration of the corneal margin, best seen on slit-lamp examination, a low blood caeruloplasmin level and increased urinary copper and often aminoaciduria. In uncertain cases a liver biopsy may be performed and show increased copper or early cirrhotic changes. Penicillamine successfully treats the condition but is a toxic drug. The psychiatric symptoms improve, but not as regularly as the other manifestations.

Huntington's chorea is inherited as an autosomal dominant genetic disorder with a virtually 100% rate of manifestation. Thus half the offspring of an affected person can be expected to develop the disorder, males and females being equally affected. The age range of onset is between 25 and 50 but it has been reported to begin in childhood and adolescence. The neurological presentation is with clumsiness or fidgetiness, facial grimaces which may be taken for mannerisms, dysarthria, and later the gross choreiform movements develop. Global intellectual deterioration develops insidiously. Psychiatric symptoms include personality change, paranoid and depressive symptoms, including suicidal acts, and sometimes a schizophrenic-like illness. In children clumsiness, ataxia, fits and intellectual deterioration are prominent. The disorder tends to present itself after children have been born, and each child has a fifty-fifty chance of developing this dementing illness for which there is no predictive test (which too would have problems; see Thomas, 1982); the emotional, family, and marital problems of affected families are therefore severe (Oliver, 1970). Martindale and Bottomley (1980) have given a helpful account of these problems and the counselling, therapeutic, and self-help assistance that can be provided.

Metachromatic leucodystrophy is a rare cause of neurodegeneration characterized by progressive dementia which can appear after several years of normal development (Corbett *et al.*, 1977). Investigations show diffuse slow wave abnormality on EEG, marked slowing in peripheral nerve conduction studies, ventricular dilatation on X-ray or computed tomography (CT) scanning and the presence of metachromatic material in urine and abnormal arylsulphatase A activity in urine and white blood cells. *X-linked adrenoleucodystrophy* (*Addison–Schilder's disease*) can also present with psychiatric symptoms and progressive intellectual deterioration in this age group, and is marked by abnormal suprarenal function and an abnormal adrenocorticotrophic hormone response to synacthen.

A large number of rare neurodegenerative disorders have been described, approximating to Heller's description of dementia infantilis, but with the onset in childhood later than the age of three or four he described. They may follow an encephalitic illness (as in subacute sclerosing pan-encephalitis) or there may be no clear-cut illness to begin with. Often the disorders remain undiagnosed. Their investigation is complex, much of it still largely experimental, and should be undertaken in collaboration with a specialist centre.

Such neuropsychiatric disorders should be suspected when there is an insidious fall-off in social and educational performance and in family relationships, prolonged or atypical psychiatric disorder which is not easily formulated in terms of psychological, social or family terms and failure to respond to treatment. The very severe mental illness which does not have the characteristic signs of schizophrenia or affective illness should be regarded as particularly sinister in this respect.

It can be extremely difficult to decide from the history and examination whether or not an apparently organic disorder is also progressive. Electroencephalographic, electromyographic, biochemical and biopsy methods may help establish the precise diagnosis (Wilson, 1972). Peripheral nerve biopsy can confirm the diagnosis of metachromatic leucodystrophy, while rectal biopsy is regarded as a reliable investigation for Batten's disease and can be used to exclude the presence of this familial dementing disorder of neuronal storage in an apparently healthy sibling. Indications for brain biopsy are few and appear to be diminishing; it is risky, often unhelpful diagnostically, and other investigations are superseding it (see Brett and Lake, 1975; Bolthauser and Wilson, 1976).

Not infrequently the results of investigations are ambiguous and conflicting and as rarer disorders are explored investigations may become prolonged. Sometimes there is no alternative to careful monitoring of progress over many months, with repetition of X-ray, EEG, psychometry, and selected special investigations at intervals, and special attention paid to the emerging picture of school and social performance and close relationships. The focus of work with the adolescent is to help with fear and sadness, which may be poorly expressed but can be assumed to be present, and with his current range of handicaps, which of course may worsen. The focus of work with the family, as well as providing information, explanation, and support, is the uncertainty of the situation and the possible, or probable, unhappy outcome, which may be death, dementia or a future largely spent in a long-stay hospital or in a severely deteriorated state at home. The clinical workers directly involved with the child and family themselves need support and help to get the balance right between equally unrealistic optimism and pessimism.

PHYSICAL ILLNESS IN ADOLESCENCE

Although adolescence is generally regarded as a physically healthy time of life, the main causes of admission to hospital for example being for overdoses and accidents, there is a large and probably growing minority of adolescents with some form of chronic or recurrent physical disorder or handicap. Some estimates, taken together, suggest that some 10% of all children are likely to be affected by chronic, disabling disorders with a large physical component by the age of 15 (Douglas, 1964; Roghmann and Haggerty, 1970; Rutter *et al.*, 1970; Pless and Roghmann, 1971) and Shirley (1963) estimated that the number of children and adolescents in the United States with chronic, disabling disorders is around a million.

Emotional and behavioural problems are related to physical disorders of this sort in a number of different ways. Thus Kashani *et al.* (1981) found depression prominent in children aged up to 12 who were admitted to hospital for long-standing orthopaedic problems, particularly when the parents were poorly adjusted to the child's handicap, showing worry, anxiety, and guilt. Chess and Hassibi (1978) have described the demoralization, denial, and depression that may be found in pre-adolescent children in relation to physical handicap, and Stearns (1959) and Tattersall and Lowe (1981) the ways in which adjustment problems of adolescence are made worse by diabetes mellitus, with negativism and rebelliousness about diet and urine tests as well as quarrelling with parents and doctors. This pattern of behaviour is usually described by physicians largely as a nuisance, but occasionally dangerous, and tends to reduce in later adolescence. A problem of a slightly different sort is described by Martin *et al.* (1982) among young asthmatics, among whom there was serious self-mismanagement of the disorder when it began in their childhood. These young adults had a poor understanding of the disorder and ways of treating attacks, restricted their activities unnecessarily and smoked heavily, the latter being positively correlated with poor progress of the disorder. The authors describe their findings in terms of the need for better health education for children and adolescents with asthma, but it is at least possible that personal and family attitudes and feelings concerning the disorder influenced poor self-management and lack of knowledge. Denial of facts about disorder in the patients (O'Malley *et al.*, 1979) and problems which tend to cause ambivalence and emotional distancing in parents and peers (Minde, 1978) seem also to affect adaptation adversely.

The misinformation, misunderstanding, anxiety, guilt, and powerfully mixed feelings about professional help already described in parents of children with mental retardation and chronic psychiatric disorder (page 244) appear to be common in adolescents and their families in the types of disorder described above. Recurring severe illness even with long spells of complete normality in between can be a major worry too. Taylor (1969), for example, has discussed the problems of coping with the epileptic fit, 'a brief excursion through madness into death', two problems for which there are elaborate social coping mechanisms, but not when the frightening experience is repeatedly followed by recovery and the person concerned wants to be accepted as a normal individual. Finally, Schowalter (1977) has described the problems of adolescent adaptation to physical illness particularly in terms of loss of autonomy, anxiety and confusion about body image and self-control, shyness and embarrassment and fear of death.

The extent to which such problems are widespread is not clear; many adolescents presumably adapt well to serious or chronic illness and hospitalization, those with overt problems coming to the attention of psychiatrists. However, the evidence of the studies quoted, the relatively unsurprising nature of their findings, their consistency with the common fears and misgivings of adolescents and their families in relation to psychiatric disorder and mental retardation, and the likely emotional impact of the threat of serious illness at a time when the boy or girl is negotiating a delicate balance between dependence and independence (of adults in general as well as of parents), all suggest that this aspect of health care deserves further attention.

Part III
Management

Chapter 16

Strategies of Intervention

INTRODUCTION

For older adolescents leading relatively independent lives, for example using university campus counselling services or walk-in clinics, help on a completely individual basis is appropriate, the focus of work remaining with what the young man or woman brings to the counsellor or therapist (see Laufer, 1968, 1980; Ryle, 1973; Newsome *et al.*, 1975).

This chapter emphasizes the importance of family and social relationships in the management of the problems of younger adolescents. For boys and girls living at home, receiving both their stresses and their support from family and school, and for whom a number of adults feel legitimate responsibility, total privacy in treatment is usually misplaced. For example it is hard to imagine the circumstances in which it would seem right to treat a 15-year-old boy or girl without the parents' knowledge and agreement. Even in an emergency, for example acute psychosis or an 'overdose' by a solitary young person seen in a casualty department, the establishment of who is looking after and responsible for the adolescent is itself an important and urgent matter. Having said this, the clinician should not to be carried away automatically on the current tide of enthusiasm for elaborate family and social involvement in all problems, particularly of older, more independent adolescents; such involvement must make sense in terms of the diagnostic formulation and the needs of management, and should take account of the young person's wishes.

For most of the problems of the younger adolescent, however, the clinician and the adolescent will need several other people to help establish what is wrong

Table 11 Strategic questions

Question	Examples	Implications
Why treat?	A 16-year-old girl of low intelligence is referred for treatment from a children's home. When seen it appears that the main problem is staff concern about her leaving school soon with few social and occupational skills and anxiety about what she will do all day	Consultation helps the staff clarify the causes of their anxiety. They come to terms with the fact that they cannot do as much for the girl as they wished and the future for her is indeed uncertain. With the question about treatment out of the way they now proceed to organize for the girl vocational and social skills training
Whom to treat; with whom to work?	A misbehaving boy is referred via a GP by his divorced and remarried mother and his natural father. His stepfather is not clearly involved in the concern about the boy nor his referral	The only remaining point of contact between the divorced parents is the boy's misconduct, and his stepfather appears to see the latter as a hangover from a marriage in which he has no part to play. It is essential as a first step to clarify for all concerned their respective roles and to face the uncertainty (and the reasons for it) in this anomalous situation
What to treat?	A highly anxious, muddled, introspective boy with poor peer relationships is referred. Family life is chaotic and anxiety-laden. The boy has major disabilities in communication and social skills and there is evidence of long-standing brain damage	The presenting problem is largely family and social in nature; its origin, however, appears not to be in the family dynamic system but in the adolescent's handicaps. He requires individual neuropsychiatric and educational assessment; and the parents, it emerges, need help with their guilt, anxiety, and misunderstanding about his problems being their fault
How to treat?	An unhappy, delinquent girl is referred for individual psychotherapy, for which a good theoretical case has been made at an assessment centre. In the centre she attended interviews dutifully. She makes it clear that she is reluctant to attend a psychiatric clinic and will not talk to the psychiatrists	A distinction must be made between her presumed need for individual psychotherapy and her ability to use it. She is found to have led an unhappy, chaotic life but was relatively happy and organized in the assessment centre. The care issue must be sorted out before treatment can be seriously considered. What can be done to make her life more stable? Can it be achieved by working with her family? If so, might this make individual work redundant?

When and where to treat?	The above girl, again	The primary need is to establish how the girl is being looked after and where she should live. Is proper care and limit-setting feasible in her home, with help? If she would be better off away from home, need this be a psychiatric unit? Possibly, or more probably a setting reproducing the care and structure of the assessment centre would be more helpful and acceptable, and against this background psychotherapy (if still needed) would be more practicable. If long-term residential care is needed, it is best if this is not in a hospital
With what authority to treat?	Over two years, an anorexic 14-year-old girl is twice admitted to hospital *in extremis*. Each time she recovers physically she persuades her parents to discharge her against medical advice. She now presents again with rapid weight loss	The girl *could* be admitted on parental authority, returned to normal weight and allowed to leave again. If there were doubt about authority to treat her the Mental Health Act would certainly be applicable at times. But the history of the girl's control over her parents, her repeated physical ill-health and the threat to her normal development are serious matters for the parents to consider. Can they assert parental authority or not? Do they want help to do so, and will they use it? Might a Care Order be appropriate and even a condition of readmission?
How to monitor progress?	Over several years a boy with conduct and mood problems matures and begins to settle down in a job and remains a long-term clinic attender; it seems difficult to discharge him	A supervision session is used to explore whether he is benefiting from his long-term relationship with the clinic, or whether this is a substitute for a normal social life. It emerges that he does not want or need to attend but is concerned that his depressed mother be properly looked after, and she gains this from her continuing contact with the team's social worker. This allows him to be more independent.

and to proceed in putting things right, and this can be a complex exercise; the more so in difficult or urgent crises, when characteristically many problems are in the form of social, legal, and ethical dilemmas.

A general framework within which to consider how to proceed in all cases, from the most complex and urgent to the apparently straightforward, is as follows:

Why treat?
Whom to treat and with whom to work?
What to treat?
How to treat?
When and where to treat?
With what authority to treat?
How to monitor progress?

This structured approach may seem cumbersome but even in relatively pragmatic and straightforward clinical matters (like, say, a tonsillectomy) all seven points would be taken care of, and in some detail too, leaving the clinician to focus on those aspects which prove difficult or unpredictable.

It is because these background factors are so important that in most of medicine they become unobtrusive routines; the surgeon would not dream of proceeding without, for example, the availability of a sterile theatre, an anaesthetist, or post-operative care. In psychiatry, however, we may sometimes proceed willy-nilly, discovering half way through that we really ought to have had the child's father there; that an urgent decision is needed but authority to proceed requires the approval of an adult not so far involved; or that what is being embarked upon (for example admission of an unwilling 15-year-old to hospital) may not be sustainable on his 16th birthday in three weeks' time.

Thinking through what to do with whom, and with what authority, is necessary not only to avoid time-wasting administrative wrangles but is an essential foundation for management and the trust of the patient and family.

The point of each question is outlined briefly in the following pages, and illustrated in Table 11 and in the chapters that follow.

THE NEED FOR CLINICAL INTERVENTION

Why treat? Sometimes those referring the adolescent are willing and able to carry on with what they are doing already, particularly with some advice, encouragement, and confirmation that there is no technical short-cut or magic solution that would make a difficult task easier. Because a referring agent initially refers an adolescent for diagnosis and treatment does not mean that consultation and the suggestion of an alternative is unacceptable; sometimes it is a welcomed possibility that had not been considered. The same applies to adolescents already taken on for treatment; further care might be carried out just as well by, for example, a school counsellor rather than a member of the clinical team, and more appropriately and conveniently too. As already pointed out, consultation is the tool with which the clinician and referring agent clarify and agree *how much* clinical intervention is needed, and this applies through out the period of clinical care. Consultation precedes diagnostic assessment, may sometimes make it unnecessary, and stands by as an available technique throughout management to monitor how much clinical management is needed and at what point others can take over.

THE PEOPLE INVOLVED

Which people?

The people involved fall into four broad categories (see Figure 28):

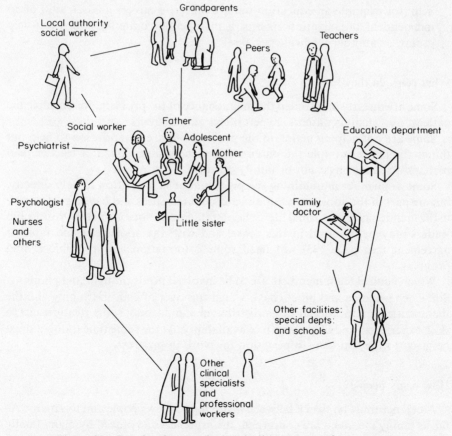

Figure 28   People who may be involved in aspects of management

1. *The patient* – the referred adolescent whose symptoms or problems are a cause of concern and will be a guide to progress.
2. *The family* – that is those with whom the adolescent lives, who are responsible for his care and who may be contributing to his problems, in a position to ameliorate them, or both. Is it clear whom the family consists of? A boy may be in a children's home, but with a family now divided into two, with natural parents and step-parents in two places, both having custodial as well as emotional ties to him. Or an adolescent may have a tenuous foothold in a chaotic family and at the same time a constructive relationship with, for example, the family of an elder sibling who has left home and married.
3. *Other adults and adolescents* involved with the adolescent as a 'problem' (social workers, family doctors) or involved anyway (teachers, classmates, friends, employers).
4. *The clinical psychiatrist and his or her colleagues.* This includes the clinical team but also 'outside' professionals who may be approached for advice or help (for example an education welfare officer, a careers adviser, staff of an independent organization such as a therapeutic community or a self-help group, or another medical specialist).

What roles do they have?

Some are directly involved in the maintenance of the problem, for example the patient, overanxious parents, hypercritical grandparents.

Some are not helping maintain the problem but are in a position to help put things right, for example the parents again, a sensible sibling, a teacher, and perhaps a school physician or family doctor.

Some are neither maintaining the problem nor in a position to help directly, but are part of the adolescent's affairs and circumstances and have a part to play in the maintenance of normal life. School staff, family doctor, friends, youth club leaders may be involved in this sense, and with the adolescent and family's agreement (see page 133) will need some information about problems and progress.

Which clinical team members are to be involved needs thought and planning. Some departments and offices have a high turnover of staff in training and the therapeutic or educational tasks distributed should bear some relationship to skill, experience, and likely length of availability. At the same time thought must be given to the source of supervision for work in progress.

How many people?

A balance must be struck between involving too few people and too many. As far as family members are concerned, the arguments advanced by many family therapists for involving all family members throughout are: (a) that all emotional or behavioural problems of one member of the family are to some extent shared by all family members and therefore no one can legitimately be left out; (b) that in any case all family members, for example younger siblings, have a right and a need to know what is happening to other family members; (c) that certain decisions cannot be taken, or sustained, without whole family agreement. To this extent the family approach is a particular way of working, not a particular form of therapy alone, and would be undermined if a family member were to be seen separately.

There is much to be said for the general viewpoint that of all systems (neuropsychiatric, psychodynamic, social) the family system is in general the single most appropriate focus for work, particularly with disturbed young people; and as described elsewhere (page 132) some work, for example aspects of assessment, and some interviews to review progress or exchange information, is best done on a family basis. However, the political dynamics of the introduction of the family approach to teams and clinics where it is not accepted unconditionally seem to require an uncompromising zealousness on the part of some of its protagonists, and even a degree of scorn towards dissidents (see Haley, 1980) and the suggestion that the family approach is useful often, or even usually, but not necessarily *always*, can generate a good deal of heat.

There is no doubt that there are occasions when useful work cannot proceed without the whole family, and times when it can. Practicality and convenience should take precedence over ideological purity in eclectic settings; what specialist treatment teams require is of course a different matter.

People involved in the wider social network, as mentioned earlier, may be needed too (see Speck and Rueveni, 1969; Speck and Attneave, 1971, 1973; Skynner, 1971; Blackwell and Wilkins, 1981). Vast case conferences can be time-wasting, with people present because they feel they ought to be rather than because they can usefully contribute, and irrelevant issues aired. Nevertheless so many professional people can be drawn into the affairs of the more worrying adolescents that meetings to determine who should do what may be necessary. Such meetings should have a chairman to clarify the focus and sum up and record conclusions and decisions. The latter should include deciding who need to remain involved, who simply need to be kept informed, and who are willing and able to disengage themselves from the case.

NEEDS AND METHODS

What needs treating, and how?

A list of provisional management goals should be drawn up; even though it cannot be completely precise it is a useful point of reference when progress is reviewed.

Social changes may be needed, for example in how an adolescent is being cared for, taught, or how limits are being set. Existing circumstances may be modified (for example a teacher may be invited to try a different approach to handling misbehaviour or academic difficulties) or a change of school or home may be required. Changes may be brought about by:

Advice and information

Collaborative work

Consultative work

Administrative recommendations (including court and other reports)

Family changes may be needed. This too may be a matter of consultation or recommendation, for example when the issue is where or with whom an adolescent should live.

Family members may simply be kept informed of progress; given specific advice; given systematic help (for example when a family collaborates in a behaviour therapy programme); or the dynamics of the family system may be identified as the problem and the focus of therapy. All this is *family work*, but only the latter is *family therapy*.

Personal change for the adolescent may be in terms of changes in:

social behaviour (for example social skills, self-presentation, coping strategies);
circumscribed behaviour patterns (for example eating habits, obsessional behaviour, tics, enuresis);
feelings and attitudes;
intellectual skills and educational ability;
physiological state in terms of physical health or physiological changes believed to underly psychiatric disorders.

Correspondingly, individually focused management may be listed in broad terms as:

the social therapies (for example social skills training; 'milieu' therapy);

the psychotherapies and counselling (for example individual psychotherapy);

the behaviour therapies (for example token economy systems, 'time out');

physical treatments (for example attention to physical health, medication);

special care (for example special arrangements to provide improved long-term upbringing);

special controlling methods (for example containment in a physically secure or highly staffed setting, providing a combination of structure, psychotherapy, milieu therapy and/or behaviour therapy).

TIME AND PLACE

When and where to meet the adolescent and family?

Timing includes the question of urgency. This chapter and chapter 6 have emphasized the importance of the careful organization of assessment and management, and this is not incompatible with high speed intervention, for example in the crisis-intervention approach taken by some clinics and teams (Bruggen *et al.*, 1973); however the practicalities of organizing work make it questionable whether the team which arranges invariably to be in a position to strike while the iron is hot can also make time for longer-term work.

The following guidelines may be helpful for the clinical team which offers both urgent and routine intervention and has to distribute time and staff for both.

If the request is for urgent removal from the home

When this is the case and immediate consultation confirms that no alternative is possible or acceptable, the choices are: admission to hospital; admission into care on a Care or Place of Safety Order (sections 20 and 28 respectively of the Children's and Young Persons' Act 1969); rarely, but an important option on occasions, being looked after by an alternative capable family or relative; also rarely, but also an essential option at times, being taken into police custody.

In a study referred to earlier (Steinberg *et al.*, 1981; and see Steinberg, 1982a), many of the most urgent requests for admission to an adolescent psychiatric unit were not because of acute psychiatric disorder but were due to unmanageable behaviour causing a breakdown in confidence and containment at home or in a children's home. The need was for urgent and effective care and control rather than for psychiatric treatment.

Psychiatrists in charge of adolescent in-patient units receive many such urgent referrals and if they wished to respond readily and competently to most of them, the in-patient unit would have to have the qualities not of a psychiatric unit but of a highly structured, highly staffed and physically secure children's home. If a unit's policy is to remain broadly psychiatric in character it must select for admission those young people with seriously unmanageable behaviour in numbers the unit's community can manage, and only when a period of psychiatric intervention is really considered likely to contribute something positive to assessment or treatment. Characteristically the adolescent's history is one of long-standing mishandling and disadvantage, and the outstanding need is for consistent, stable, reasonably long-term security, care and control. A psychiatric unit is not the most appropriate place for providing this, not least because the child will often need two or three years of stability and security of relationships and should not spend the remaining years of his or her childhood in hospital in order to get it; and in any case he or she should not be regarded as psychiatrically ill. My own approach to such referrals is to offer urgent consultation to whoever is currently responsible for the adolescent and recommend that if the need being demonstrated is for care and control, it be met by the social service department; and to propose a meeting with those involved to help plan a long-term strategy for the child's care and education and to see what part if any the psychiatric in-patient unit can play on a planned basis, for example by offering short crisis admissions if necessary with a rapid return to the setting designated as home.

Which children do need urgent admission to hospital? Adolescents who have attempted or threaten suicide or serious self-injury may need urgent admission if they cannot be effectively supervised by the adults looking after them and they show evidence of serious suicidal intent or depression (see page 185). Acutely psychotic youngsters, with acute manic, depressive or schizophrenic illness should be admitted urgently because of the clear need for psychiatric nursing and treatment. Anorexia nervosa is a special case. A rapidly falling weight can be a cause of very great anxiety among all concerned, but it should not be taken for granted that urgent psychiatric admission is automatically the right course (see page 134).

If the request is for urgent out-patient appointment

In this case it is as well to check first what is meant by this; sometimes a referrer means an appointment in days or weeks rather than months. Sometimes a referrer means the same day or the next. Again, a precipitate 'fire brigade' type response to a request for an urgent domiciliary visit, disrupting several hours' work and perhaps resulting in the postponement of other people's appointments, can result in one being shown into the house by the laconic focus of the emergency who is eating sweets and watching TV, and unsure of what all the fuss is all about. ('Mum'll be back at 7.') The most helpful general approach is to operate an adaptable service which can:

(a) see (or admit) urgently the very few adolescents who really need rapid intervention;
(b) make a consultative service readily available so that the *nature of the referral* can be discussed urgently with the referring professional; this is a practical and effective way of differentiating the urgency of newly referred adolescents, who can then be given appropriately timed diagnostic assessments over the next few days and weeks.
(c) make the latter service available for seeing parents and sometimes families urgently for a preassessment visit (for example at home) in which the anxiety and sense of crisis is specifically coped with, and detailed and comprehensive psychiatric assessment postponed until things have cooled somewhat, and for which adequate time can be made available. This approach is particularly

important when acute anxiety recurs around a chronic problem (for example autism, epilepsy, severe obsessional disorder) where from time to time parents feel they will never get adequate help; yet a careful, planned assessment is a precondition of adequate help.

As to *place*, there are arguments for seeing families at home or at the clinical team's offices. Skynner (1976a) has pointed out that families labelled 'uncooperative' by various services may best be engaged by a visit to the home; and the atmosphere and resources of the home and neighbourhood can be grasped in a way not possible at the clinic. On the other hand, Bentovim and Gilmour (1981), among many others, refer to the advantages of the hospital setting, including clarification of the authority and boundaries of the clinic team and the availability of the hospital's technical resources. It is tempting for clinical workers to regard the clinic as relatively neutral territory, and it is easy to be sceptical about this view. However, while a visit to a hospital can be daunting at first, there are ways of making the setting pleasant, friendly, informal, and reasonably private, a consideration which should apply to the reception and waiting area too. Once again, practice should be adaptable, so that a clinician is in a position to see adolescent and family at their home or at the clinic depending on needs, wishes, and mutual convenience. While there is certainly no special reason for always seeing people in their homes, there is a need for a psychiatrist to be as familiar as possible with the places from which his clientele are referred; it is important to spend time out and about and become familiar with the local neighbourhood, schools and headmasters' offices, social work departments and children's homes, to acquire a realistic conception of what life is like for the boys and girls referred, and for their parents and teachers too.

As a further guide to practice, one should be prepared to have a sense of territory in deciding where to hold a meeting. A consultation with, say, school or residential staff about whether or not to refer an adolescent to the clinic, is best held at the school or children's home. Similarly, it can help to hold a preassessment meeting to discuss the urgency of a referral (as on page 274) in the home. A discussion with another clinician (for example a family doctor) who may well be continuing with a child's or family's case should be held at his surgery, to affirm his clinical role. Correspondingly, when it is likely that assessment will be followed by the psychiatric clinic's involvement it makes sense to make the psychiatric clinic the setting. Such considerations are not crucial but if the clinical team has the choice it is worth considering how best to fit the meeting-place to the focus of work.

AUTHORITY TO PROCEED

The importance of authority and responsibility in adolescent development and therapy has already been discussed (page 6, 7). There are four forms of authority to consider:

legal authority
parental authority
the adolescent's authority
medical authority

Legal authority to proceed with treatment is not always clear. The bare legal bones are straightforward enough; for example up to the age of 16 a boy or girl must accept the treatment his or her parents want him or her to have, and on the 16th birthday the adolescent may consent to treatment himself or herself, or withhold consent. In practice, while few clinicians would have qualms about, say, insisting with parental backing that a boy or girl attends a family meeting or stays in a hospital unit, the legality of enforcing medication on a 14-year-old, even with parental consent, is not absolutely clear. In an emergency to prevent someone getting seriously hurt, I would not hesitate to sedate a highly disturbed young person if I felt it was clinically correct, and of course an adolescent detained under the Mental Health Act may be treated against his or her will. But it is quite another matter to insist upon routine medication or a behaviour therapy programme if an adolescent makes quite clear his or her dissent.

The clinician (with parental approval to proceed) must make his own judgement about the case, taking into account the degree of dissent (for example obstinacy and ambivalence, as opposed to clear refusal); the seriousness of the problem and the reasonable likelihood of treatment being effective; the discomfort and risks of the treatment being contemplated; and the feelings of all the other staff involved, taking care that key groups (for example night staff in a residential unit) are not left out. Having weighed these matters up, the clinician should make the decision; it cannot be left vaguely to the team consensus.

If the clinician does not have *parental authority* to proceed he cannot treat an adolescent under the age of 16. Either the adolescent would need to be treated under a section of the Mental Health Act, which is relatively rarely indicated, or on a Care Order. This too can be a difficult decision (see page 162) unless the boy or girls is quite clearly mentally ill. There are certainly cases where a section of the Mental Health Act may seem appropriate for dealing with psychiatric emergencies in an uncooperative adolescent with a schizophrenic illness, while insistence that he or she takes part in a longer-term educational and social therapy programme might more appropriately be the responsibility of the parents or those acting *in loco parentis.*

Problems can also arise when separated parents, with custody undecided, differ over whether or not their child should be treated. In such circumstances legal advice should be obtained; I would be guided by the recommendation I would make on present evidence if a court were to have sought advice on the child's custody.

Where the law is unclear, as it quite often is in the grey areas and loopholes adolescents seem so adept in finding, the advice is: (a) seek a competent legal opinion; (b) be guided by what seems kind, sensible, and ethical; what 'feels right' and would probably seem right to the general public is how a hospital administrator described it on a particularly difficult occasion; (c) discuss the problem openly but not endlessly with colleagues, adolescent and family; and (d) make a decision (record it) and proceed. Psychiatric practice is often risky and largely unpredictable, and in the end one can only balance the risks of various alternatives, including the possibility of doing nothing, which may carry the highest risk of all.

The *adolescent's own authority* for all or part of treatment is important too. A boy or girl may be well enough, mature enough or sensible enough to come to an informal agreement about a treatment programme. In many cases this is not only appropriate but desirable; in other cases the boy's or girl's wishes may be properly overridden by adults. In either case the facts of the situation should be made explicit, and the reasons given. An adolescent may not be allowed a choice because the adults responsible for his or her care believe that harm would result. Alternatively a treatment programme may be entered into on the understanding that the boy or girl will take it seriously, and if the adolescent does not do so it will be abandoned. A delinquent youngster may be offered the opportunity of using psychotherapy, for example, and thereby offered the alternatives of voluntary treatment or accepting the authority of a court to challenge his or her conduct in other ways.

Medical authority does not replace parental or individual authority except in exceptional circumstances where the Mental Health Act is used to insist upon treatment. In the sense in which it is used here medical authority refers to the extent to which medical recommendations are accepted because of the physician's real or presumed technical skills. For example, a psychiatrist may diagnose mental illness and recommend admission and treatment, advice which may be taken; this should be distinguished from admission on the authority of the family and in the absence of a medical diagnosis on the grounds that the family (or community workers) cannot manage for the moment, the approach taken, for example, by Bruggen and his colleagues at Hill End Hospital (Bruggen *et al.*, 1973). The focus for work is then not correcting disorder, but helping those responsible for the adolescent manage him or her in the community. This can be a team's whole style of work, or a way of working at a particular stage in treatment: see page 212.

Thus medical authority is largely to do with identifying *disorder* and treating it; other people's authority, including the adolescent's, is needed for dealing with *problems*. The clinical team should help distinguish their responsibilities from those of the family, allowing also for those that are shared. Medical authority, for example, to prescribe medication for an adolescent day patient with schizophrenia, parental authority to ensure attendance, and shared responsibility to encourage normal social behaviour.

In summary, there are three particularly important aspects of medical compared with parental or patient authority and responsibility:

1. If an adolescent has the symptoms and signs of psychiatric disorder, the clinical psychiatrist should be able to say so, and recommend treatment. Whether this advice is accepted is another matter.
2. If the problem requires considerable motivation on the part of the patient or substantial support from the parents (for example, in treatment of conduct problems) then *either* the adolescent must make a contract with the clinical team to try to cooperate in treatment *or* the parents should do so on their child's behalf. This need not be in writing, though this can help, but simply makes explicit the reality that clinical authority in such problems has major limitations.
3. In some cases it is appropriate to negotiate a shift in authority and responsibility.

> *Example 11*
> An anorexic girl is admitted to a psychiatric unit on the advice of a psychiatrist (with hesitant parental compliance) because from his clinical assessment and knowledge of the syndrome he can predict serious mental and physical problems ahead. After a few weeks the girl is no longer in any physical danger and is generally improving; she and her parents ask if she can now be discharged. In the first few weeks the psychiatrist would have very firmly advised against this. But now the family are asked to consider how they will be able to feed the girl adequately and whether they feel confident about doing so; if not do they want to continue learning in family meetings how to prevent relapse, and at the same time sort out whatever problems lay behind the disorder? Authority and responsibility are now explicitly passed to the family to decide how to use the clinical team to best advantage. The task ceases to be a technical, clinical one to do with diet, nursing and operant techniques, and becomes an understandable, common-sense issue of parents having difficulty feeding their child. The clinician still has the responsibility to point out difficulties and evasions and to predict the likely outcome of various patterns of family and individual behaviour, but authority to proceed (and decide on a sensible discharge date) rests with the parents.

Much the same transfer of informal authority and responsibility can helpfully take place with other disorders where management began with the psychiatrist taking a more traditional, authoritative medical approach. If this transfer of authority is adopted it must be undertaken explicitly and clearly at a meeting with patient and parents; it is an important occasion and should have impact.

MONITORING PROGRESS

The importance of listing aims for management has already been referred to. They are usually necessarily tentative, and should be pragmatic rather than idealistic or theoretical. For example, 'explore usefulness of working with school' may make more sense as a first step than 'improve patient's self-esteem'.

It is useful to plan a meeting to review progress with those involved right from the start; this includes fixing the time and place and gives a sense of purpose to the proceedings. On the one hand, distressed adolescents and their families need a sense of being given all the time they need; there often seems to them too much to sort out, get used to and say, and a fear of being rushed before seemingly insuperable difficulties can be faced and coped with. On the other hand, allowing plenty of time is not incompatible with fixing a date for progress so far to be reviewed; it gives a sense of structure and predictability to an unknown and possibly frightening future. It also means that medium-term goals for particular forms of management can be set, and alternatives explored if necessary in a reasonably systematic way.

A not uncommon dilemma is the problem of the particularly skilled staff member who is exactly the person to take on a particular aspect of management but who is soon to leave the team. This too can be explained, and short-term goals (including the difficulties involved in changing therapists) set.

If possible note-taking should be supplemented by videotape or audiotape recording, with the family's permission and full explanation of how the recording will be kept and used. This records information in a way with which even the best notes cannot compete, and in a form which leaves room for future reinterpretation. It is particularly useful for helping to monitor slight changes occurring over a long period, for example in psychotic illness or suspected neurodegenerative disorder.

Systematic recording of behaviour or other observations (for example mood, weight) which are the focus for work is always valuable, because it demonstrates what is going well as well as areas that need more attention. The skills of the clinical team's psychologist should be used to select the mimimum useful number of observations to be made, and their timing. Overinclusive charting will be done poorly or not at all and is hard to interpret.

From time to time clinicians turn their attention to the problems of the routine notes which so often become a bulky and not very useful repository of miscellaneous scraps rather than the useful working log they should be. The medico-legal need for a record of everything said and done is one motive for obsessive note-keeping but no doubt there are others. What is striking, however, is that when matters need recording on paper for definite purposes such as charting progress or recording material for research, supplementary notes have to be made. Efforts have been made to bring sense and order into note-keeping (see page 8) and have not been widely successful. The nature of the records we keep needs more attention; they consume a great deal of time, energy, effort, paper, and space to no proportionate advantage, and writing clear, comprehensive, and concise clinical notes is a skill which deserves more teaching than it receives.

Clinical work in progress requires supervision. Even the most experienced practitioner gains enormously from discussion and consultation sessions with colleagues. This is time-consuming, but unsupervised, unmonitored work is a false economy. As always, things can go to the other extreme and a style of work can develop in a clinical team where nothing can happen and no decisions are taken without supervision piled upon supervision and much preoccupation with mutual checking-up. Should this chronic, fulminating condition show signs of developing it indicates a need to review working relationships; the problem often lies in areas of overlap between the functions of different disciplines.

A SYSTEM FOR MANAGEMENT

Special techniques and management strategies cannot be a substitute for a style of working which helps the unhappy adolescent and his apprehensive family to have enough confidence in the clinician to proceed. It is probably impossible adequately to imagine what it must be like for a patient and family to expose to unknown professional workers the muddled hopes, fears, aspirations, misunderstandings, areas of ignorance, mistakes, weaknesses, and failures that in some incomprehensible way have led the adolescent and family, often reluctantly, to seek psychiatric help. It is important for the clinician to remember that his first duty is to put the people who come to him at ease and to try to help, and in a polite and relaxed way. Sometimes a beginner in clinical psychiatry, anxious about psychiatry's woolly and sentimental reputation, will be unnecessarily crisp and brusque. It is important also to accept that anger, hostility, and complaints on the part of adolescent and parents are usually due to anxiety; it is a real blunder when the tyro mistakes this for arrogance or, still worse, confidence, and in his own anxiety tries to put worried people in their place. He must also allow people time for what they have probably prepared themselves to say by way of explanation, and he should explain how his team goes about assessment and what is going on, because not without justification people have no idea what a psychiatrist may or may not do; if he fell asleep they might think it some sort of a test. He must decide for himself what to say about his assessment but it is essential to explain something in plain language and whether what he has found seems to be, for example, an illness, a set of emotional problems and worries, misbehaviour that will really have to stop, or family misunderstandings that are getting everyone upset. People worry about madness, and brain disorder causing it. If the psychiatrist is absolutely certain of a diagnosis, for example a schizophrenic illness, my own view is that he should say so, and allow time for explanations and questions. If it is impossible to give the problem a clear name, he should say this too and explain that he will try to help and keep everyone in the picture, as, together, problems and possible solutions are clarified. It is worth mentioning the very different ways in which psychiatric terms are used even in the best regulated circles, and inviting adolescent and family to discuss with him anything frightening read in books, newspapers, or heard on television.

With this reminder that in clinical interviews form is no less important than content, the following list may be helpful, not as a clinical *vade-mecum*, but as a guide to thinking in adolescent psychiatry.

1. What needs to change, in the adolescent?
   What if anything is wrong, in his physiology, his pattern of behaviour, his thinking and feeling?
   What needs to grow and develop, in his social skills, his educational and creative abilities?
2. What needs to change in his circumstances? What needs to stay the same?
   How should his family change? Are there things they can do to help the adolescent with his problems? Are there ways they can assist the clinician? What do they need to know, as parents and as participants in treatment? What skills do they need to learn? Are there more fundamental changes needed in the way the parents respond to the adolescent, for example do the parents appear to have problems as individuals or in their marital relationship? What skills and strengths need to be affirmed and encouraged?
3. What else needs to change? What else, outside treatment, needs to be done?
   What do other significant people in the adolescent's life have to know and do? School teachers for example? And again, what resources and skills need recognition, affirmation, and encouragement?
4. What else does the clinician need to know?
   Diagnostic monitoring continues throughout therapy. What does the clinician need to know now (for example about the adolescent's present state and circumstances) and at what intervals should re-evaluation take place? Psychological testing or information from school, for example, may be needed now, in a few months' time and in a year. When will progress be reviewed? Should a date for reviewing progress be made now?
5. Is it clear who will be doing what?
   Individual treatment, the exchange of information, work with the family and consultative or collaborative work with other professionals may be planned; who is going to undertake these areas of work? Is it clear to family and team who is responsible for what? Are any proposed roles considered difficult or incompatible (for example individual psychotherapy with an adolescent and family therapy with his family)? Should someone be identified as a key worker to help liaison and coordination between the people involved? How will they keep in touch? How will the referring professional and family doctor be kept informed?

6. How will change be monitored?

How will information be shared and difficulties resolved while work is in progress? How will change and development be anticipated and matters arising coped with (for example symptoms and behaviour changing, the adolescent leaving home or school and seeking work or changes in the ways in which the family perceives and responds to events). When will meetings to review progress be held? With whom? Should the clinical team's involvement be seen as indefinite by the family, or should a time limit be set? Which is therapeutically appropriate? How will ending treatment or any foreseen change of therapists be anticipated and worked with? What will adolescent and family understand by progress, or lack of it?

7. Supervision, support, and learning

How experienced and skilled in the tasks set them are the clinical workers concerned? What supervision and support is planned? What problems can be foreseen and by what machinery will they be coped with? How will knowledge about the problems (from the literature; from the team's experience) be fed into meetings? What can other colleagues learn from progress with this case? By what means?

Chapter 17

Psychodynamic, Social, and Behavioural Approaches

INTRODUCTION: PROBLEMS IN PSYCHOTHERAPY
WITH ADOLESCENTS

The various schools of psychotherapy and social therapy have their rules and internally consistent theories and most psychotherapists are quite definite about who they will see, with what frequency, in what circumstances and what limits they will set on themselves as well as on their clientele.

The rules the psychiatrist or psychotherapist may quite properly adopt for a piece of psychotherapeutic work with adults or older independent adolescents, however, will often fail to fit the requirements of clinical work with the younger adolescents discussed in this book.

There are four main reasons for this. First, there is so much else to be done with other people. It is certainly possible for an adolescent to be seen for individual psychotherapy with the rest of the family receiving no advice, progress reports, or other liaison with the therapist; but that is unusual, and once the therapist engages in some sort of work with other members of the family this affects the psychotherapeutic relationship with the adolescent. It is not, in my view, necessarily incorrect for the individual psychotherapist to have a relationship with the parents too, though some would say so. But it does affect the psychotherapeutic relationship, and this requires thought and the anticipation of possible problems, for example anxieties about confidentiality, parental intrusiveness or the psychotherapist becoming too closely identified with the parents. If an adolescent is in a residential unit, this poses other problems; if an adolescent confides to his psychotherapist his wish to run away or hints at suicide or self-injury how much should the psychotherapist share with the residential care or nursing staff? Provision has to be made, explicitly, for what is or is not confidential when a team as opposed to an individual is responsible for overall care.

Second, and related to this, there is almost always work to be done with other issues, for example to do with social life and school. An adolescent may need advice to get his hair cut for an interview for a job; this sort of thing does not come readily to most psychotherapists who might be quite startled at the proposal that they take an authoritative, parental line with patients. Either the psychotherapist must be prepared to offer this sort of comment, or there must be someone else to do so, which brings us back to the first point again.

But it is not only a matter of ensuring that sensible, practical advice is available, and this leads to the third point. Most people who work with adolescents find they must engage in active conversation with them, being prepared to offer comments and criticisms, answer (or refuse to answer) personal questions, and express opinions. The stock rejoinder 'I wonder why you ask' will be taken as phoney, which in a sense it is because the adolescent's style of talk will often be exploratory, circumstantial, even experimental, negotiating for a relationship with the psychotherapist; there is no enduring reason with psychodynamic implications why he asked. The psychotherapist who assumes (or still worse, interprets) Oedipal conflict, for example because an adolescent asks if he or she is married, may well become thoroughly diverted into insignificant issues and, probably, uncomprehending silence. The adolescent's psychotherapist must, first and foremost, be a real person whom the adolescent can take on. This is consistent with the models of emotional development discussed on page 76, and also with Anna Freud's views (1958) of the adolescent characteristic of using a range of defensive manoeuvres. Like Lorand (1961) and others, she has commented on the difficulty of establishing a therapeutic alliance with many adolescents.

One of the fundamental principles of psychodynamic psychotherapy is that in the therapeutic relationship past feelings and fantasies are resurrected and re-enacted so that the adolescent might perceive in the therapist, for example, a punitive and critical father, or a seductive and undermining mother. But the development of such internal models of past relationships is not so well established in the developing adolescent; perhaps in adult psychotherapy the adult unconsciously consents to have an anal fixation or Jungian dreams to meet the psychotherapist's and his or her own needs for a relationship. Adolescents tend to be more exploratory, to have less guile and sophistication, and their inner feelings and images are still in transition. Moreover, just as the adult patient often has adolescent-type problems, the adolescents seen by psychiatrists quite often have immature, infantile needs and reactions. It is not that 'straight' psychotherapy cannot be undertaken with adolescents, but it needs considerable spadework first, and this lengthy preliminary work is to do with establishing mutual roles, clarifying that the therapist is neither parent, teacher, policeman nor peer, but adult, human, interested, professional, expert, non-patronizing, non-seductive and friendly.

Fourth, those who take a friendly, interested, and informal approach to adolescents, particularly if they do things with them rather than try earnestly to engage them in 'meaningful, ongoing relationships' will very often be chosen by the adolescent as someone to confide in. One of the recurring disappointments of adolescent psychotherapy and counselling is the trained professional worker abandoned in an office, reading journals, while the boy or girl regales a less formally experienced member of staff with confidences and complexes. The point is not simply that the latter detracts from 'proper' psychotherapy; it may do, or it may also become useful psychotherapy if the person selected is provided with supervision and support; it may well be a useful relationship anyway. The adolescent, partly because of the state of his psyche and partly because of his social circumstances, 'spills over' into a range of relationships which may include proper psychotherapy, quasi-psychotherapy, and ordinary adolescent–adult relationships. From any or all of these relationships the adolescent may gain a great deal. The clinician's task is to know what is going on, to nurture what seems helpful, to discourage what seems positively unhelpful, and to leave alone what is unhelpful but inocuous. There are times when an adolescent must be expected to deal with certain issues at the time and place provided and with the person available, and there are times when this is inappropriate.

Example 12
An adolescent in an in-patient unit has fears of homosexuality which he will not discuss with his psychotherapist, but which he feels able to discuss with a female nurse. At a case conference one proposal is made that the nurse must refuse to discuss the topic, and tell him to bring it up at the psychotherapeutic session. Another suggestion is that the nurse should take over, with therapeutic supervision, this aspect of the boy's problems. The suggestion which is adopted and which works is that the nurse (supervised by her senior nurse, not by a psychotherapist) helps the boy explore why he has trouble taking the topic to his psychotherapist, and ways of doing so.

Much of the above is true of other forms of work too, and arises from the point made earlier that in work with children and adolescents one is concerned with care, education, and upbringing as well as with treatment, and they influence each other in ways that do not intrude to the same extent in work with adults.

The implications for the clinician are:

(a) to strike a reasonable balance between clarity about clinical goals and methods while encouraging normal life with all its untidiness to proceed for the adolescent and family;

(b) to know what is going on without interfering unless one sort of help is undermining another;

(c) to be consistent enough without being inflexible, and professional without being pompous;

(d) when problems and dilemmas arise, to be honest and explicit, for example 'We're meeting you all as a family especially to talk over these difficult worries together; but, Mrs B., You only talk about them with the nursing staff. That doesn't help Mr B. or the children. What do you think? What do you think we should do?'

THE PSYCHOTHERAPIES AND RELATED WORK – ATTEMPTS AT DEFINITION

In *psychotherapy*, a relationship which is mutual, interacting, and sustained and involves both feelings and cognitive processes (Hinde, 1979; 'perception and love': Wyss, 1966) is actively and systematically used by the psychotherapist to enable change in the patient. The goals for change may be the correction of disorder, emotional and personal development, or usually both. This may happen in other relationships too, but not systematically. An adolescent may overcome fears and gain confidence through playing games or in group activities, but this is educational or social therapy rather than psychotherapy in so far as it need be regarded as therapy at all.

The method by which psychotherapy proceeds may involve primarily talk; but in children and adolescents the medium may be play, art or other forms of activity. Again, art, music, and drama are educational in the widest sense, essential for development in their own right, and are essential for all adolescents. They are psychotherapeutic when used specifically and systematically to encourage development or correct disorder in a disturbed boy or girl.

In group therapy, group feelings and relationships are used to bring about emotional and behavioural change. Group therapy with adolescents overlaps with *social therapy*, where personal and social skills and conduct are modified by experiencing social obligations and expectations. Most residential adolescent units, emphasizing the importance of using peer–peer and adolescent–adult relationships in clinical management, are socially therapeutic ('milieu therapy'). But the *therapeutic community* (see page 39 and Figure 29) is a specially organized setting which relies primarily or entirely on such social relationships to bring about change and growth.

Complete precision about these different types of approach to adolescents is impossible; some are clearly primarily therapeutic (systematic treatment aimed at correcting disorder) while others are better regarded as primarily educational and creative, enhancing normal growth and development. Is it worth trying to make broad distinctions between *therapy* (treatment) and the rest? I feel it is, because in adolescent psychiatry we are dealing with young people's emerging

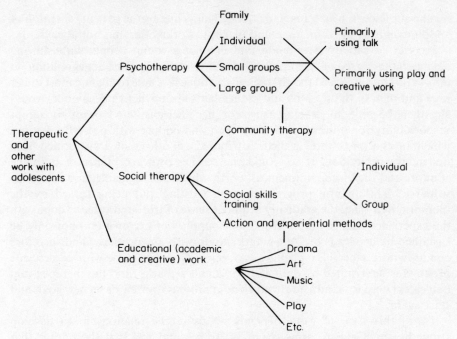

Figure 29   Psychotherapies and other work with adolescents

individuality, autonomy and responsibility, and it matters whether the person concerned is a patient or a pupil because his or her status, self-image, and self-esteem are affected by such things.

Individual psychotherapy

Individual psychotherapy is a difficult task with adolescents; it is time-consuming, and requires considerable commitment from adolescent and thera-pist. Accordingly it should not be entered into lightly, but prescribed with the care and selection with which one would prescribe a drug.

First, it is important to make sure that there is a broadly definable task for psychotherapeutic work; a task can be reasonably clearly defined without needing precision about detail. (For example, a preliminary task for an isolated, articulate girl with a long history of family and institutional instability and persistent suicidal attempts, was to see if she was able to express her anger and self-destructiveness in an individual psychotherapeutic relationship instead of in her behaviour.) Implicit in the recognition of the task is to show that it (and therefore the adolescent) is taken seriously; establishing a regular, predictable time and place for work in itself takes the boy or girl seriously in a way few adults may have done before. This can produce mixed feelings of security and anxiety for the adolescent, who refuses to attend. This is met by the patient repetition of appointments at the same time and place; it works often but not always.

Second, in rapidly developing and changing young people with shifting defences the goals of therapy will require reaffirming or renegotiating at intervals. Thus, if indeed the girl refered to above was able to confine most of her rage and pain to the sessions and reduce her self-destructive behaviour, would she then be able to develop trust for her therapist, and begin to accept responsibility for possessing, dealing with and coping with powerful feelings which in the past were evaded, attributed to others or transformed into destructive behaviour? If so, could she see her own acceptance of both the comfort and the disappointment as worth while, then valuable, and herself as valuable? This painful progress through trusting and being valued by the therapist, and using the gradually acquired sense of trust and value to cope with the experience that she must grow some supplies of her own and not only be sustained by his, leads on to new tasks to do with independence and therefore coping with further loss, change, and gains. Often in work with adolescents progress is interrupted by dramatic crises and setbacks, and the therapist and adolescent need to stand aside from work in progress, review its set new goals and start again.

Third, this style of work depends on using the relationship to develop strengths; in Kleinian terms (page 84) to see and feel that the notion that oneself, someone else or things in general are neither totally bad nor totally good but both, to live with resulting disappointment and find that this is all right; in Eriksonian terms (page 91) to advance through paranoia and mistrust to hope, through lack of control to self-control; in terms of Winnicott and Bowlby (page 108) to feel safe enough in an attachment to experiment, explore and play – in this case exploring new feelings and new ways of being, and learning that a competent adult can stand firm, be himself or herself and survive and thereby refute the patient's implied or explicit proposal that 'it' (and the patient) is all a waste of time. Again, in terms of attachment theory, learning to play the dangerous game of being a new sort of person with new ideas and new feelings *and* with the potential for new and different attachments and relationships. What the adolescent's psychotherapist in general should not do is to strip away defensive structures, try to rework previous experience, or attempt new insights or to reorganize the personality (Weiner, 1970a).

Reflecting (perhaps unconsciously) Jung's view, Miller (1959) and Laufer (1964) recommend encouraging rather than challenging the adolescent's concern with present and future rather than the past. These approaches taken together reflect the reality that in the psychotherapy of developing young people one is not simply reworking past material; the therapeutic relationship is a real and new relationship which contains elements of care and nurturing as well as therapy.

This is another reason why adolescent psychotherapy is so demanding, and leads to the fourth point: individual psychotherapy with adolescents requires experience, and all but the most experienced should have either supervision or consultative sessions to help keep on course and to provide support.

Fifth, the 'overflow' already referred to (page 285) must not be ignored or wished away but dealt with. In the case already referred to (an in-patient) the psychotherapist explained to the girl that she would have to leave to him (that is entrust to him) what material to keep confidential and what to share with nursing staff (for example the expression of suicidal wishes). The same applies to entreaties 'not to tell my parents'. The honesty and concern expressed by this approach override any theoretical interference with the psychotherapeutic process.

Sixth, again for the reasons given by A. Freud (1958) and Weiner (1970a), interpretations should be used with care. This statement needs slight qualification; the bald 'you are expressing X' when the adolescent has said Y is likely to be taken as impertinent and incorrect, and if it happens to approach the truth the more unhelpful anxiety and denial it can generate. As Dare (1977) points out, there are many sorts of interpretation. For example the therapist can speak for the young person's feelings at being seen in a psychiatric clinic, or comment on links between how the boy or girl feels or what he or she is drawing or playing and current events in his or her life. Reference to psychoanalytic hypotheses should in my opinion be avoided. They almost always make no sense to the adolescent, but they are often useful to guide the psychotherapist's approach.

Example 13

The psychodynamic part of the formulation for a fearful, overcompliant boy is that his tension and overconscientiousness are derived from earlier fears of challenging an angry and punitive father. In psychotherapeutic sessions (using art) the therapist, with the idea of castration anxiety in mind, but not interpreted to the adolescent, engages the boy in a trusting relationship and proceeds to confront him about his work, an argument which their relationship readily survives. It is neither here nor there whether at some level of cognitive and affective integration the boy really fears loss of his genitals; it is a convenient symbol for a punishing, undercutting retribution following self-assertion. The therapist leads the boy into increasing self-assertion which he discovers is safe.

I am not sure what to make of the paradoxical intervention, a technique which has generated much enthusiasm recently. Evans (1980) points out its relationship to that notorious *bête noire* the double-bind, and proposes that intrapsychic double-binding is possible and different, and is part of the ambivalence which plays so prominent a part in adolescent intrapsychic functioning. The power of ambivalence is its intensity; it is not merely doubt about choice, but the attempt to hold two important and completely opposing wishes. Evans gives as an example a girl displaying her cleavage while pretending that she is not; he comments on her showing the hairs on her chest 'as a means of noticing what she is doing, expressing interest in her general development and also simultaneously ignoring the central feature, namely her wish to flaunt her sexuality in an inappropriate manner, by labelling as positive an irrelevancy' (Evans, 1980).

The paradoxical intervention appears to interfere with the power of ambivalence by presenting a proposition that acknowledges one side of the ambivalence without encouraging it; it destabilizes ambivalence, and the impotence or stasis that goes with ambivalence. Evans reminds us that it is best received against a background of affection and concern rather than preoccupation with control, and a light-hearted provocative style is more helpful than solemnity; he emphasizes that it is not the function of the therapist to score points off clients or offer sarcasm to meet his own needs. Paradoxical intervention can be particularly helpful in letting patients know how difficult the problem they present seems to be, and how much time they will need to overcome it. Often there is a confusion between the intensity of feeling to get through, round or over a problem, and the emotional investment (for reasons of safety) in hanging on to it. Stressing the time that will be needed acknowledges the size of the problem while assuming its eventual resolution; the patient is encouraged to acknowledge and experience the troublesome emotion, and this undermines the intrapsychic opposition to the emotion that in fact is just sufficient to help perpetuate it, as a weight on one side of a set of scales sustains the other.

These styles of responding to and supporting adolescents and seeing them through painful periods happen not only in psychotherapeutic relationships. The notion that some problems are big and special and complex and need big, special, complex treatments represents a reification of intrapsychic problems that is not justified by our knowledge about them. Of course people are complex, but we do not know and perhaps cannot know how much of an individual's complexity is contributing to that particular knot that has brought him or her to the psychiatric clinic. An adolescent's oddity or idiosyncrasy may become a major disability or emerge as a rewarding, interesting aspect of his or her personality with good schooling, good relationships, and good luck. So before raising the size and status of a problem to one needing psychotherapy it is as well to be sure that there is not a simpler way, perhaps one already begun with a teacher or another adult, or a new friendship formed or hobby adopted, that might not achieve much the same result or better. To emphasize again a recurring theme in this book: before embarking on treatment, it is important to see if there is a more natural, ordinary alternative, perhaps one that can be encouraged through consultation with an adult (such as a teacher) who is in a position to provide it. If this does not work, or works partially leaving a core of special difficulty which needs treatment, properly conducted consultation will reveal this too.

Individual work

This imprecise term refers to all the non-psychotherapeutic work which an adolescent may experience with, for example, a nurse, care-worker, teacher or indeed the psychiatrist, and which in many circumstances is an alternative to psychotherapy and may be preferable to psychotherapy. It includes friendly interest, discussion, support, shared activities, games, outings, and some talking over of confidences and problems. What matters is that its existence is recognized, its usefulness acknowledged, and its effect kept under review in whatever way the professional worker normally keeps work under review. An example is that given on page 285 of the nurse, taught and supervised in the ordinary way by a senior nursing colleague, who undertakes a skilled piece of nursing which enables an equally skilled piece of psychotherapy to continue.

The point has been stressed because so often an adolescent will generate a number of 'helping' adults, none of whom is sure of his or her respective roles and goals, and as a result the adolescent effectively distributes problems, collects assorted responses, and integrates nothing.

Counselling

Newsome *et al.* (1975) have pointed out that the distinction between psychotherapy and counselling is hard to make. She emphasizes that counsellors should be clear that their main area of concern is with normal developmental difficulties rather than personality problems. I have suggested elsewhere (Steinberg and Yule, 1983) that counselling as described by many of its practitioners has much in common with the process and methods of consultation (see page 350). In counselling, as in consultation between professionals, the emphasis is on normal coping, not disorder; it is not about giving advice, persuading, convincing or otherwise trying to change behaviour; it should not involve interrogating; it is a shared enterprise in which the counsellor helps the client to define and clarify problems and review them, establishing new aims and approaches (Newsome *et al.*, 1975). The implication, also, is that the client retains autonomy and responsibility for using counselling. The Rogerian model Newsome advises with its triad of warmth, empathy, and unconditional regard, and the encouragement of self-reflection, encourages personal growth (Rogers, 1951; Adams, 1965).

A firm distinction cannot always be made between psychotherapy, other individual work and counselling not least because practitioners differ about their aims and methods. But the emphases of them are different; thus an adolescent who requires psychotherapy for an emotional difficulty may also require counselling, for example for social behaviour or sex education or in clarifying vocational ambitions. The *individual work* referred to earlier, and which may be indicated instead of or as well as psychotherapy, will sometimes take the form of counselling. The term *supportive psychotherapy* is often used; I have always felt support to be something worth while in itself and kind to offer to people during periods of difficulty, and its elevation to a therapy unnecessary.

Whatever the therapy, what do you do if the adolescent will not attend, or will not stay? The psychotherapist should not despair. As already mentioned it is worth continuing to make appointments and repeatedly remind the adolescent of the psychotherapist's existence and of the expectation that he or she will come. Even if the adolescent will not come, he or she will gain something (though not enough) by at least having the experience of being taken seriously. In an in-patient setting more immature boys or girls may need to be taken firmly by the arm to psychotherapy to remind them that the therapist wants to help and means business; the boy or girl does not have to be made to stay, but reminded that this is the time he or she should see the staff member who will be there next time too. This rarely turns out to be time-wasting. At best, the adolescent will sooner or later want to see what it is that this persistent, boring adult has in mind (a grumbling 'you're *always* saying that' is something of an accolade and can represent a modest breakthrough in a relationship). Persistence in a friendly but firm, concerned but non-anxious way is often a new experience for an adolescent in chronic difficulties, and demonstrates one of the most important things the professional working with adolescents must learn, namely not to accept the characteristic adolescent proposition that the adult is useless. This is one of the most potent of the disturbed adolescent's methods of checking whether the adult world is safe enough to challenge. Middle-class professional workers, vulnerable to their own liberal-intellectual doubts about themselves, psychiatry or the world may fall into this trap and thereby let boys and girls down.

Creative and activity therapies

Creative work has very special qualities; it requires and in turn helps to develop many capacities which recur when we consider young people's abilities or disabilities, such as imagination, initiative, drive, hope, and the ability to learn and plan, play and use language (for example see Rosenblatt, 1980), to see something through to completion, meet the challenge of new exploration (see page 112), cooperate with others, cope with disappointment, and use partial failure as a base for further effort and learning. Powerful feelings are involved in creative effort, and particularly in group work such as trust exercises, role play and psychodrama where self-assertion, performance before an audience, and self-exposure challenge trust of self and trust of others. Aspects of the creative process have already been touched upon (see pages 73 and 84 and, for example, Freud, 1908; Hudson, 1966; Koestler, 1969; Vernon, 1970; Storr, 1972; Cobb, 1977; Viorst, 1980). It is too wide a subject to be reviewed here, and occupies only a marginal position in child psychology, yet creative imagination and activity are, for all their elusive qualities, of central importance in the process by which an infant becomes a competent adult.

Difficulty in such activities can be immensely painful, and even modest success enormously encouraging. The importance of the capacity to conceive of some form of aesthetic production, see it through, use it in a way as a transitional object (page 88) as a medium for a piece of personal development, and the enormous difficulties in such areas experienced by many troubled or disabled adolescents, have led to a wide range of psychotherapies which use creative work, of which art therapy is perhaps the most established (Kramer, 1978; Weaver, 1981; and for an illuminating practical account, Waller 1978). Weaver stresses that interpreting a patient's art work is an erroneous view of the practice and use of art in therapy. It is the shared process of artistic production rather than inner fantasy or the piece of art finally produced that is the most important thing; both therapist and patient relate to the artistic work which becomes the object, or alternative or additional object, of the transference. In work with many adolescents this intermediate focus for experimentation with powerful and sensitive sexual, tender, loving, aggressive or destructive feelings can provide a safe basis for therapeutic work with boys and girls for whom a direct person to person approach is too seductive or otherwise threatening.

This applies to other activities which adolescents engage in and which can enhance their development: putting on a play, as well as psychodrama; painting for fun as well as formal art therapy; fun and games and sport as well as 'activity therapy'. The distinction is that already referred to between formal therapy as treatment for a problem, and creative activity as a natural educational, developmental, and social experience. Some adolescents need creative therapies, but all adolescents must experience art, music, drama, play, and fun. While the clinical psychiatrist may prescribe one or other therapy for selected adolescents, he must also ensure that these normal things are also present in the lives of all the children he sees. Often they are not available or not being used. In relation to art therapy, Weaver (1981) suggests that 'art therapists as artists perhaps try to maximize the occasions when it is the creative work rather than the therapy which leads to dispelling neurosis'.

FAMILY WORK AND FAMILY THERAPY

The distinction already made between individual psychotherapy and individual work applies here too. There are many ways, other than family therapy, of working with the parents or families of adolescents, for example when an adolescent on a behaviour programme has the prescribed schedule applied at home by his parents. In this wider sense there is family or parental work to be done in the case of every adolescent in treatment, even if the work is simply to keep the adolescent's mother and father informed and involved in decisions.

It may emerge that one of the parents needs individual help in his or her own right – counselling or psychotherapy – and this should be kept explicitly distinct from the work with the adolescent. Similarly there may be marital work to be done with the parents. The boy or girl should know when this has been arranged. This is not to say that if the parents wish the matter to be kept private from the adolescent that this should not be respected. On the contrary, the adolescent should be told that the parents have something that they wish to discuss privately; almost invariably the boy or girl will know this anyway, and it helps to see his or her parents assert this wish and have it respected, and know that they are looking after themselves, being looked after, and their authority acknowledged. This is responsible adult behaviour, unlike embarrassed avoidance of difficult issues, and adolescents need to see adults coping reasonably competently with difficult situations. Being grown up should seem a feasible objective and a potentially enjoyable one. Adolescents can be helped considerably by seeing adults enjoying life, even though they may appear scornful of some of the means by which they do so.

Family therapy: indications and contradictions

One of the issues already mentioned is how far to work with the family when an individual adolescent is referred. This is partly a question of what the prospective patient wants, partly how the problem is formulated, and partly how far the clinician can proceed without exchanging information and clarifying responsibilities and authority with other members of the boy's or girl's family. The latter two aspects are particularly important but the first should not be ignored.

Although in a recent review Lask is right to regret the lack of adequate studies of the outcome of family therapy (Lask, 1979), and in particular notes some reports of spectacular results with minimum evidence to confirm them (Minuchin *et al.*, 1975; Liebman *et al.*, 1976), there have been some helpful and cautiously encouraging reports (Alexander and Parsons, 1973; Sigal *et al.*, 1976; Lask and Kirk, 1979; and in an adult population Langsley *et al.*, 1968, 1969). However, family therapy, according to Haley (1975) and many others, is not a treatment method alone but a particular orientation that includes many different treatment approaches. The challenging proposition of many family therapy practitioners and which is as much an ideological and conceptual position as a claim for therapeutic effectiveness, is rather like this:

> Given that concern about the way an adolescent is growing up is a family matter, and always has at least some family aspects in its causation and correction, family assessment *always* and family therapy *often* are the proper responses (Whitaker, 1975); it is the case for individual work, or work with the adolescent and one or both parents, that must be made, not the case for family therapy.

Thus the proponents of family therapy take the view that it is not possible to work properly without a family perspective, at the very least in the initial assessment. Whether one agrees with the position or not, it is not an unreasonable one for a specialist team to take. My own objection to an invariably family-orientated perspective is that individual (behavioural, physiological, or psychodynamic) or social perspectives are also reasonable and rational, and clinical work must be pragmatic and adaptable, take account of what the patient and family want (and find convenient) and must recognize that there is no reason to suppose that family therapy will not, like every other therapeutic advance, reach a peak of enthusiasm for a time and then retreat, leaving behind something well worth integrating with psychiatry and child care as a whole, and enlarging common sense.

On the question of indications and contraindications, Walrond-Skinner (1976, 1978) distinguishes between the *exclusive approach* (no contraindications), the *last resort* position (when all else has failed), the *diagnostic aid* position (family interviews as an adjunct to assessment or monitoring or maintaining progress with another treatment), and the *differential treatment* approach where practitioners endeavour to select family therapy as the treatment of choice. She confirms that at present this is a clinical judgement as to what seems to work, rather than a scientific conclusion. Her own list of indications include:

1. Symptomatology which seems embedded in a dysfunctional system of family relationships.
2. Problems presented as difficulty in a family relationship.
3. Separation problems – noting that in helping an adolescent separate from a family (and vice versa) individual treatment may be indicated alongside family therapy (Byng-Hall and Bruggen, 1974).
4. Where family members are functioning at immature levels in terms of ego psychology with paranoid–schizoid functioning, lack of ego boundaries and excessive use of denial, projection and splitting (Skynner, 1969).
5. Where family disorganization occurs at a practical, social level. Walrond-Skinner gives as examples poor, culturally disadvantaged families with poor verbal skills for whom some have contraindicated family therapy, but whom many including Minuchin *et al.* (1967) have been able to help by directive problem-solving methods.

As might be anticipated from an experienced family therapist, Walrond-Skinner's contraindications are more to do with circumstances than theoretical objections. Thus she suggests as contraindications (a) the absence of key family members or appropriately experienced family therapists, (b) when the situation has been presented too late, or (c) where another agency is involved and expects special attention or commitment to one family member (for example request for a court report). She also points out that some families have reached a point of precarious equilibrium that is best left alone, while in some cases severe illness (physical or mental) may contraindicate family therapy. In my own clinical team we have often used family therapy in this last group, recognizing (and arranging for) the individual help needed by the affected member.

In practice, I feel that *some* work with both parents, involving siblings when possible is always indicated if the adolescent is under 16 or lives at home. Family therapy is indicated if the problem, or a substantial part of the problem, makes sense in largely family dynamic terms, and if it is a practical proposition. If it is not a practical proposition (for example, if a family member will not attend) the clinician must decide for himself whether to refuse to offer a treatment approach which for this case he considers second-best (a position where principle and posturing can come rather close) or to compromise and do the best he can. My own approach is the latter except where it is quite clear that a boy's or girl's problem is serious and persisting because embedded family behaviour is undermining treatment.

Example 14

A boy of 13 with conduct problems at home and school is referred to a succession of psychiatrists all of whom see the problem in terms of parental disagreement and inconsistency in the boy's handling and the encouragement of unhealthy competition between siblings. The father, a busy executive who is often away from home for days at a time, and the mother, who refers to some marital problems but refuses to allow them to be tackled, both insist that the boy is abnormal and that only individual treatment, preferably on an in-patient basis is acceptable. From every point of view there is no reason for individual treatment; there is no psychiatric abnormality in the boy and the family pattern is clearly maintaining his behaviour in the way it is. The father is too busy to attend even an assessment interview having had enough of 'all this family nonsense'. The parents are told that regrettably there is no way the clinical team can help on these terms.

Family therapy: approaches

Bruggen and Davies (1977) distinguish between the *psychoanalytic perspective*, with the individual experience of family members as the focus, and the *systems perspective* with family behavioural systems and subsystems, rules and boundaries, as the focus, the two representing end-points on a continuum of theory and practice. The primarily psychoanalytic worker will offer observations and interpretations, for example to do with projection and projective identification, while the primarily systems-orientated worker is more concerned with the behaviour of the family members to each other and to the therapist, and the way this behaviour is part of a dynamic maintaining members in particular roles, including the sick role. Thus the systems therapist actively intervenes, directing attention, confirming some roles (for example the parents' authority and need to support each other), challenging others (for example refusing to see an anorexic teenager as a young woman but as a particularly infantile child), intervening in seating arrangements and behaviour, and acting as a model for behaviour and for the general mood of the proceedings (Minuchin, 1974; Minuchin *et al.*, 1980).

Dare (1975) has helpfully categorized interventions in family therapy as follows:

1. *Those used to establish the overall strategy*, acknowledging that the choice of treatment (family), the setting (clinic), the frequency of attendance proposed, the importance of father being present, all communicate something important and therefore constitute interventions.
2. *Prescriptive interventions*, which are medical model interventions whose implications may need to be qualified by other interventions. Thus prescription of a bell-and-pad for an enuretic child, for example, conveys an impression that the whole problem is in the bladder control of the child, which may not be the case.
3. *Contractual interventions* which establish the nature of the treatment alliance and the focus for work, which is affirmed by the therapist's comments and general approach. Thus a family may want to use a session to lecture a wayward adolescent, which the therapist points out is not what they are there for.
4. *Establishment of a mutual language*, for example to point out ambiguities and muddle and clarify and confirm what is being communicated to whom.
5. *Interpretations* which Dare distinguishes from verbal interventions in general, and limits to unconscious significances in speech and behaviour which the therapist infers and points out.
6. *Establishment of anamnesis* to put current events and experiences in a family historical context.
7. *Active interventions*, for example using role-play, psychodrama or enacting or rehearsing certain tasks.

Family therapy and the clinical team: some conclusions

In the sort of clinical practice envisaged in this book family therapy will have an important place alongside several alternative styles of treatment. Other sorts of intervention may be used instead of or as well as family therapy, or family therapy may take place during a stage of management, for example when a separation problem is coped with by family therapy giving way in due course to individual therapy for the adolescent and marital therapy for the parents. The eclectic approach suggested here may cause the team unease. If the clinical team can be flexible and adaptable without being inconsistent, use good ideas from a number of sources pragmatically, make rational cases clearly for one approach or another while recognizing that ideology and feelings are in general more powerfully motivating, and have disputes that do not become destructive, it will provide a good group dynamic model for its clientele and indeed its trainees, and one within which learning and development can take place. But note that such disputes are real, not ritualized, and will continue while the family approach finds its proper place in child care and child psychiatry.

For useful short reviews of family therapy see Bruggen and Davies (1977), Walrond-Skinner (1978), and Breunlin and Breunlin (1979).

SOCIAL AND GROUP THERAPIES

Much in the systems approach to family therapy seems to be social therapy rather than psychotherapy, in that it manipulates social relationships to bring about change in the social system and in the members of that system. The same can be said of much of group therapy.

Elsewhere with colleagues I have described the development of small groups first at the adolescent unit at Long Grove Hospital and subsequently at Bethlem (Steinberg *et al.*, 1978) For the mixed group of adolescents admitted to both units, varying widely in psychiatric disorder, intellectual level, and verbal skills, the emphasis in these groups has been to use social expectations and opportunities primarily to extend social skills, with the assumption that the acquisition of such skills has a secondary effect on emotional maturation. Whether progress in the groups causes or results from progress outside them, and how much of what is acquired in the groups persists beyond them, is difficult to assess; the first step, and currently the subject of an operational study, being the development of means of monitoring group events reasonably objectively.

Despite the uncertainty of effect, however, we felt small group work to be justified in any case because boys, girls, and staff tended to function in small groups anyway, and setting time aside for regular, systematic, and supervised group work became a useful setting for learning about interpersonal relationships, and provided a focus for activities (for example outings, games, farewell parties) additional to those of the school and ward. Each small group has acquired a time, territory, and quality of its own, with, for most of the children, a sense of belonging which has seemed distinct from 'belonging' to their family, school, or the hospital. Although some children and some groups have often enough done particularly important work (for example determination to cope with, befriend and help a particularly seriously disturbed or disabled member, or deal with the loss of individual members, patients or staff), the basic sights have always been set at a modest level, to provide as common a denominator as possible for groups which include young people who may be of low intelligence, autistic, seriously misbehaving or acutely schizophrenic, as well as those with conduct and emotional problems who are bright and articulate. Thus staff new to the groups have learned to appreciate elementary achievements such as recognition by adolescents of the expectations that they should be at the groups; arriving on time and staying to the end; behaving reasonably to other members; talking and listening, and later sharing with and showing concern for others, and showing initiative, all as important social skills in the approximate order one

Table 12 Examples of goals for small group work based on Erikson's developmental model

Stage in epigenetic chart (Erikson, 1965)	Taylor's (1972) reinterpretation of Erikson (slightly modified)	Erikson's 'favourable outcome'	Interpretation of favourable outcome in terms of group goals
Trust versus mistrust	I am loved versus I am not loved	Drive, hope	Turning up; staying in room; experiencing the group as trustworthy; the group being trustworthy
Autonomy versus shame, doubt	I am free versus I am dependent	Self-control, will-power	Listening; trying to join group; asserting and setting own limits; the group being assertive, setting limits, contemplating acceptance of newcomers
Initiative versus guilt	I will versus I will not	Direction, purpose	Trying to take part: contemplating using the group; the group members contemplating making plans
Industry versus inferiority	I can versus I cannot	Method, competence	Experimenting with planning: finding that plans can 'come off'
Identity versus role confusion	I am versus I am not	Devotion, fidelity	Experiencing self as a group member; experiencing group as a body to be joined, avoided, left, returned to; sense of past and future for group and for self in group.
Intimacy versus isolation	We are You are versus I am not	Affiliation, love	Sharing; cooperating; liking; involvement
Generativity versus stagnation	I can create and give versus I must hold on	Production, care	Suggesting doing things for group, for group members, with other groups, sharing
Ego integrity versus despair	We have been versus I have been robbed	Renunciation, wisdom	The group has been worth while for us; giving to the group

might hope an immature, disturbed adolescent to achieve them. We have used goals derived from Erikson (page 91 and Table 12), a system which of course goes beyond adolescence and into late maturity. Our adolescent in-patient groups have, of course, included many young people who had so far failed to negotiate many pre-adolescent stages of emotional maturation in that many were immature, demanding, impulsive and untrusting, and for many we considered even modest advances as described above as representing significant progress. Thus a quite different standard has been set compared with that for group work with, for example, articulate people with psychoneurotic problems. For young people with autism, mental retardation, major conduct disorders or psychotic illness, it is an important step to grasp that they are taken seriously enough by a group of peers and adults to be expected in the same place and at the same time, twice a week; it is a further step to arrive there and on time, without undue peer and adult pressure; it is a further achievement to stay for the duration of the session and another to begin to use the group and, later, to begin to experience and reflect about feelings in relation to others, take responsibility for his or her own behaviour, share feelings and ideas and experiment with making individual and group plans. Many boys and girls have made progress in the groups without even achieving the traditional group ideal of sustained reflective talk.

The principles we have used are very broadly adapted from the experience with adolescent groups of Evans (1965, 1966), Acton (1970), and Bruce (1975, 1978) with the addition of an emphasis on group activities, both spontaneous and planned. These authors pointed to:
1. the importance of the adolescent group therapist being active, not passive;
2. the necessity to set firm limits on behaviour;
3. recognizing that adolescents preferred to learn from peers, so as much work as possible should be done with and through peers;
4. the difficulty adolescents have with feelings about the therapist, so that in groups boys and girls feel less vulnerable;
5. the importance of the recurring theme of the adolescent's challenge to adults: that they are not good enough, strong enough, caring enough or competent enough to deal with the adolescent's anger or despair, or to convince the adolescent that anything (the adolescent, the unit, psychiatry, life in general) is worth while. As pointed out earlier, this challenge to adults, which at its most fundamental asks if it is really worth growing up, can feed readily into normal adult self-doubt and vulnerability, with the staff member wondering if the adolescent might not be right.

Bruce in particular (1975, 1978) emphasizes the importance of staff survival and sees the group as a 'play area' in which what he describes as the 'murder game' can be played safely. This is a useful model for groups of young people with maturational problems, and relates closely to the attachment model (see page 106) in which a secure bond with trusted others provides a safe base from which to explore. Baby animals need to play with their parents and sibs at being ferocious in order to learn to assert themselves without doing damage or being damaged. Young people need much the same experience, and if they have not learned this fine balance in earlier childhood, they are not so finely tuned to deal with adolescence, when the realities and social implications of their verbal, physical, and sexual power make them so much more potent; and adults correspondingly more vulnerable, and therefore less able to cope with the boy or girl who still needs a good deal of looking after.

The groups at Bethlem are used as an adjunct to the therapeutic aspects of the unit community; all in-patients go into groups, with no selection by diagnosis. Only totally destructive behaviour in the group, making it quite impossible to do any work while that boy or girl is present, results in the adolescent's temporary suspension from group attendance; instead the boy or girl stays in his or her room, where the group visits him or her from time to time and awaits his or her return. From time to time in the lives of each group there is a period of much walking about, visiting and pursuing errant members. Groups tend to wax and wane; change, loss, and the arrival of new participants disrupt group life and provide valuable foci for work.

Small group work with adolescents tends to be regarded generally as theoretically desirable, extremely difficult to sustain except where groups are very highly selected, and uncertain in outcome (Kraft, 1968; Frank and Zilbach, 1968; Berkowitz, 1972; Meeks, 1974; Abramowitz, 1976). Almost universally the goals are similar: to support, assist, and confront the adolescent through peer interaction; deal with current issues; provide a forum to learn new ways of dealing with relationships; reduce feelings of isolation and replicate a family-type setting to do work not achieved by the family (Evans, 1965, 1966; Berkowitz and Sugar, 1975; Weisberg, 1979; Heacock 1980c).

There is varying opinion on selection for groups. In general the view seems to be that in in-patient small group work the attempt is worth making to work with mixed diagnostic groups, despite the problems, and not to be embarrassed about excluding an individual from time to time; and for out-patient groups, to be more careful to select those who might best fit together. Whatever the ideal approach might turn out to be in this respect, it important to remember that any treatment in an in-patient setting has a quite different impact from that for out-patients. Living at home and living in hospital are totally different experiences and each treatment is embedded in its background in a different way. Coming home from school, having tea and going up the street to an out-patient group (perhaps accompanied by a friend or two who will wait in the waiting room) is quite different from attending a group which is composed entirely of people with whom the boy or girl lives and who are involved in other aspects of the treatment and care.

Social skills training has less emphasis on patient–therapist feelings, although of course they are there. The setting may be individual or in a small group, and the techniques used may include role play, psychodrama, role modelling

(Sarason, 1968) or simply rehearsal, for example of an interview for a job. Although some adolescents are extremely vulnerable in such experiential situations, many enjoy the experience and benefit from it, especially when the occasion is reasonably well structured with adults firmly in charge. With a group it is particularly important to help boys and girls feel safe enough to take part by having present an adequate number of adults who trust each other, and who proceed with confidence. Disturbed adolescents are highly vulnerable to anything like a vacuum; often they will become very anxious about lack of adult confidence and control, and either withdraw or fill the gap with useless and disruptive behaviour.

BEHAVIOUR THERAPIES

The difference between the focus of the behavioural approach and that of other treatments is its concern with observable individual behaviour rather than inferences about intrapsychic processes. There is no theoretical reason why the difficulties of an adolescent with problematic behaviour (for example enuresis, conduct problems, or phobic or obsessional behaviour) should not be understood both in terms of the psychodynamic processes by which a pattern of behaviour becomes established, and the behavioural and circumstantial processes that perpetuate it and which may be more significant aetiologically at the time the adolescent is seen, and more amenable to change. The simple model given in Figure 20, page 123, can be applied to many adolescent and family problems.

Correspondingly, behaviour therapy alone or in combination with family therapy or individual psychotherapy may be helpful. In intractable problems such as certain obsessional states we have found at Bethlem that a combined approach is helpful; management then has three components:
1. Definition of the problem and setting up a behavioural approach to cope with it.
2. Teaching the adolescent's family to implement the behavioural programme.
3. Using the family's inability to work effectively on the behaviour programme as a focus for family therapy. For example, the parents may be unable to work together, act consistently, give clear messages, support each other, or behave with both affection and firmness to their children.

This dynamic–behavioural model is consistent with that of attachment theory (Figure 16, page 110). Experiences and behavioural responses become incorporated into the memory and behavioural repertoire of the individual. The child who has to throw a tantrum to gain the attention of his depressed mother may incorporate this internal working model, to use Bowlby's phrase (page 108), and resort to it in certain circumstances; in adolescence, if he fails to secure adult attention by social techniques he has acquired and adopted over the years (for example asking, hinting, nagging, whining, threats) he may in his rising state of arousal and distress resort to what used to work, namely a tantrum, which is one way of conceptualizing the phenomenon of regression.

This mechanism may operate within a family and be responsive to directive family therapy; or it may be largely determined by the adolescent's inner image of his teacher, say, as an unresponsive mother, and at least in theory be responsive to counselling and psychotherapy; or there may be no functionally significant inner image and outbursts of impulsive, aggressive behaviour follow frustration in certain circumstances as a complex behavioural response. While it is usually impossible and always difficult to give different weights to different aspects of a formulation, if a significant component seems behaviourally determined it is reasonable to begin with a behavioural approach, though bearing in mind Dare's advice about the inevitable attribution of some form of significance to any authoritative prescription (page 297).

According to Yule (1977) what distinguishes behavioural methods from other treatment is their dependence on a scientific, problem-solving strategy of intervention. This requires four steps:
1. Objective definition and description of what exactly the problem consists of, which includes the circumstances before and after the problem behaviour as well as details of the problem itself.
2. Setting up hypotheses to account for the observation in terms of what is sufficient and necessary for a particular piece of behaviour to occur and persist and what enables it to be extinguished. This is termed a functional analysis of behaviour.
3. The hypothesis is tested, which means that a systematic programme is implemented and systematically monitored, so that any small changes that occur can be detected and used, if necessary, to modify the programme.
4. Evaluating the outcome by using research designs to demonstrate connections between treatment and outcome.

Yule points out that the two basic principles which guide behavioural treatment are that behaviour is responsive to particular stimuli, and to its consequences; and that both aspects include social factors in the environment, that is other people and how they behave and respond. These principles are embodied also in social learning theory, which is concerned with the development of behaviour within interpersonal and social relationships, from which it follows that (a) a proportion of problematic behaviour is likely to be due to failure to learn acceptable behaviour, including failure to be taught, and (b) that the mechanisms for learning unacceptable or otherwise problematic behaviour need not be in themselves abnormal (Patterson, 1969; Yule, 1976; Brown and Christie, 1981).

The careful, systematic approach adopted by behaviour therapists can be helpful in ways not directly connected with behavioural theory.

Example 15
An enuretic boy of 12 is referred to a child psychiatric clinic for psychotherapy because the bell-and-pad prescribed in a school health clinic has not worked after a trial of several months. The boy and his

parents are as unhappy about being seen in a psychiatric clinic as they are worried about the persisting bed-wetting; there is no psychiatric disorder the clinical team can find, and the family appear to be functioning quite normally. The battery on the bell-and-pad machine, however, is not. Careful questioning, probing beyond the referral letter (which states that the bell-and-pad has failed after prolonged efforts), reveals that on only two or three nights in the past three months has the equipment been set up properly or worked properly. Whatever may or may not be wrong with the bladder, child or family, attempts at a simple and effective treatment have clearly not yet begun.

Precisely the same can happen in an in-patient unit, school or children's home when an effort is made to ensure that a particular response always follows certain behaviour (for example social reinforcement every time an incontinent adolescent uses the lavatory properly, or an easily angered boy manages to contain his temper). Again and again the psychiatrist or psychologist may be informed that 'it' is not working, and as many times find that 'it' is not in fact being carried out as agreed. The method may not have been properly planned; not properly taught; if properly taught to senior nursing, teaching or care staff, not properly passed on to their colleagues; not properly supervised; progress poorly documented, so that there is inadequate evidence for change or lack of change (and therefore a source of encouragement or opportunity for modification is missing); or there may be misgivings or organizational difficulties about implementing the treatment programme which are not adequately appreciated by the clinician. Maintenance of an effective therapeutic programme is hard work, requires imagination and is full of pitfalls. The difficulties listed above should not be seen as examples of awkward colleagues frustrating a sound treatment programme; on the contrary, sound treatment requires skilled teaching, supervision, consultation, and feedback between clinician and colleagues as an integral part of the programme.

Behavioural methods

The consequences of behaviour affect whether or not the behaviour subsequently occurs more or less frequently. In *operant training*, for example, social reinforcement (attention and encouragement) or a token which will give prestige or privileges is given every time desired behaviour (for example attending school) occurs. *Punishment* means doing something unpleasant to a child and invites connotations of pain and cruelty. It is often ill-timed, inconsistent and retaliatory, tends to replace rather than supplement reinforcement for good behaviour, provides an aggressive model for behaviour, and tends not to have lasting effects (Brown and Christie, 1981). On the other hand some form of punishment may be appropriate when immediate effect is crucial, for example in a case quoted by Corbett (1975) where every other measure failed to prevent a mentally retarded child's severely injurious head-banging. Some forms of punishment are used to represent clear-cut social disapproval, for example the immediate expression of anger by an adult who has been made angry by an adolescent's behaviour, or being made to pay for damage done to someone else's property. Probably this represents the normal imposition of social rules rather than behaviourism, but none the less should be applied consistently and with the rules made clear in advance.

In *negative reinforcement* a punishment (for example being sent to a bedroom) is removed when the boy or girl makes amends, for example an apology. In *time out* a positive reinforcement is removed, for example instant removal of a misbehaving young person from the scene of his or her misbehaviour. What is important in *time out* is that it is immediate, effective (that is boring) and inevitable, and each time out session should only last a few minutes. (*Seclusion*, where an adolescent is kept apart from other in-patients because of dangerous behaviour, is not the same as *time out* and fulfils a different (protective) purpose. Some legal authorities have pointed out that as time out necessarily involves seclusion – namely the boy or girl is made to stay in a particular room, if only for a short time – it requires the same scrupulous attention to ethics and legality as does seclusion, including clear prescription by a responsible person and a record kept of the event.)

An obvious point, but one to bear in mind when advising adults on the handling of children, is how often children's misbehaviour is unwittingly reinforced; thus a misbehaving child may increasingly receive attention in the classroom largely when monkeying about, and receive no attention when behaving and working well; sometimes an unhappy, neglected boy or girl may paradoxically prefer being hit and shouted at to being ignored. Or parents will eventually give in to persistent nagging; though perhaps this particular adult weakness can also reflect one of the battles young people sometimes need to win; in some forms it may represent the first stirrings of a capacity for negotiation.

Shaping refers to the way in which a behaviour reinforcement programme is gradually applied. Yule (1977) gives as an example a hyperactive child being immediately reinforced even for very brief periods of sitting still so that, step by step, a piece of behaviour present in the child's repertoire is systematically encouraged. Very careful timing and selection of reinforcers that work is as important as identifying the behaviour to be reinforced. Smiles, praise, and huges may be effective for some children, and tokens, food or sweets for others. We once found the use of Mars Bars to be a powerful reinforcer in shaping an encopretic boy into the habit of using the unit lavatory.

Modelling, in which anxious or socially inhibited children watch how more confident, competent peers and adults deal with situations can be an extremely effective therapy (see Rachman, 1972) and can speed up desensitization techniques (see Yule's review, 1975). Adolescents are sometimes reluctant to acknowledge what they learn from adults, particularly if they perceive their mentors as intrusive, patronizing or overconfident; but like younger children they mimic none the less, and some imagination and sensitivity on the part of adults is needed to enable modelling to take place without making a boy or girl self-conscious. It is also important to remember that it will happen anyway, and to see that what is available for modelling is also desirable.

In *desensitization* the boy or girl is exposed by a graded approach to a feared situation *in reality* (for example by being taken to school) or *in imagination*, in either situation with the child in a relaxed state by being in the company of a trusted person and if necessary having been taught relaxation techniques (Wolpe, 1958; Lazarus 1960; Marks, 1969; Rachman, 1974; Yule, 1977). In this context it is worth mentioning that the relationship between adolescent fearfulness about leaving home and going to school is often not as clear-cut as some clinically defined phobic states in adults. It would perhaps be convenient to differentiate between true phobic states and other problems, but as Berg (1980) has pointed out this is not easily done.

Thought-stopping, and other *cognitive behaviour therapies* and *response prevention* techniques have been used in treating some phobic and obsessional–compulsive disorders, and *self-monitoring* of progress can be effective alone or as a supplement (Stern, 1970; Kumar and Wilkinson, 1971; Meichenbaum, 1977; Mackay, 1982).

Behaviour therapy training for parents and teachers

Yule has reviewed some of the issues involved in training non-clinicians, for example an adolescent's parents or teachers in the use of behavioural methods (Johnson and Brown, 1969; Howlin *et al.*, 1973, Yule, 1975, 1977). This enables children with behaviour problems to spend more time in normal circumstances, and those in constant contact with them can put behavioural programmes into practice round the clock, and feel more competent as a result. It also goes some way towards dealing with the situation specificity of many behaviour problems of young people; thus a boy or girl may misbehave or be socially withdrawn only with certain people or in particular situations. Yule points out, however, that many parents have difficulty in putting these principles into practice and, particularly with chronically handicapped children, may need long periods of contact with training therapists;further, that training methods have not been properly evaluated; that the argument for involvement or otherwise of other siblings in the family is so far inconclusive; and that the emphasis on behavioural methods may be precisely the approach most likely to reinforce guilt in parents who feel that their behaviour towards the child has led to his or her difficulties. These difficulties can be met (see Howlin *et al.*, 1973) but require specific attention, and with these qualifications the principle of clinicians teaching effective methods to be used in normal settings is an important one. A promising development in recent years, for example, has been the application of home-based behaviour programmes for the problems of children with antisocial and aggressive behaviour from which it has emerged that aggressive children who also steal are harder to treat (see Patterson, 1973; Walter and Gilmore, 1973; and reviews by Yule, 1975, and 1978). Work with autistic children in particular has demonstrated the importance of extending behavioural and social learning programmes out of the clinic or residential unit into the home and school setting where the child will actually be spending his or her time, since improvements often remain linked to the settings in which they are brought about (see review by Rutter, 1977b).

Chapter 18

Aspects of Residential Treatment

INTRODUCTION: THE RANGE OF RESIDENTIAL CARE

Adolescents arrive in residential institutions for a variety of reasons: for treatment, for example when psychiatric treatment is unsafe or impractical on an out-patient basis; for short-term or long-term 'looking after', when the boy's or girl's natural home has broken down; for special care or education in residential schools or therapeutic communities; for safe custody, training or punishment or a combination of these things, when an adolescent's behaviour is socially unacceptable or self-destructive; and they go also into the reception, remand, and assessment centres to which local authorities in the United Kingdom have access, in which children and adolescents can be held until plans are made about where they should go next. Usually the young person arrives there as a result of intervention by social workers or police officers, sometimes at parents' request, sometimes because the breakdown of family life is already known to the worker or department concerned, sometimes because the child is simply found, literally, on the streets and is taken to a place of safety (the official term) by the police. Legal authority for taking this action is usually an interim Care Order or Place of Safety Order under the provision of the Childrens and Young Persons Act 1969.

The development of this range of provision has already been discussed (Chapter 3) and the steps in independence an adolescent is allowed by law were outlined in Table 4, page 98. The distinctions between facilities primarily for the treatment of disorder, primarily for care and development, primarily for education, and primarily for control have also been discussed; this applies equally to residential resources, and it is particularly important to clarify what precisely is needed, and whether the service selected will meet that need, when removal of a child from home is contemplated.

What can we say about these residential facilities? First, they provide a home for a very large number of young people; at least 275,000 boys and girls in England and Wales at any given time (Moss, 1975). Second, as shown in page 49 they form a most complex, vast, and variegated system with many areas of overlap and many gaps, and much controversy about what is most appropriate for whom (Tizard et al., 1975, Millham et al., 1978 a, Rutter, 1979 a; Steinberg 1981 c, 1982 a). Third, they are expensive, largely because of the high number of staff needed for the children who are there, and where they are not particularly expensive a case can almost always be made quite easily that they are in urgent need of more and better trained staff and radical material improvement. Fourth, their effectiveness and usefulness is hard to establish. Clearly a homeless boy or girl must have somewhere to live and this cannot always be provided by fostering; it is also true that some adolescents emerge successfully from psychiatric units, children's homes, and other special communities with hopes fulfilled and goals met. Between these two fixed points, however, there is a very large number indeed of children and adolescents whose selection for one or other form of residential care has been rather arbitrary and whose experience in it has on the whole not been good. Finally, systematic study of this area, with its ever-changing staff, children and practices, and the difficulty of clarifying how progress is judged, is problematic.

Rutter (1979a) points out the important distinction between the question of how an institution affects children's behaviour within, and how it affects subsequent behaviour. We know that different institutional methods result in different behaviour among the residents (Sinclair, 1971; Clarke and Martin, 1971; and see Tizard et al., 1975) and although various approaches in the residential care of delinquents have not had an appreciable effect on subsequent reconviction rates (Gibbens, 1977; Clarke and Cornish, 1978), some behavioural methods (Davidson and Seidman, 1974; Wolf et al., 1975 a, b, and review by Yule, 1978) and some general styles of staff behaviour seem to affect different delinquent boys differentially, though we have yet to determine which specific approaches help which young people. The overall picture is a relatively gloomy one, yet there are areas of progress with some young people in some regimes and this may lead to more effective selection and management.

In children's homes too, there is evidence that children's behaviour is influenced by the way staff work (Tizard, 1974) but as far as outcome is concerned many boys and girls in long-term care experience high and persisting levels of emotional and conduct problems, and this tends to be particularly true of young people with antisocial behaviour who also, and perhaps not surprisingly, experience the highest changes in care staff (Wolkind and Rutter, 1973, Wolkind and Renton, 1979; Wolkind, 1977; and review in Tizard et al., 1975).

As shown in Chapter 3, there have always been displaced children, and their history and that of the provision made for them often make unhappy stories.

Among the many factors that need consideration, such as prevention of displacement in the first place, staff training and methods in children's homes, and alternatives to living in institutions, there is the question of prestige. If a boy or girl must live away from home it seems to me that a residential school carries less stigma and indeed has a certain attractiveness compared with the image of the children's home. Possibly the concept of the boarding school at least in Great Britain carries with it sufficient ambiguity to gain something from the status of the better known independent schools; probably the overt primary aim of education conveys a less stigmatizing purpose than the need to be looked after professionally. Some of the therapeutic communities, too, have developed a style and status that helps the young people in then feel that they are somewhere special, a feeling, and a quality of such establishments, to be encouraged.

SELECTION FOR RESIDENTIAL TREATMENT OR CARE

The issue of adolescents leaving home for alternative management arises in three main ways as far as the clinical psychiatrist is concerned. He may be asked to advise upon 'placement' of a boy or girl who has committed an offence or is being assessed in a children's reception centre; he may be considering (or asked to consider) admission of the adolescent to hospital; or the boy or girl, already an in-patient, may be too young to live independently on discharge and for one reason or another the home from which he or she was admitted may be considered an unsuitable place to return to. In our experience at Bethlem two-thirds of boys and girls admitted return to the home from which they came (Turner and Bates, in preparation), although the experience of others seems to be that most adolescents admitted to hospital go on to some other kind of special facility (Barker, 1974a; Rutter, 1979a).

The special characteristics of in-patient units and, correspondingly, what is gained by admission have been described by Robinson (1957), Barker, (1947b), Hersov and Bentovim (1977). Gruber (1980), Steinberg (1982a) and elsewhere in this book (page 47). The wide range of alternatives overlap, and what distinguishes in-patient psychiatric care from other forms of care is primarily the 24-hour service provided, usually 7 days a week, with resident doctors available and shifts of psychiatric nursing staff (awake at night) who are trained to supervise adolescents, to implement treatment programmes, and to monitor changes in adolescents' mental and physical states and behaviour. This definition does not apply to children's homes, where clinical skills are not needed and night care staff 'sleep in', an arrangement which is quite satisfactory for their resident children. Nor does it apply to therapeutic communities and custodial establishments where supervision, again, does not and need not include clinical skills. The availability of psychiatrically trained nurses and doctors for adolescents who may be on medication (or who may, occasionally, need urgent medication); who may injure themselves; and who quite often have complex psychiatric, neuropsychiatric or psychosomatic problems which general physician and psychiatrist alike can find daunting, represents a specialized but essential form of care for a relatively narrow but particularly difficult spectrum of need.

SELECTION FOR IN-PATIENT CARE

The following points should be considered whenever the suggestion is made that a boy or girl in difficulties should be treated in hospital.

1. *Given that a case for psychiatric treatment has been made, can it be provided with the adolescent living at home?*

In the consultation that should be the first step in assessment it may emerge that the referring professional had not been aware of all the possible alternatives to admission, including those that the adolescent unit team can undertake. This might include the ability to take an informed and carefully calculated risk in the light of the wider experience of particularly difficult problems in-patient teams will usually have, and the capacity to admit the adolescent quickly if necessary under the care of the same workers. In practice the risks are not high, and the dangers of precipitate admission because of adult anxiety rather than because the boy or girl need urgent residential treatment are in general greater. It is true that there can be considerable disagreement in child and adolescent psychiatry about who needs admission, and where the machinery for consultation is not properly established there can be embarrassment on both sides when an experienced clinician considers only admission to be practicable and the in-patient team knows that more can in fact be done on an out-patient basis. Where such consultation is possible, however, a very useful liaison can be set up between residential unit and out-patient clinic with the latter focusing on what is needed to help the boy or girl at home and school in the knowledge that plans are in hand for urgent admission if needed.

The experience of the teams developing intensive out-patient work for adolescents and their families, rendering admission, and particularly urgent, unplanned admission unnecessary, deserves careful evaluation (see Bruggen *et al.*, 1973; Bruggen and Davies, 1977; Bruggen and Westland, 1979; Bentovim and Gilmore, 1981; Hildebrand *et al.*, 1981; and reviews by Steinberg, 1981c, 1982a).

2. *What are the positive reasons for admission to an in-patient unit?*

Using the social crisis model (Bruggen *et al.*, 1973) the reason for admission is the family's (or community workers') acknowledgement that they cannot cope with the boy or girl concerned, and this is used as a focus for family or group work, the ideal outcome being the adolescent's return to a setting now able to meet his or her needs. This is a most appropriate model for dealing with social crises and is based on quite different assumptions about the role of clinical psychiatry from those made in this book. For example, as pointed out earlier, teams taking this approach tend to prefer not to make clinical diagnoses or recommend treatment or admission on *medical* authority. It does not seem to me that this approach needs to be primarily psychiatric or hospital-based, and it could, for example, be interesting to evaluate its use as a component of a social service department's children's reception centre.

Using the clinical psychiatric model, the reasons for admission are largely to do with the need for 24-hour monitoring and management by a primarily medical and nursing team practising psychiatric assessment and treatment as defined on page 52. Although pressing a point to its logical conclusion is not always consistent with common sense, it is nonetheless worth bearing in mind that the crucial distinction between an in-patient unit and every alternative (including day-patient care) is quite simply having trained psychiatric nurses available and awake at night (many child care staff, of course, 'sleep in') with a duty psychiatrist available if necessary.

Admission is appropriate where effective assessment, or management, or both, requires particularly *medical* skills (for example medication, monitoring physical health), core *psychiatric* skills (monitoring and managing mental state) or *psychiatric team skills* (integration of physiological, psychological, and social approaches) *and* it is impractical to provide this in the home and on an out-patient or day-patient basis. This may be because the boy or girl is too hard to handle, at risk, too distressed, because he or she has individual characteristics that have proved impossible to assess adequately as an out-patient (sometimes because of a rapidly fluctuating state) or because treatment needs particularly careful titration against psychological, physiological or behavioural changes.

Psychotic illness, either acute, relapsing, insufficiently investigated or requiring a review of management is perhaps the example most fitting the above description. Individual disorders of uncertain psychological and physical origins, or with psychological and physical consequences, are other examples. Thus the management of some young people with anorexia nervosa, some hysterical states, epilepsy and other neuropsychiatric disorders and young people who injure themselves persistently or seriously, or who appear at risk from suicide are best managed in hospital for a time.

An unfortunate group of young people, small in number but cumulative, remain dependent on residential psychiatric care for a long time; some autistic, schizophrenic, or retarded children, and some with particularly chaotic disorders of personality, turn out to be quite unmanageable in settings providing specialized care and training alone. For them a combination of the need for constant and adaptable treatment and, as time passes and development proceeds, repeated attempts at physiological, behavioural, psychological, or social forms of management, requires long periods in hospital, and during this time work must be maintained with the rest of the family and such peer relationships and education as the adolescent can use must be provided. As many of such young people as possible should be found places in special communities if they cannot be looked after at home, but for a minority a long-term hospital place seems the only practical alternative, and there is a shortage of hospital units that can meet these needs, particularly for those in their teens and young adulthood. These boys and girls and their families are always hard to help. Occasionally it is possible to back up transfer to a non-clinical setting (for example a therapeutic community or children's home) by the offer of urgent readmission when necessary, but many children with these problems cope particularly badly with change, and the arrangement can fall down in practice. The problems of these young people, particularly in the 15 to 25 year age-range, deserves greater attention.

Sometimes assessment, treatment, and the monitoring of treatment require a round-the-clock approach, for example in treating enuresis, encopresis, tics, and some obsessional and phobic states when out-patient treatment has failed. A short period of intensive in-patient work is then worth trying, and is then an option rather than a last resort.

Most adolescents with conduct problems who cannot be managed at home need the medium-to long-term care and control that is best sought other than in a hospital. But the problems of some of these adolescents and their families can be complex and the special advantage of a hospital setting for their treatment is so that individual assessment can proceed while a further (or first) attempt to work with the family is made. A psychiatric unit may be the only place where psychological and developmental assessment can be made, conclusions reached about the possible benefits of behaviour therapy or psychotherapy, and, in parallel, family work undertaken with a view to *either* a return home *or* assisted separation. But there are very large numbers of young people with conduct problems, and their admission to residential units other than as a small minority can cause very serious difficulty indeed for the unit community as a whole. The admission of these boys and girls should be on a planned basis, not as emergencies, unless the particular unit is orientated especially to dealing with their problems, which general psychiatric units for adolescents as a rule are not. The in-patient team should help plan the adolescent's long-term care in close liaison with the family, social service and education departments, looking ahead to the several years' care these young people need, and the limited goals for short-term psychiatric admission carefully thought out and agreed. The adaptability of this approach, where neither the value of the psychiatric contribution nor the place the adolescent will return to (including home) may be clear at first, makes it useful for some boys and girls with such problems as drug misuse and school refusal.

As a general rule for all admissions it is worth adopting the principle that the in-patient unit is for treatment, and that the boy or girl must still have a family and home to go to at weekends, on discharge, and to regard as his or her own. If the uncertain nature of the adolescent's problems and future needs makes their future home uncertain too, it is particularly important for regular meetings to be held with family members and a social worker from outside the unit to review progress together and arrange future care as soon as it is possible to make realistic plans. With adequate individual and family support and a suitable day centre to attend even quite disturbed children can be managed at home.

3. *If an adolescent must be away from home, what are the alternatives to psychiatric care?*

On discharge, or as an alternative to admission, the most normal setting that can meet the boy's or girl's needs is the one to recommend. *Ordinary boarding schools* can cope well with some adolescents with emotional and conduct problems, particularly those who have shown a capacity to improve on admission to the unit with little more than exposure to normal social expectations. Good *children's homes* for those who need more nurturing, and *special boarding schools* where the adolescent is capable of a little more independence and has a home to go to in holidays are probably next on the spectrum of normality. The *therapeutic communities* are for those who need a combination of total care and social therapy or psychotherapy over a long enough period for major advances in emotional development to be achieved, and there is a range of *hostels* for older adolescents, some of them tending towards being group therapeutic, others expecting more independent behaviour and perhaps out-patient treatment as the main source of supervision and therapy. *Community homes* are particularly variable in nature. Young people who need more control with educational and vocational training provided and who are less able to use a primarily psychotherapeutic setting may do best in a community home with education available (a'CHE'). The communities guided by the principles of Rudolf Steiner provide long-term (if necessary lifelong) homes for emotionally and intellectually handicapped children and their emphasis on stimulation and achievement through art, music, crafts and active involvement in a warm, self-supporting community is exactly right for some young people with chronic social and emotional difficulties. A small number of young people with very severe personality problems and persistently dangerous behaviour need containment in secure conditions in the hope that while they and the community are kept safe they can also be held for long enough to make use of social or behavioural therapy or psychotherapy. The youth treatment centres, community-orientated secure units for young people, and for a few the adolescent units in the special hospitals (for example at Broadmoor and Moss Side) are necessary for some (see also page 36).

Knowledge of the broad range of services and residential settings available can only be a rough guide. They tend to change over the years and there is no substitute for up-to-date knowledge of the various alternatives; visits to such different centres by members of the clinical team should be part of its teaching programme and form a particularly informative way of following up patients who have been discharged to them. The transfer of young people from the psychiatric unit to any institutional home should be preceded by careful selection of the best available place, detailed discussion between representatives of both sets of staff, and some meetings where the boy or girl, with past and future key workers, can talk over feelings, questions, and plans to do with the change. Some effort should be made to provide a sense of continuity; even though the adolescent's family cannot provide all the care needed, their presence in the background and availability for visits, holidays, anniversaries, and other regular contact is important for child and family, and may need special attention and maintenance.

THE FUNCTIONING OF IN-PATIENT UNITS

It will be clear that different adolescent units operate in very different ways. If there is a single particularly important distinction, it is probably the extent to which units operate primarily as therapeutic communities, with other ap-proaches being supplementary, or as a clinical unit with the focus on individually-planned treatment, the social mileu then being supplementary. For the reasons given in preceding pages the unit at Bethlem works on the latter principle. Which approach is 'best' is an extremely difficult question to answer: best for whom? It is a question which should be as much concerned with community needs as with whether or not a given unit is effective for the boys and girls it admits. As was pointed out in the earlier chapters, the range of adolescent problems is so wide and variegated, and psychiatric practice so polymorphous, that any group could set up a specialist service and be reasonably sure of a suitable clientele emerging from the pool of chidren's difficulties, and one that it could help. Undoubtedly the question is a philosophical and political one too; the number of adolescents who *must* have residential psychiatric treatment, simply be away from home, or kept away from the rest of the community in reasonable security is very small. For the majority, the ideal form care should take is controversial, and the history of children's problems, care, and psychiatry gives no reason to think that clear answers are around the corner. A picture is emerging, however, of the sort of problems present in the child and adolescent community, and the raw material of what different units and services do is available too, though not adequately evaluated. Although the various residential units have many differences, they also have much in common, and just as a careful classification of children's problems has been a valuable step forward, a systematic categorization of what adolescent units actually do, the sorts of question they ask in making their assessments, and their working methods, may be a useful step towards clarifying who should do what for whom (see review by Steinberg, 1982a).

What in-patient psychiatric units have in common is a clientele which has upbringing and educational needs as well as treatment needs; whose members are developing differentially and rapidly; who cannot be treated entirely as individuals but whose family and social connections outside the residential unit are important and insistent; and who (for these reasons) need the help of a team with more than one sort of professional skill.

This requires the members of the treatment team to have different training, backgrounds, and inevitably different ways of conceptualizing problems and solutions, and they will be members of different professional hierarchies too. In Britain at least, team members may be employed by educational as well as social service and health authorities, and within the latter belong to different professional groups with quite different emphases in their work and responsibilities; thus the psychotherapist's special interest and prime commitment to a particular form of treatment will differ fundamentally from a nursing officer's responsibility to distribute staff on a rota around the clock to ensure that there are trained people on duty every day of the year. On paper, such professional differences are easily set out; in practice, setting up a coherent working philosophy for a multi-professional team, and consistent treatment programmes for individual adolescents, reveals the major differences in attitudes, thinking, and priorities between psychiatrists, psychotherapists, social workers, family therapists, teachers, nurses, psychologists, occupational therapists, administrators, and others. Making the most of this necessary range of skills and attitudes in the interests of teaching, treatment, and research means that the team and its leadership must inevitably cope with organizational and interpersonal problems. These problems can be quite difficult at times, but they should not be allowed to occupy unit 'blind spots' or regarded as merely troublesome side-issues. It is not possible to use the skills of different professionals with different backgrounds and personalities without controversy and conflict emerging, unless the team or unit is run on rigidly autocratic lines or has become institutionalized, in which case the conflicts will still be there but causing diassatisfaction and ill-will and almost certainly adversely affecting the adolescent's care in some way. Moreover, conflict represents both misunderstandings and the strongly held convictions of experienced people; understanding the origins of arguments, and ways of resolving them constructively, is important in staff training and professional development, a model for adult relationships and debate, and crucial if a team is to remain imaginative, creative, and capable of development. What tends to catch some new staff unawares is that such confrontation is not the same as the contrived confrontations of some experiential groups, but real, and to use Winnicott's words again in a slightly different context, 'it will not necessarily be nice.'

The functioning of organizations is a complex subject. Argyris (1960), Katz and Kahn (1966), Goffman (1968), Menzies (1970), de Board (1978), and particularly the review by Ryle (1982) and the literature on the functioning of therapeutic communities (page 39) provide ways into this wide-ranging field. The following are aspects of special importance in the functioning of adolescent units, and can only be touched upon here:

Questions of authority, control, and leadership
Rules and decisions
Roles, goals, and responsibilities

Competition

Communication and support

Development and change

Authority and control

The importance of adult authority in relation to the normal development of adolescents has already been discussed (page 6, 7) as has its importance both in practical management and in psychotherapy (see page 275 and also Eisenberg, 1975; Skynner, 1976 a, b; Miller, 1974; Lampen, 1978; and Bruggen, 1979). In any potentially difficult, risky, painful or uncertain enterprise authority is vital, but in psychiatry decisions must frequently be taken in ambiguous and controversial circumstances, where no course of action is unequivocally known to be right. Admission, approaches to assessment and treatment, the unit's rules and sanctions, and the timing of discharge are all subjects ripe for dispute. An adolescent can easily pick holes in an adolescent unit's rules about smoking, for example, and inexperienced staff may readily find themselves seeing the point in the boy's or girl's argument and starting to take his or her side against other members of staff. Leadership and authority are to a considerable extent arbitrary when it comes to questions of rules for living, and senior members of staff will often have to stand by what they believe to be right, and use undemocratic arguments like 'because I say so'. Staff must be careful that, as good liberal intellectuals, they are not drawn into irrelevant arguments about democracy; they are running a treatment team, not a state, and many of the community's members are disturbed and immature and, among its staff, relatively in-experienced and there for training.

Each unit must resolve questions of authority and leadership in its own way. At Bethlem, because of the high proportion of transient staff in training, the unit is run by a core of senior staff of all disciplines whose style is to allow plenty of time for listening to junior staff and discussion, but whose decisions are taken by the responsible member of staff, not by consensus. The senior staff have both formal administrative meetings at which to take (and when necessary review) decisions, and regular meetings taken by an outside consultant at which to face their own differences and deal with ambiguities about role and responsibility. In a psychiatric unit, the final word on unit administration and patient care rests with consultant psychiatrist and senior nurse; the nature of the task makes it impossible formally to give either precedence in every conceivable circumstance.

What is important is that uncertainties are worked out between senior doctor and senior nurse, not left to their juniors to wrestle with. An adolescent unit's school too must have its own real autonomy recognized, with the head teacher in charge. Senior staff should be skilled and mature enough to be able to distinguish the rational and irrational components to disputes about authority, and to allow that where responsibilities overlap the work of the clinical team requires them to reach a decision, agreeing to disagree if necessary. Patient care can then proceed and disputes can be dealt with separately in the staff groups as matters between staff members, not as arguments about how to proceed clinically.

The functions of the different meetings which deal with the running of the unit must therefore be clear too. We have found a need for the following:

1. *Ward rounds or case conferences*, which are for making clinical decisions.
2. *Administrative meetings* for the unit's policy decisions.
3. *Staff meetings* at which feelings and working relationships are discussed but at which decisions are neither made nor revised, although as a result of the meeting proposals may be made to the administrative meeting.
4. *Community meetings* between staff and children are similarly about feelings although proposals for action are taken up by staff members or referred to the administrative meeting, and may of course be delegated back to the boys and girls.

Rules and decisions.

Lampen (1978) has discussed the various pressures on the leader of a team to be lenient or authoritarian, often from many sources and in conflict with each other. Psychiatrists tend to be particularly vulnerable to the request to be decisive, like a proper doctor. Of course there are times for decisiveness but the clinician should also be aware of the expectation for an immediate decision when a team member feels he or she is in a tight spot, perhaps mistakenly, and hopes to be helped around it by an arbitrary decision from on high. To respond in the requested way can be appropriate, but not invariably, and circumspection is needed.

Example 16

A new staff nurse asks a new psychiatric registrar if a boy can go home early this weekend; his stepfather on a rare visit is offering to take him out for a special treat on Friday afternoon. The request is followed up by an urgent telephone call from a plausible stepfather, 'I need to know before the weekend.' The nurse says the boy, who has recently settled down after weeks of misbehaviour and wrist-cutting, has strongly hinted that he will get worse again if his request is not met. She feels he deserves a reward for doing so well these last few days. The registrar agrees, and the boy returns from his treat only to break up his room and then the ward before absconding. The nurse and doctor had not sufficiently appreciated that the boy's improvement had followed weeks of patient work to set firm limits on the boy's meetings with a stepfather who intermittently and unpredictably came and went from the boy's life, bearing gifts and then vanishing for a time.

This is a relatively crude example, but the newcomer to adolescent psychiatry must be warned not to be rushed into unnecessary decisions and to be familiar with the many different facets of a patient's care. In the cold light of day it may seem foolish to be hurried into taking steps that may undermine what others are doing, and, in theory, the doctor should know anyway what is going on. In practice such mistakes can easily happen, and in this context it is worth remembering that the types of decision made in adolescent psychiatry about such apparently mundane matters as relatives' visits and trips out can be just as difficult and complex as decisions made about a patient's blood pressure or metabolic state and often more so.

Discipline, too, is a difficult subject. It is very important to anticipate misbehaviour and plan for it, rather than simply react to it in whatever way the person on the spot feels is most appropriate. As a general guide:

1. There should be a limited number of definite 'house rules', for example about smoking, alcohol, violence, and school attendance. These are made by staff.

2. There should be areas where responsibility should be shared with adolescents, for example, in ward community meetings. 'Nuisance behaviour' should be responded to by peer pressure, guided by staff; but where boys and girls cannot take responsibility the staff should take it for them. On these and other occasions staff can also demonstrate that they can disagree in public and resolve disagreement in a friendly way. Physical damage and graffiti should be put right swiftly; indeed, the unit premises and furnishings should be attractive and in a good state of decoration and repair. Not to give this priority is a false economy.

3. Staff should set the threshold of expected behaviour well on the reasonable side of average. It is unnecessary to make a fuss about the occasional swear word, and some staff do not mind the informality of being called by their first names. But it is better to deal very firmly with, say, verbal abuse or threats, than to let physical violence happen before the staff react. Damage should be paid for by the perpetrator; few are so confused and disorientated as to be excused this. Physical threats, bullying, and violence should be nipped in the bud and treated with extreme gravity.

4. Each unit will have its own ultimate sanctions, when attempts to understand the origins of unacceptable behaviour and confrontation both fail. A very naughty adolescent, however big, may have to be sent to his or her room, and perhaps kept in pyjamas for a few hours or a few days. This is punishment and a firm expression of disapproval and not to be confused with time out. At the

same time it is important to continue other treatment programmes and not allow a boy or girl going through a bad patch to become scapegoated as the unit villain; efforts to improve behaviour should be looked for, recognized, and encouraged. Opportunities to make amends, for example by an apology are important.

Persistence is important. Adults should have more patience than disturbed immature young people, and should continue with the same approach in a consistent fashion for a reasonable time even when the boy or girl seems not to be changing and junior staff are beginning to press for dramatic changes of direction. Keeping a record of how an adolescent is behaving over a few weeks demonstrates what changes are taking place (or, indeed, if they are not).

5. Those outside the unit who share authority with the staff (parents, or the social worker for a child in care) should be involved in meetings to repeat the message that the adolescent is cared for but that certain behaviour is unacceptable, and to affirm what authority the staff have in applying sanctions. If an adolescent is over 16, or parents will not allow the staff appropriate authority, the boy or girl may have to leave. This may take the form of temporary suspension while return on a more constructive basis is planned. It is worth considering in advance, when a 16 (or nearly 16)-year-old is admitted, what action can be taken about seriously negative, aggressive or destructive behaviour. *Either* some form of contract (for example about taking part in the unit's programme) must be agreed to *or* the unit team must have alternative ways of coping with gross misbehaviour. What chance will the unit's usual system of limit-setting have? Will medication be appropriate or not? Will suspension or discharge be appropriate or not? Will the Mental Health Act be applicable or not? Such considerations may be regarded as inappropriate in a case conference dealing with an apparently compliant 16-year-old, anxious to get away from the assessment centre where he has been repeatedly involved in fights, and who expresses earnest agreement with the report that describes his need for 'deep psychotherapy'; but psychotherapy at any depth, or any form of care, will need to be viable and sustainable, and once again questions of authority and responsibility are crucial and should be considered from the beginning.

Roles, goals and responsibilities

Different staff members will have quite different professional obligations and aims. It is both difficult and important for members of different professions to recognize this; it is not easy for a nurse to see a patient and his parents from the social worker's perspective, nor a social worker to appreciate the problems of, say, a senior nursing officer trying to preserve reasonably consistent work among 20 or 30 staff. Where one staff member cannot experience another's position (for example by working in his or her role for a time), the staff member must take on trust from senior staff members in that discipline what their work is like, and what the possibilities and limitations actually are. Inevitably, many boundaries are blurred, and roles overlap, and senior staff should focus on how they are going to deal with ambiguities of role when they cannot be defined neatly.

Competition

All experienced staff will have made their own intellectual and emotional adaptations to the powerful feelings evoked by working with deeply troubled adolescents and their families; these will differ from person to person and may clash. There will be competition about who is taking the 'right' approach to a particular person or problem, and often the strongest feelings will be generated about seemingly mundane matters. An adolescent who regularly sees his father and stepmother may also have regular visits from his natural mother, and a social worker may feel concerned about how the natural mother is received on the ward, believing that she is being handled clumsily by the nurses. The nurses may feel that the social worker is incorrect and that the way the boy's mother is received on the ward is their business and that there are no difficulties; and that perhaps the woman is 'playing off' one member of staff against another. By now the staff are in danger of using the woman unwittingly as a focus for interprofessional and interpersonal rivalry about such taboo subjects as who is the most sensitive, experienced, and perceptive member of staff. When such feelings surface they need to be faced so that they do not get in the way of reaching rational conclusions about how different situations are best handled. If they are not faced and worked with, mutual doubts between people and between professional groups turn into mistrust, and even asking questions and offering constructive criticism becomes anxiety-laden and difficult, which is a nutritious culture for the development of fantasies about what other people are up to.

Communication and support

Support is an elusive notion. It is to be hoped that everything a team does is emotionally and intellectually sustaining for its members, and this applies as much to day-to-day relationships and teaching sessions as staff groups. Team members should be perceptive and responsive to each other, and able to seek and use help and advice as well as offer it. Limits should be set, too, on how much help staff should expect from within the team. Anxiety and sadness in relation to work is a proper matter for the staff group or for a supervisor or colleague. But if it is persistent or recurrent and interferes with work, and particularly if it is related to matters outside work, the staff member who steps in to help should advise that help be sought from an independent source. His or her role may be supervisory or consultative, but should not be therapeutic. Support, however, is not only to do with problems; there is something wrong if members of a team cannot find things about which to congratulate or encourage each other, and fairly often too.

Communication of information is a recurring difficulty. Some therapeutic communities try to deal with absolutely everything on a group basis so that everyone is in the picture all the time, but this brave effort is impracticable for large clinical units using a range of treatments. Memos, notices, and circulated lists of decisions have their place but have their limitations too and vigilance should be exercised about any excess of circulating pieces of paper. Key information, such as decisions taken in conferences and 'handover' notes between staff and nursing shifts should be clear and concise and a focus for teaching and supervision.

Work with disturbed adolescents is widely recognized as being particularly demanding and stressful and is vulnerable to weakness in communication and support. Unresolved staff difficulties can impair staff members' therapeutic skills and ability to communicate as well as leading to fatigue, minor and major illness, disillusionment, and high staff turnover (see Freudenberger, 1975; Maslach, 1976; Levinson and Crabtree, 1979; Cornfield and Fealing, 1980; Thompson, 1980). Staff support is a much-used term but strategies of support are variable, largely untested, and often insufficiently effective, for example they may help staff get by without really helping staff development. For the purposes of this brief outline, a number of approaches that may be helpful include the following:

1. Regular staff meetings to explore working relationships and feelings, taken by an outside consultant, and in which senior, decision-making staff take a full part (see Skynner, 1975).
2. Clear leadership from the senior members of the staff and reasonable stability of the senior group.
3. As clear role-definition and delegated responsibility as possible, with adequate occasions for asking questions and clarifying ambiguities.
4. Leadership which can get the balance right between stretching staff reasonably yet being perceptive and responsive to strain, anticipating it rather than reacting to it later. The psychiatrist in charge of an adolescent unit must in particular control the demand made on the unit from the community; there are times when even the most urgent admission must be held off.
5. Recognizing the importance of staff teaching, supervision, and professional development. In some settings teaching is treated as a luxury; it is of course a necessity, and includes self-management skills (for example in organizing personal work programmes and work load) as well as learning technical skills. Basic teaching about child and adolescent development, and even the occasional reminder that not all patients get better and not all staff feel competent and cheerful all the time, is helpful. Attendance at conferences and courses and visits to other clinics and units are reassuring in this respect; as is the reception of visitors from elsewhere.

Above all, adolescents need not merely technically competent adults looking after them but people who, though tired and upset at times, also enjoy their lives and their work. Those responsible for a residential unit's administration and organization have an important responsibility for the latter, and a proper education programme is an important aspect of this.

Development and change

Individuals and institutions, having adapted as best they can to the demanding requirements given in the previous pages, tend to resist change: stability is seen as desirable. However, the dynamics of adolescence and the personalities of staff, the young person's need for education, experimentation, and growth, the constant change at every level in the community at large, and the need for innovation, change, and development in psychiatry, mean that stability can turn into institutionalization even in the most progressive circles.

Krohn et al. (1974) have pointed out how staff organization, attitudes, and relationships can reflect patients' problems both in rigid institutions and in periods of change; certainly organizations to a greater or lesser extent find change difficult (see Crabtree and Grossman, 1974; Krohn et al., 1974; Heal and Cawson, 1975; Steinberg et al., 1978; Ellis, 1980). Staff, especially newly appointed senior staff, can sometimes perceive the need for radical changes without fully appreciating that such changes may be feasible largely because of the stability of existing aspects of the system; some staff members perceived as resisting change may also be contributing to the unit's stability in ways that are not recognized in the formal administration of the unit or made explicit in its meetings. Innovation means change, which in turn means loss as well as gains, and the senior clinical staff should recognize those aspects of a unit's informal organization that contribute to its strength; exactly the same applies to the parent hospital of an adolescent unit, which sometimes develops a mutual relationship with its adolescent department not dissimilar to that of a parent with its troublesome offspring.

Chapter 19

Medication and Other Physical Treatments

INTRODUCTION: SOME GENERAL PRINCIPLES

Medication has a limited but essential place in adolescent psychiatry. There is often unease about its use with young people primarily because it is difficult to distinguish illness from those anomalies of emotional development and behaviour for which the hope, or wish, is that psychotherapy, special care, and education alone will help. The use of drugs is then perceived as second-best treatment, a substitute for skilled interpersonal care, and this view can be reinforced by the tendency for some of the most ill adolescents, for example those few with psychotic disorders, not to be the focus of interest of psychiatrists whose approach is primarily psychodynamic.

Our understanding of psychiatry does not justify the suspicion that some may feel that medication necessarily represents an alternative to more effective or more civilized care. There is no doubt that drugs can be and are misused, over-prescribed and given for inappropriate reasons. Equally, the possibility that among miserable or misbehaving adolescents and their families in chronic personal, social, and educational difficulties there might be even a small proportion who would be significantly improved by medication, is not something that should be ignored; and in the absence of systematic studies of the indications and contraindications for medication in this age group there is a special obligation on every psychiatrist to be alert to evidence that medication might help. The relative lack of interest in this aspect of child psychiatry by a high proportion of trainees (Garralda, 1980) is a cause for concern.

Apart from the better known indications for medication, such as the schizophrenic and major affective illnesses, it is reasonable to take into account such evidence as there is for some other problems having a physiological component. A boy or girl whose misbehaviour or misery does not seem sufficiently accounted for by his or her circumstances (long term and situational); in whom a psychodynamic formulation does not seem to fit; where physiological disturbances such as changes in appetite, sleep, weight, and arousal (particularly if shifts between arousal and withdrawal seem to underlie or replace finer changes in emotion); and in whom there is a family history of similar problems, particularly if they were helped by physical treatment, may be helped by medication.

The decision to use medication is a clinical judgement which is based also on urgency. It can be very difficult to differentiate a drug-responsive illness in an adolescent from one which may respond to other methods. If a boy or girl is intensely distressed, at risk (or putting others at risk) as well as in considerable emotional pain, one may know in a few days if not hours whether medication might help, while it may take months to know whether other approaches might be effective. On the other hand, it is also true that once drugs have been tried this identifies the problem in a way that may make other help difficult, for example psychotherapy requiring the adolescent to accept his or her feelings and take responsibility for his or her behaviour.

It is therefore necessary to consider the following:

1. Wanted versus unwanted pharmacological effects of the drug.
2. Wanted versus unwanted psychological effects of the use of drugs on the family, on the clinical team, on the boy or girl, and therefore on other aspects of management.
3. The degree of urgency in relieving emotional pain or alleviating risk by use of medication.

In the discussion on diagnosis (page 143) the significance was stressed of asking who is complaining of what, and why? This question applies here too; if it is held that a boy or girl needs medication because of his or her distress, the anxiety being raised in others too (for example parents or member of the clinical team) can play a part in the suggestion. What one clinical worker considers reasonable and tolerable distress or danger may not be what another can accept; it will also depend on different professional workers' understanding of the nature of the distress and the way it is being responded to. One may insist that *of course* the adolescent is furious or depressed, given the circumstances, and that psychotherapy is holding the child's pain and containing his behaviour adequately; another may doubt this. There is no simple way of resolving such differences in diagnostic appraisal nor the ability to cope with powerful feelings in oneself and others, but these different perspectives on the use of medication should be considered when the decision is made whether or not to prescribe drugs.

Emergency sedation is a special case. Bruggen and Davies (1977) have described giving an injection of chlorpromazine to an extremely aggressive boy 'because the staff were anxious about further things like that happening'. This is an honest attempt to deal with integrity with the reason for giving the medication, but it is not the whole truth; if it were, the logical course would have been for the staff to take the medication themselves. I have suggested elsewhere (Steinberg, 1983) that in such circumstances the primary reason for giving medication is to control wild behaviour, and that the proper need for frankness is not entirely met by talking in terms of allaying perfectly appropriate staff anxiety, but by making it clear that the drug is being given as a safe and effective way of stopping aggressive behaviour, not as a treatment that is expected to achieve more than that.

A drug may be used for any of the following reasons:

1. *Because it has a more or less specific therapeutic effect*, in so far as any psychotropic drug does so. Lithium carbonate comes closest to fulfilling this function, and antidepressants do in some forms of depression. Chlorpromazine and similar drugs can be powerfully effective in schizophrenic states.

2. *Because it is a way of controlling distressing or dangerous symptoms*, for example when a sedating drug allays painful levels of anxiety or inhibits aggressive behaviour, either of which seems uncontrollable by other means. It is reasonable to use drugs to stop dangerously aggressive or self-destructive behaviour:
   (a)   in emergencies, when all else fails;
   (b)   when no other methods prevent recurrent dangerousness:
   (c)   to help contain an adolescent in a setting where it is hoped that in due course the boy or girl will be helped by other means.

Despite our relative ignorance of the nature of psychiatric disorder, it is reasonable to assume that those physiological changes with which drugs interfere are only part of an interacting cycle of processes (for example, see page 66). Medication may or may not be sufficient to correct the interactive process underlying symptoms. One adolescent may be profoundly depressed because of an abnormality in nervous transmission; another because of a profound sense of loss following bereavement; another because of a separation aggravating a largely unconscious vulnerability to loss, with its origins in earlier childhood; while another adolescent's depression may be compounded of more than one of these. There is no theoretical or practical reason why medication may not be appropriate in some patients' cases in addition to whatever psychotherapy, social therapy or social changes are needed. This is not to say that prescription of a drug cannot undermine other efforts in one way or another; it is important to recognize that it can. The point is that a general policy of never prescribing medication if an adolescent also needs, for example, psychotherapy is unsound.

Like psychotherapy, drugs are costly, inconvenient and their administration involves risks and side-effects. They may interfere with the learning process, and may therefore adversely affect the other therapy and education (page 236). They can have paradoxical effects in some young people (page 330), may affect growth (page 329), and can cause illness, disability, including dependence, and death. Parkin and Fraser (1972) have described 31 children under five years of age who died between 1962 and 1969, and 22 who were poisoned but survived, having presumably accidentally ingested tricyclic antidepressants prescribed for a parent's depression or their own enuresis. In older age groups the dangers of drug misuse and overdose are well known (page 184). On the other hand untreated or inadequately treated psychiatric disorder is disabling and potentially dangerous too. As in most decisions the clinician must make, there are few absolutes, and conclusions are reached not by applying rules of thumb but by weighing advantages against disadvantages.

Some general conclusions:

1. Drugs have a small but important place in the range of adolescent psychiatric disorders.
2. They are preferably used for relatively specific therapeutic effects, but it is legitimate to use them
   (a) symptomatically, to relieve distress;
   (b) to prevent destructive or self-destructive behaviour when nothing else works;
   (c) to help contain a child in a setting that is educational, caring, or therapeutic, if nothing else will do so.
3. Physical side-effects should be watched for by the clinician, explained to patient and family and other involved professionals, particularly the adolescent's teachers. Warnings should be given about disabilities the drugs may cause.
4. Psychological side-effects are not always beneficial; they can undermine patient's, family's and indeed the therapist's other efforts.
5. All patients on long-term medication should have occasional blood counts performed, for example twice a year, and there should be properly made plans to review their need for medication, and the dose, at least as often.
6. Who should look after a supply of drugs? This is not only a matter of the adolescent's safety from overdose, it is also a matter of the patient's medicine being left around the house or the garden, flushed down the lavatory, taken occasionally, or shared among friends and relatives. Responsibility to look after his or her own medicine should be part of the wider responsibility a boy or girl is expected to take. For some the psychiatrist will want to emphasize that the adolescent is still young and needs looking after, so that parents and teachers should look after the medicine. For many, the responsibility should be the adolescent's own. Extra caution is indicated where there are younger children in chaotic, poorly supervised households. Not only is it well established that psychiatric patients very often do not take the medication prescribed (Willcox et al., 1965) but even in the more orderly and controlled atmosphere of general teaching hospitals it has been shown that there is many

a slip between prescription and ingestion (Vere, 1965). Nursing staff in units that do not use medication very often may need reminding that patients may pretend to swallow medication, later throwing it away, or, worse, saving it up for a rainy day. Some drugs are available in syrup form (for example chlorpromazine and amitriptyline) but they also contain usually unwanted calories, and are bad for teeth, which should be brushed after the syrup is taken.

7. Resistance to taking medication is often based on fear or misunderstanding that the drug may be a substitute for the therapist's interest; that it may be harmful, even deliberately intended to be; that it is not likely to help, not enough to justify its bad taste and the 'muzzy' feeling it induces; that it is intended not to help but to restrain and sedate; that the drugs are the same as a relative or another patient has been given, and means that the boy or girl has the same problem. All this requires a sympathetic hearing and a full explanation to patient and parents.

8. It is extremely difficult to give detailed guidance on the dose of drugs in adolescence. Some of the adolescent psychiatrist's patients are quite young, small children of 11 or 12, others are bigger and heavier than many adults, and their developing physiology may have unexpected metabolic effects, for example in the paradoxical effects of barbiturates and amphetamines in children (page 330) or the higher dose of lithium some adolescents may need and tolerate (Berg *et al.*, 1974, and page 338). Thus the rate of absorption, metabolism, and clearance of a drug will vary with the child's size and other developmental factors, and in any case there is considerable variability between individuals in their reactions to different drugs (Shaffer, 1977c). The best general guide is to begin with a small, safe dose and gradually increase it while being aware of (a) the maximum safe dose, taking account of the child's general health, and size, using surface area calculations if in doubt for small adolescents (see Butler and Ritchie, 1960), and (b) being clear, making clear to the team, and recording both desired and undesired effects.

9. Record clearly in the notes the drugs and dose currently being prescribed; the patient's family doctor should be kept up to date on this and, when writing, explain briefly and simply *what else* the clinical team is doing, to keep the use of drugs in perspective.

STIMULANT DRUGS

Sympathomimetic amines such as dextroamphetamine (Dexedrine) and methylphenidate (Ritalin) have been used in a wide variety of childhood and adolescent problems over the years but have resulted in few systematic studies (Conners and Werry, 1979); the most consistently recommended indication is for hyperactive children as an adjunct to other treatment (Chess, 1960; Fish, 1971: Cantwell, 1975 and page 199). Hyperkinesis is a descriptive term for problems of conduct involving chaotic, impulsive, overactive, and aggressive behaviour accompanied by short attention span and distractibility; it may or may not be accompanied by developmental delay or evidence of brain dysfunction. Its relationship to conduct disorder in the wider sense is unclear, and diagnostic practice varies considerably. Thus very few cases were identified in the Isle of Wight Study (Rutter *et al.*, 1970), to the extent that, in the United Kingdom at least, it may be considered a relatively rare disorder while in many United States child psychiatric clinics it has been regarded as common. In adolescence, moreover, the clinical presentation of the child who has been hyperactive begins to change, with educational retardation, antisocial behaviour, depression and low self-esteem replacing the clinical picture of excitable, overactive, impulsive behaviour (Cantwell, 1977).

The disorder is a good example of one which needs careful diagnosis and the use of methods other than medication, yet where drugs can be immensely helpful. Shaffer (1977c) suggests that stimulant drugs are most helpful where the clinical picture is dominated by: (a) poor attention span; (b) overactivity and disruptiveness in the classroom; (c) psychological and neurological or EEG evidence of brain dysfunction, although when brain damage is marked, and particularly in epilepsy, depressive reactions may occur (Ounsted, 1955). The undesirable effects of these drugs include insomnia and anorexia, irritability and depression and there have been reports of psychotic reactions (Lucas and Weiss, 1971). A number of studies have reported retardation of growth in children on long-term medication with stimulants (Safer and Allen, 1973) and also a compensatory acceleration of growth when the drug was discontinued (Safer *et al.*, 1975). As far as interference with growth is concerned, methylphenidate at dosage less than 20 mg daily appears to be the safest choice, and Shaffer (1977c) in his review of the literature quotes Werry and Sprague's finding that there was no therapeutic advantage (and more side-effects) in using doses greater than 0.3 mg/kg/day (Werry and Sprague, 1974). Toxicity results in restlessness, tremor, ataxia, confusion, hallucinations, cardiac arrhythmia, hypertension, hyperpyrexia, and the latter or intracranial haemorrhage can lead to death. Treatment for overdose includes chlorpromazine to control hyperpyrexia and a rapidly acting α-blocking drug such as phentolamine to control hypertension (Shaffer, 1977c).

In a very full and helpful review of stimulant drugs in hyperactivity, Barkley (1977) concluded that three-quarters of hyperactive children given stimulant medication are subsequently judged to be improved, particularly in the short term, but drugs do not seem to help with longer-term social, academic, and psychological adjustment, confirming the views of, for example, Eisenberg (1966), Werry (1970), and Fish (1971) that these drugs alone are not sufficient for treating this group of disorders. These drugs appeared most likely to help where inattentiveness was prominent (Barkley, 1976) which is consistent with the primary psychopharmacological effect of these drugs of increasing concentration and attention span and reducing impulsiveness in responding.

MINOR TRANQUILLIZERS, SEDATIVES, AND HYPNOTICS

It is rarely necessary to prescribe minor tranquillizers and sedatives for anxiety and other states of emotional discomfort in adolescence, even though they are very common. The indications recommended on page 326 are not usually met, the symptoms not usually being extremely distressing or handicapping, at least not for very long, and they are normally understandable and readily treatable by other means.

The main drugs in this general category are the *benzodiazepine minor tranquillizers* such as chlordiazepoxide (Librium), diazepam (Valium), lorazepam (Ativan), and nitrazepam (Mogadon); *barbiturate sedatives* such as amylobarbitone sodium (sodium amytal) and phenobarbitone (Luminal); and *non-barbiturate hypnotics* such as dichloralphenazone (Welldorm). Antihistamine drugs such as promethazine hydrochloride (Phenergan) are occasionally used for sedation too. The number of such drugs is very considerable and the distinctions between anxiety-reduction, sedation, and hypnotic effect are largely due to speed and length of action and relative strengths rather than to fundamentally different actions. Most of these drugs have been tried in emotional and behavioural problems although systematic studies in childhood and adolescence are scanty (Shaffer, 1977c; Connors and Werry, 1979). Such evidence as exists suggests that they are as likely to make behaviour worse, adding drowsiness and sometimes disinhibited aggression to behaviour problems, as can happen in adults (Dimascio, 1973; Salzman *et al.*, 1974). Phenobarbitone, too, is believed to increase activity and difficult behaviour and impair cognitive function in children, although according to Shaffer (1977) this has not been adequately demonstrated.

The only generalization about the use of these medicines in adolescence is not to do so except in unusual circumstances. Occasionally a generally competent adolescent in a normal family setting presents with disabling anxiety or phobic symptoms, with physiological evidence of high arousal such as sweating and tachycardia, that is a clinical picture very similar to adult-type anxiety neurosis. A small regular dose of chlordiazepoxide (for example 5 mg BD or TDS) or diazepam 2 mg BD or TDS) may be useful, or a single occasional dose (which may need to be slightly greater) an hour before a feared anticipated situation may be helpful. Use of such drugs in such circumstances should be accompanied by strong support and encouragement to maintain a normal school and social life, and accompanied by simple behavioural methods like advice about graded exposure to anxiety-making situations and self-monitoring of progress on an uncomplicated chart. Such drugs must, therefore, not be prescribed casually, but as part of a firmly recommended and supervised treatment regime; they should be used not as a means of avoiding normal life but as assistance in taking part in it, relying on the capacity of patients protected from disabling anxiety by chemical or placebo medication to develop effective coping mechanisms

(Steinberg, 1972; Tyrer and Steinberg, 1975). Side-effects of these drugs include aggressive disinhibition, as already mentioned, tiredness and ataxia. Sudden withdrawal may provoke fits. Long-term use of higher doses may produce dependence and the risk of abuse.

Two special and unusual uses of non-specific tranquillization seen have included a 16-year-old boy with long-standing cerebral dysfunction, dysphasia, and high levels of tension and anxiety who became relatively and helpfully disinhibited and fluent on small, regular doses of lorazepam; and a 15-year-old son of West Indian parents who presented in an acute paranoid psychotic state which resolved with the prescription of diazepam.

Using sedatives to induce sleep should also be avoided except in most unusual and special circumstances, for example high levels of fear and arousal at night which cannot be resolved by other means. In such cases nitrazepam or dichloralphenazone may be effective.

In all such cases the clinician should be firm about reducing and then stopping medication after a period of treatment, which is likely to be more difficult if the drug has been allowed to become the sole form of management; it should always be explained that the medication is an adjunct to whatever else is being done – the latter should be seriously sustained therapy which the adolescent should increasingly use as the medication, after a few weeks or a few months, is gradually withdrawn.

MAJOR TRANQUILLIZERS AND ANTIPARKINSONIAN DRUGS

Three important groups of major tranquillizers or antipsychotic drugs are the *phenothiazines* such as chlorpromazine (Largactil), trifluoperazine (Stelazine), thioridazine (Melleril), and fluphenazine (Moditen and Modecate); the *butyrophenones* such as haloperidol (Serenace) and pimozide (Orap); and *thioxanthenes* such as fluphenthixol (Depixol). All are sedating, relieve schizophrenic and other psychotic symptoms, tend to have long-lasting effects (several days), bring about changes in cerebral excitability and can cause fits in high doses, and cause extrapyramidal symptoms. The latter include facial immobility, excessive salivation, general muscular weakness and lack of movement; *acute dystonia*: painless spasmodic involuntary contraction of muscle groups producing tongue protrusion, neck and spinal muscle spasms and oculogyric crises; *tardive dyskinesia*; grimacing movements of face and tongue, which is unusual, slow to develop, and often irreversible and may be predisposed to by brain damage; and *akathisia*, an apprehensive, agitated, restless state which may resemble the very symptoms the clinician is trying to control. It takes some days to develop.

Important side-effects of chlorpromazine are weight gain, skin pigmentation, vulnerability to cold weather (frostbite and hypothermia), and photosensitivity. The latter is prevented by shade and the skin cream Uvistat. Chlorpromazine also interferes with metabolism in the liver of morphine, pethidine, and tricyclic antidepressants and in large doses can mask pain and fever making diagnosis of some physical disorders difficult. Phenothiazines can cause hypoglycaemia. Because of these and other wide-ranging effects chlorpromazine must be given with caution when physical illness is present and it goes without saying that any other physicians involved should be aware of the patient being on the drug (for example, in the investigation of the acute abdomen, or the treatment of an overdose of drugs).

Thiordiazine (Melleril) does not cause photosensitivity, but doses above 600 mg daily can cause pigmentary retinopathy and blindness; it is less likely to cause extraphyramidal symptoms. All of these drugs may cause hypotension and depression, and the phenothiazines (like tricyclic antidepressants) reduce circulating growth hormone levels and their long-term use may affect children's growth (Sherman *et al.*, 1971).

The major tranquillizers also interfere with aspects of learning, for example in attention, concentration, reaction time, and fine motor skills. Emotionally and behaviourally disturbed children characteristically have educational problems too and moreover the help they may need (for example social skills training and behaviour therapy) relies on learning capacity. In prescribing this medication it is important to weigh its advantages against these disadvantages.

The main indications for these drugs are in the following conditions:

1. Psychotic illnesses such as schizophrenic disorders and mania.
2. Incapacitating and distressing anxiety, aggression, arousal, and excitement in some adolescents with autistic disorder and major disorders or personality development, including their intermittent use in emergencies; and in children and adolescents with severe conduct disturbance including hyperactivity (Barker and Frazer, 1968; Werry, 1978).
3. Occasionally small doses of a major tranquillizer (for example haloperidol) deal more effectively with anxiety than one of the benzodiazepines.
4. Haloperidol is one of the more useful drugs for Tourette's syndrome, reducing the incidence of tics and vocalizations (Connell *et al.*, 1967) – a treatment which has some biochemical rationale (Cohen and Young, 1977) and which may be true of other antipsychotic medication used in this condition too (Ross and Moldofsky, 1978).

What general conclusions can be drawn about the use of this wide range of drugs in this wide range of disorders?

1. *Chlorpromazine* is a safe, widely used drug with marked sedating effects. In high levels of arousal, anxiety, and aggression it is the drug to be tried first. Low doses may be effective (for example 25 mg orally), while highly aroused, normal-weight adolescents in acute manic or schizophrenic states can benefit from high doses (building upto 800 mg a day), experiencing dramatic reduction of psychotic symptoms with relatively mild sedation.
2. *Trifluoperazine* is more likely to produce extrapyramidal symptoms but is less sedative. It is more appropriate to use it when apathy and withdrawal rather than excitement is the problem. There has long been a general impression that

it is particularly helpful in paranoid states. If so, and it has not been clearly established, it would be consistent with paranoid disorders having a particular prominent cognitive, ideational component and possibly being more amenable to self-appraisal and reality testing in the absence of heavy sedation. It too has a wide dose range of 2 mg to 15 mg daily in divided doses.

3. *Fluphenazine* is a particularly potent phenothiazine, weight for weight, and may be given as a depot preparation (Modecate) of 25 mg every two, three or four weeks, after an initial test dose of 12.5 mg. Extrapyramidal side-effects can be troublesome and respond to antiParkinsonian medication (see below) or by giving half the dose twice as often. The temptation with depot preparations is to see the boy or girl less often; the only advantage of depot preparations is to make sure that the drug is getting into the patient, and convenience for the patient too. As emphasized already, other aspects of supervision and treatment should continue with the necessary care and frequency. Charting the fluctuation of improvement helps demonstrate the frequency with which the injections need to be given.

4. *Fluphenthixol* may be used orally or as a long-acting depot preparation and may control mania where other drugs have failed, but is best avoided in younger adolescents. Again extrapyramidal symptoms are a problem and the British National Formulary (1981) recommends periodic blood counts when high doses are given. The test dose is 20 mg, followed by 20–40 mg every two to four weeks.

5. *Haloperidol* is a useful drug with an extremely wide range of dosage, helpful at low dose in anxiety states (0.5 mg BD) and effective in controlling high levels of overactivity and excitement at doses of up to 10 mg per day or more. With all but the heaviest, well-built adolescents it is best to begin with a dose calculated by weight at 0.025 mg/kg (low dose), and 0.05 mg/kg (high dose). Although widely recommended for psychotic disorders where apathy, inertia, and thought disorder are prominent, it can make mania or hyperactivity worse and induce excitement and aggressive behaviour.

The anti Parkinsonian drugs

The anticholinergic drugs procyclidine (Kemadrin) and orphenadrine (Disipal) control drug-induced extrapyramidal disorders. The most widely held view about when to prescribe them is on the emergence of substantial side-effects, rather than in advance, because they may interfere with the therapeutic effect of phenothiazines and mask the early signs of tardive dyskinesia. It is important to explain what they are for when prescribing them, in case patient and family do not appreciate the specific reasons for giving both types of drug. Anticholinergic drugs may cause drowsiness and nausea, dry mouth, constipation, urinary difficulties and, in high doses, delirium, confusion, and hallucinations. They can precipitate acute glaucoma.

The dose of procyclidine is 2.5 mg to 5 mg TDS gradually increasing if necessary, with 5–10 mg given intravenously or intramuscularly in acute dystonic reactions. The equivalent doses of orphenadrine are 25 to 50 mg TDS gradually increasing if necessary, with 20–40 mg by intramuscular injection for acute dystonic reactions.

ANTIDEPRESSANT DRUGS

The two main groups of antidepressant drugs (leaving aside lithium – see page 335) are the tricyclic antidepressants such as imipramine (Tofranil) and amitriptyline (Tryptizol), and the mono-amine oxidase inhibitors (MAOI) such as phenelzine (Nardil). The MAOI group are particularly toxic, with well-known dangerous interactions with a wide range of foods (for example meat and yeast extracts and many cheeses) and sympathomimetic amines including those, like ephedrine, found in proprietary medicines for coughs and colds and as medication for bronchospasm. I have not used them in children and adolescents and they are not reviewed further here, but they are potent drugs in the treatment of some depressive and phobic states and should not be forgotten in the case of intractable disorders in older adolescents (see Frommer, 1967, 1968; Tyrer, 1976).

Imipramine and amitryptilline are similar to each other in every way with the exception that amitryptilline is more sedative, and preferable when considerable agitation and anxiety is present; both are available as tablets and syrup, and for both the dose range is 75–150 mg daily in divided doses. Amitriptyline can also be given as a sustained-release single dose capsule of 50 mg or 75 mg at night. Side-effects such as drowsiness, dry mouth, constipation, blurred vision, postural hypotension appear quite rapidly, and toxic effects tend to emerge later; weight gain, limb tremor, hypomania, hallucinosis, and fits may occur. They may exacerbate glaucoma. The antidepressant effect may take two or three weeks to begin to work. Absorption varies from individual to individual, and blood levels of the drugs should be estimated before assuming that the drug is not effective.

It is because of their cardiotoxicity that the tricyclic drugs are particularly dangerous in overdose; 200 to 400 mg (as few as eight tablets) can be fatal in small children (Conners and Werry, 1979) and treatment is difficult and hazardous.

The antidepressant drugs are used in:
depressive illness
phobic disorders
behaviour disorders
enuresis
obsessive–compulsive disorder
Gittelman-Klein and Klein (1971) found improvement is school-phobic children in a controlled trial of imipramine, and Weinberg *et al.* (1973) demonstrated improvement in mood disorder and academic problems in

children with a family history of depression who were given imipramine. Winsberg *et al.* (1972) and Rapoport *et al.* (1974) found that imipramine significantly reduced aggressive and overactive behaviour, although in the latter study methylphenidate (see page 328) had been more effective. Only one study of the drug treatment of hyperactive children has demonstrated the superiority of imipramine over methylphenidate, and the authors (Werry *et al.*, 1980) considered this due to the relatively moderate degree of disorder in the study, and the low dose of methylphenidate prescribed.

Imipramine and other tricyclic antidepressants reduce the frequency of bed-wetting in most patients (Shaffer *et al.*, 1968; Blackwell and Currah, 1973) but while there is little doubt about the drug's helpfulness while it is being taken, relapse tends to occur when medication stops. The dose is 25–50 mg at night in the ordinary (not sustained release) preparation. It is not clear how the drug works in the control of enuresis. It is effective too rapidly to be accounted for by its antidepressant effect, and in any case, there are no grounds to regard the disorder as a 'depressive equivalent' (Graham, 1974; Werry, 1976). Possibly a local effect on the bladder itself is significant, or its central stimulant effect on motor activity and possibly cognitive function may be relevant (see Werry *et al.*, 1975; Shaffer, 1977c). The possible benefits of combining tricyclic treatment of enuresis with other methods such as the bell and pad deserve systematic study.

Clomipramine (Anafranil), a tricyclic antidepressant closely related to imipramine has been reported to be helpful in obsessive–compulsive disorders (see page 183) although in one careful double-blind study in adults it improved only those patients who initially had a depressed mood. The helpful effect of the drug diminished after a few months and patients relapsed when the drug was stopped (Marks *et al.*, 1980). The authors discuss the complex possible relationships between obsessive–compulsive and depressive disorders and conclude that the likelihood of clomipramine being effective in obsessive–compulsive disorders depends upon the degree of depression also present, and the drug's continution for over a year in combination with other treatment (see also page 180).

LITHIUM CARBONATE

Lithium (Camcolit; Priadel) is well established in adult psychiatry as an effective drug for the control of manic states and the prevention of manic and depressive phases of depressive illness. It has a wide range of biochemical actions whose precise relationship with its clinical effect is not known. It may reduce synaptic catecholaminergic activity which is possibly overactive in manic states, or it may affect calcium, magnesium, sodium and potassium metabolism, and cell membrane transport, in a way that underlies physiological changes in abnormal mood states. It may have similar effects on carbohydrate metabolism and corticosteroid rhythms. The whole question of mood disorder in children and its aetiology, symptomatology, description, and treatment is far from clear (Rutter,

1972c; Hersov, 1977c). Manic-depressive illness, 'endogenous' depression, and variations on normal states of unhappiness have an unclear relationship with each other (Kendell, 1976; review by Bhanji 1979; and page 225). The situation is complicated in child and adolescent psychiatry because the evidence of emotional development is that it takes a reasonable degree of maturity to be able to experience and express what we recognize in adults as characteristic depressive illness.

Can a biochemically and physiologically based depressive psychosis exist in children? If the illness as such does not exist, because the young child is physiologically and cognitively incapable of being depressed in this way, can an equivalent physiological disorder exist, perhaps expressed behaviourally rather than emotionally, and if so could it be responsive to treatment with lithium carbonate? The particular band of chronological age and development seen by adolescent psychiatrists, extending from very immature 11-year-olds to young adults, makes it uncertain in the case of the individual adolescent whether adult-type disorders are to be anticipated or not.

Against this uncertain background the following can be said:

1. Adult-type manic-depressive illness makes an unequivocal appearance in the adolescent age group, although it remains very uncommon, and is unknown in younger children (Wertham, 1929; Barrett, 1931; Campbell, 1952; Sands, 1956; Anthony and Scott, 1960; Perris, 1968; Winokur et al., 1969; Youngerman and Canino, 1978).

2. Lithium treatment is as effective in adolescent manic-depressive disorder as it is in adults (Brumback and Weinberg, 1977; Horowitz, 1977; Youngerman and Canino, 1978).

3. Some disorders of adolescence not typically manic-depressive in type appear to respond to lithium (Annell, 1969a, b. Dostal and Zvolsky 1970; Youngerman and Canino, 1978; Kymissis et al., 1979; Stein et al., 1982.)

The latter category contains a most heterogeneous group of problems, including behaviour disorders, anorexia nervosa, schizophrenic illness, and problems of mood and behaviour in mentally retarded young people. A recurring theme in the adolescent psychiatric literature on the use of lithium carbonate is the boy or girl diagnosed as schizophrenic on first presentation and who is later reassessed as having a manic-depressive illness which responds well (produces a normal mental state) with lithium treatment. In immature adolescents and in inarticulate young people of limited intelligence it is always important to recognize that many psychotic states accompanied by muddled thinking and ideas of reference are not neccessarily schizophrenic; high levels of arousal and anxiety and severe mood disorder can produce a similar clinical picture, and a proportion may be responsive to lithium treatment (see page 226).

The proportion of young people with major disturbances of conduct (including those with other diagnoses such as autism) who may be responsive to lithium treatment is likely to be small; after all, the incidence of manic-depressive illness in the adult population is low. Nevertheless such problems can be grossly disabling, not least by preventing the boy or girl ever settling down in a place where he or she can be looked after and in certain cases (see below) it is worth considering whether lithium might be helpful (see review by Steinberg, 1980).

The clearest indication for using lithium is when the adolescent's mental state has the typical characteristics of adult manic-depressive illness: elation, pressure of speech, flight of ideas with rhyming, punning and other jokes, and sometimes frenzied overactivity with incoherent thinking and increasingly bizarre delusions and hallucinations; a family history of manic or depressive illness; and a cyclical course to the disorder. In the depressed phase there is agitation or retardation, profound despair with ideas or delusions of unworthiness, guilt and persecution, and suicidal ideas or plans.

The variation on this pattern seen in adolescence approximates to the clinical stereotypes drawn up by Anthony and Scott (1960) and Youngerman and Canino (1978): a mental state resembling the adult disorder; a family history of similar illness; an early tendency to mood swings of increasing amplitude and length; and an extroverted personality; recurrence with little evidence of a relationship with external events; and the absence of organic or schizophrenic illness.

The third set of indications is where there is no real clinical evidence of mania or depression, but an intractable and disabling disorder, unresponsive to other efforts to help, and with (a) periodicity of symptoms not apparently connected with external events, (b) a family history of affective illness, and (c) arousal or withdrawal being prominent in the boy's or girl's history and mental state.

In summary, I would suggest as the symptom cluster to make lithium worth considering: severity, intractability, and periodicity; a family history of mood disorder, especially if the mood disorder in the relative amounted to manic or depressive illness and if it responded well to drugs or ECT; and particularly if the adolescent's symptoms include arousal, excitement and impulsive aggression *or* withdrawal and apathy.

Taylor (1979a) has pointed out that among mentally retarded people manic-depressive psychosis is regarded as less common than in the general population, but it does occur, and increased agitation, hyperkinesis, withdrawal or obsessional behavioural may indicate it.

Another interesting aspect of the possible indicators for using lithium is Campbell's observation (1976) that excitable, aggressive or self-mutilating retarded young children were more likely to improve with lithium treatment when its use decreased focal EEG abnormality, or caused diffuse slow activity and slowed alpha rhythm in normal EEGs.

When considering these indications it is important to balance the considerable hope for a 'magic cure' from all concerned against the fact that while at first a disorder may seem quite unrelated to external events, closer acquaintance with adolescent and family can reveal previously unsuspected situational pressures.

Also, lithium is a toxic drug, and reasonable stability of circumstances and effective supervision is necessary to prescribe and monitor it safely.

It is prescribed at dose levels between 500 mg and 1,000 mg daily, with the aim of achieving reasonably steady blood levels of 0.6 to 1.4 m mole/litre of plasma, with 2.0 m mole/litre as the upper limit for safety. There has been considerable discussion about the relative merits of plain and sustained release tablets, the problem being to maintain a blood level which is both safe and effective. The advice given by Crammer *et al.* (1978) is to use a plain preparation, beginning cautiously with 250 mg 12 hourly, increasing to 500 mg twice a day while monitoring blood levels. These should be estimated several times in the first two weeks, noting the time of the last dose and the time the blood is taken, but when stability is reached estimation every month or two is sufficient. High salt (sodium chloride) intake increases lithium excretion, and vice versa, so anything likely to upset electrolyte balance (low salt diet, vomiting, excessive sweating for example) requires a period of particularly careful monitoring of blood level. The use of tetracycline and diuretics can also raise blood lithium levels by the effect of these drugs on renal function (see also Crammer *et al.*, 1974, 1978; Crammer, 1977; Johnson, 1979). Some adolescents, by virtue of a higher renal output, may need higher than usual doses (Berg *et al.*, 1974).

Lithium causes a wide range of side-effects, including reversible neurological, thyroid and renal disturbance (see Table 13). There is divided opinion about it

Table 13   Side-effects and toxic effects of lithium

Early side-effects
Nausea
Fine tremor of the hands
Dry mouth
Thirst and polyuria*
Loose stools

Early or late toxic effects
Diarrhoea and vomiting
Ataxia
Clumsy, uncoordinated limb and hand movements
Slurred speech
Muddled thinking

Severe toxicity
Worsening disorientation
Epileptic fits
Coma leading to death

* Which may also occur as a *late* side-effect, does not worsen, and reverses one to two weeks after the drug is stopped.

causing irreversible renal damage, with opinion largely against this as a serious risk, although this question is an open one for the time being; there is also uncertainty about whether lithium can cause brain damage, although it seems that it may do so if given with haloperidol (see Cohen and Cohen, 1974; Loudon and Waring, 1976; Thomas, 1979). Reports of the use of lithium in adults suggest that it neither aggravates nor controls epilepsy (Crammer, 1977). Animal studies show that it can inhibit bone growth (Birch, 1979).

Any adolescent given lithium should first have a thorough physical assessment, with special emphasis on electrolyte balance and renal function. Baseline cardiac, EEG, thyroid and cognitive tests should also be performed, and a growth chart maintained throughout treatment. Although the evidence for lithium causing renal damage is at present scanty, pre-existing renal dysfunction or water and electrolyte imbalance (as may occur in anorexia, severe depression or uncontrolled mania) can cause lithium in ordinary doses rapidly to reach a toxic level.

Table 13 summarizes the unwanted effects of lithium carbonate, grouped into: (1) early side-effects that warrant only particularly close monitoring of physical symptoms, signs and blood lithium levels; (2) those indicating toxicity and that the drug should be stopped immediately; (3) the results of severe toxicity. Toxicity requires hospital treatment as a medical emergency, with increased sodium intake.

As with other forms of treatment, careful monitoring is not only for reasons of safety; all forms of treatment are expensive and inconvenient and, in psychiatry, of uncertain effectiveness. Some means of systematically charting progress as well as side-effects should always be undertaken, and this need not be an elaborate and sophisticated exercise.

ANTICONVULSANTS

In addition to their anticonvulsant effects in epileptic disorder, and the significance of their side-effects, the anticonvulsant drugs are also of interest to child psychiatrists because of their possible effects on some forms of conduct disorder.

The most commonly used anticonvulsants are phenytoin (Epanutin), primidone (Mysoline), phenobarbitone (Luminal), carbamazepine (Tegretol), sodium valproate (Epilim), and sulthiame (Ospolot), all of which are used to control tonic–clonic (grand mal) and partial (focal) seizures; while sodium valproate and ethosuximide (Zarontin) are used in absence seizures (petit mal). All are sedative to varying degrees, especially phenobarbitone; sulthiame is only mildly so, although the latter drug can cause hyperventilation. Stopping anticonvulsants too rapidly can cause fits. Epanutin causes acne.

Phenobarbitone is well known for its reputation for causing cognitive impairment and behaviour problems in children but as Stores (1975) and Shaffer (1977c) have pointed out, there are many questions still unanswered about the cognitive and behavioural effects in children of the whole range of anticonvulsants (see also Stores, 1978). In addition to the less obvious psychological impairment these drugs may cause, such as impaired verbal learning and vigilance in the case of phenobarbitone (Hutt *et al.*, 1968), and impaired concentration and coordination with phenytoin (Idestrom *et al.*, 1972), confusion and psychotic states have been reported with primidone, phenytoin, carbamazepine, and sulthiame (Stores, 1975).

There have been a number of studies of the use of anticonvulsant drugs for behaviour problems in children and adolescents, whether or not they have epilepsy too. Careful studies of phenytoin by Conners and his colleagues have shown this drug to have no advantage in this respect over a placebo (see Looker and Conners, 1970; Conners *et al.*, 1971; Conners and Werry, 1979). Sulthiame, on the other hand, a drug which is pharmacologically distinct from the other anticonvulsants, has had more promising results in tests on hyperactivity and aggressiveness whether accompanied by epilepsy or not (Al-Kaisi and McGuire, 1974; Stores, 1975, 1978). Many of the patients in the study by Al-Kaisi and McGuire were adolescents, half had epilepsy, and all had an IQ level below 50.

Carbamazepine is another distinctive anticonvulsant drug, chemically related to the tricyclic antidepressants, which has been recommended for use in behaviour disorders, but its usefulness has not been established. (see Dalby, 1971; Stores, 1978).

As with lithium, the anticonvulsants are powerfully effective and toxic drugs with a number of additional therapeutic possibilities that are as yet unconfirmed. This can result in great expectations on behalf of young people with longstanding, difficult behaviour problems, especially if they have epilepsy too. The relationships between behaviour problems and the disorders that cause epilepsy and result from it, the effect of antiepileptic medication, and epilepsy's psychological, social, and family consequences are immensely complex (Taylor, 1969, 1972). Whatever anticonvulsant medication may or may not be able to do for young people with conduct disorder, it is important (a) to take a careful clinical history to separate, as far as possible, situational from physiological phenomena, (b) to make sure that the boy or girl is not on too much medication at high dosage, (c) to make use of recent developments in measuring blood levels of anticonvulsants in the latter exercise (d) to measure as precisely as possible cognitive, motor, behavioural, and mood problems as a baseline with which to compare the effects of changes in medication, (e) not to neglect the very considerable feelings of anxiety, anger, depression, and guilt that epilepsy generates in children and their families and others, and the effect of this on the child's mood, behaviour, and educational and social progress.

ELECTROCONVULSIVE TREATMENT (ECT)

Electroconvulsive treatment (ECT) receives little mention in the literature on adolescent psychiatry; it is rarely indicated, and currently causes public disquiet even when used for consenting adults. Clare (1979) provides a helpful review of ECT (and psychosurgery) in adults, discussing ethical aspects too, such as the problem of clarifying degrees of risk (such as permanent memory loss, learning impairment and death, which are very low but present none the less) in order to obtain truly informed consent. Probably those who feel most strongly that ECT should *never* be used, particularly in adolescents, do not see the occasional young person in a profoundly withdrawn and depressed state which persists and worsens over many weeks and perhaps months despite every effort with psychotherapy, social measures, and medication. It is reasonable to consider using ECT in such circumstances, if the history and mental state include those factors associated with a good response to ECT in adults such as relatively sudden onset, pronounced retardation and self-reproach (Hobson, 1953), weight loss, early waking and somatic delusions (Carney *et al.*, 1965). There is no satisfactory evidence of its value in manic illness or schizophrenic states (Clare, 1979).

Should the question of using ECT arise, the psychiatrist should explain to those responsible for the adolescent (parents, social worker) the reasons for considering the use of ECT and such risks and disadvantages as there are; he should also explain to the boy or girl what the treatment would involve (the anaesthetic, temporary confusion, etc.) because the boy's or girl's attitude to the treatment is important even if his or her consent could be overridden by parents. It is important not to let the question remain in the air for ages; in the short term it is equally important to set aside adequate time for those involved to understand the *pros* and *cons* of the matter. There should no inhibitions about seeking other psychiatrists' opinions, because the situation arises too infrequently for any single psychiatrist to have extensive experience of its use in adolescence; thus at the Bethlem unit, where admission policy is geared towards giving priority to the most unequivocally and severely ill young people, with the correspondingly relatively large minority of patients with affective illness admitted, one consultant has used ECT only once and another twice in the past seven years.

DIETARY CONTROL IN ANOREXIA NERVOSA AND OTHER CONDITIONS

Management of feeding is so specific to the problems of anorexia nervosa and obesity that it is discussed under those headings on pages 210 and 215. Nevertheless any psychiatrist who finds himself looking after children, sometimes as the only doctor taking an active long-term interest in them, should make sure that they are having a good, balanced diet and a pleasant one. The state of their teeth, general health, and growth should be his concern, especially in residential settings, as should the consumption of alcohol, drugs, cigarettes, and excessive refined carbohydrate.

Although the hyperkinetic syndrome is not prominent in adolescent psychiatry, it is worth mentioning attempts to control it with diet. Taylor (1979b) has reviewed this thoroughly, and concludes that the scanty evidence for following an arduous diet does not justify its routine use in clinical practice, and makes the important point that if a family want to try it the clinician's job should then be to supervise an experimental treatment, monitoring change with sufficient care to allow sensible conclusions to be drawn. We do not know what part allergies to food or other substances may play in hyperactivity or indeed in other conditions. There is no reason why some foods might not cause or exacerbate mood or behaviour problems in some people, and Taylor's advice is to be preferred to simply dismissing the possibility too readily; though always bearing in mind that who feeds what to whom is a powerfully emotive matter between adults and children.

Chapter 20

Collaboration, Consultation, Teaching, and Learning

INTRODUCTION: PROBLEMS

The theme of this chapter is not what professional workers do with the patients and families they see but how they work with each other. Interpersonal, interprofessional, and organizational problems that intrude in clinical work, and the reasons why they are important, have been discussed in preceding chapters, and may be summarized as follows:

1. The various professions involved with children have quite different histories and historical connections, having grown out of the churches, the legal and law enforcement professions, medicine, science, philosophy, teaching, and both charitable and reforming aspects of welfare work.
2. The personalities and aspirations of individual men and women who choose to enter the professions that come together in clinical work with adolescents are likely to be very different; certainly their training, salaries, and status are very different and their professional aims and the conceptual framework they use have as many fundamental differences as similarities.
3. An adolescent's needs can rarely be met by a single person. At the very least one clinical worker can guide a family, but even then the boy's or girl's teachers will have important information to provide and parts to play. One of the important advantages of a family approach is that for many problems it may enable one professional worker to replace several; but for many disturbed young people and in particular those who make up the clientele of clinical psychiatry, the skills of a number of different people with different backgrounds and ways of working have to be brought together.
4. They are brought together in a wide variety of very different ways. Two family co-therapists working together with a family have a very different relationship to, say, a psychiatric registrar and a consultant surgeon discussing an

adolescent who has taken an overdose of drugs and is in one of the latter's beds. Correspondingly, discussion between a community psychiatric nurse and a head teacher about whether a boy or girl can manage (and be managed) in a school, soon reveals the very different perspectives of the two professional groups. Even within a single clinical team the angles of vision of the different groups represented can be remarkably different.

5. Regardless of formal training, different professionals have very different skills, interests, and personal capacities, different ethical attitudes to their work, different motivations and aspirations, even different amounts of time and energy they are able to or willing to devote to it.

6. This much can be broadly true of any group of people whether brought together in an office, a factory, a dramatic company, a surgical unit or a battleship. But in all of these the nature of the job and the training and supervision needed are more or less clearly established, roles reasonably clear-cut, the hierarchy fixed and within limits the organization or unit is regarded by the wider community as knowing what it is about; the public may criticize the motor industry for one thing or another, but does not profess to know how to put a gearbox together. In psychiatry and its allied professions the nature of the job and the training needed is not clearly established, roles are not clear-cut, the hierarchy is often in question and most people are prepared to express a view about how best to deal with troubled adolescents and indeed are often willing to do so. Parents, teachers, prison officers, newspaper editors, the surgeon arguing with the psychiatric registrar will all have their own views about adolescents and psychiatry and sometimes they are right.

7. The nature of the problems and the tasks involved are not clear for two reasons which are not directly to do with professional background. First, description, prediction, and methods of intervention in child and adolescent psychiatry are poorly established, and although in recent years some progress has been made in the first two, there is still a great deal that we do not know about when and how psychiatry should usefully intervene. Second, some of the matters with which child and adolescent psychiatry deal will always be nebulous and changeable; concepts of right and wrong, good and bad, normal and abnormal are eternally arguable, and changes in cultural attitudes, social policies, economics and politics will always directly influence children's development and the way families and schools function and professionals respond.

8. Finally, there are inherent difficulties in working with disturbed adolescents and their families; unhappy, anxious people who feel unsafe for whatever reason will tend to test the safety of any setting and relationship which sets out to offer help, sometimes in a most challenging way. This is an everyday experience in work with disturbed adolescents and is consistent with the attachment model described on page 129.

The ways in which this is done and the precise reasons in each young person's case will vary considerably, but the theme is a constant and familiar one. It may be expressed most obviously by an attempt literally to break out of the unit or clinic; it may be expressed in a more subtle way, by persisting withdrawal, helplessness, and silent unresponsiveness; it may be expressed intellectually or philosophically, for example when adolescents challenge adults' right to teach them their skills, their right to make rules, and the genuineness of their interest in them.

Disturbed adolescents will also challenge the support adults seem to provide each other, to see if they really are competently united in the child's interest. The adolescent may treat some staff members as if they were 'ideal' and others as if awful, which may cause staff misgivings; and if efforts to elicit a satisfying response do not succeed, then more immature efforts may be made, a conceptual view consistent with Kleinian theory, Winnicott's work and the attachment model (see pages 87 and 106). In this context, it is important not to dismiss the child's efforts as 'manipulative' and 'attention seeking'; they may be, descriptively speaking, but both terms have unnecessarily pejorative connotations. The human child needs to attract adult attention and response, and the anxious, developmentally impaired child can be expected to do this in an anomalous way, that is if he or she has not given up.

For these reasons teamwork with disturbed adolescents is complex and difficult, and different professional workers will inevitably have their own styles of response partly determined by their personalities, partly by their training and experience so far, and partly by the system (for example professional hierarchy) within which they work. Yet for reasons described in other chapters it is important for adults to act together, consistently and with authority for the sake of the patients. The best way to describe how team relationships can be challenged is to give an example.

A SOURCE OF CONFLICT IN A CLINICAL TEAM

Example 17

A consultant psychiatrist decides to treat a seriously depressed boy on an in-patient unit with individual psychotherapy supervised by a consultant psychotherapist whose work is largely outside the team. The senior registrar begins to see the boy twice a week, and work proceeds painfully but constructively in what the psychotherapy supervisor and the psychiatrists consider is the right direction. The nursing staff have grave doubts because the boy is reluctant to attend sessions and is extremely disturbed after them. Sometimes this is quite serious, and the observation of the nursing staff is that he is far worse than he was, more actively threatening suicide, injuring himself more, behaving extremely aggressively and sometimes appearing paranoid to a psychotic degree. Nevertheless the psychotherapy supervisor believes progress in the sessions is being made.

The nursing staff, who look after the boy for 166 hours of the week outside the two psychotherapy sessions, are divided in their views, some (including senior nurses) feeling that treatment is proceeding as it should, half (including other senior nurses) believing it is quite clearly making the boy worse and their job more difficult, and the remainder are uncertain. The night staff are experiencing particular difficulty and one 'rotating' nurse is reluctant to work on the ward, which is a particular source of anxiety for the nursing administration.

From among those nurses who believe the treatment is wrong, the boy, between outbursts, selects one or two to confide in, and explains that he feels much better chatting to Nurse X and Nurse Y, and that will help him much more than awful Dr Z who does not really know him, does not understand, does not say anything, is just like a psychiatrist, etc. Soon the staff are in two teams: the 'good' team (from the boy's point of view) perceive an adolescent who is just holding his own despite psychotherapy because he is able to confide in a few nurses; the 'bad' team are pressing ahead with psychotherapy because they see in the present state of affairs an exact replication of the child's experience with his family, with foster parents, with a series of children's homes and with the clinic that referred him, all finally giving up in the face of the boy's 'manipulation', rage, disturbance, and threats.

In the case conference the psychotherapeutic point of view is that the situation is exactly as expected and the clinical duty is to press on; the nurses' view is that they have to look after an increasingly disturbed boy whom psychotherapy is making worse. They are angry, anxious and overstretched and, like the boy, are also testing out the system for 'good' and 'bad', 'strong' and 'weak' areas. The solution is as follows:

1. The consultant explains that the treatment is right and will continue.
2. A teaching session is used to supplement previous discussions (which many nurses had to miss) on the theoretical basis for the treatment approach, and plans are made to enable senior nurses to attend the psychotherapy supervision group when they can; thus far they have been too busy looking after the boy to free colleagues to attend.
3. In staff meetings the division of opinion is discussed, and the way in which the boy has classically split the staff revealed. All the staff know about 'splitting'; it is one of their commonest expectations. But once personally involved in a 'split' it can be extremely difficult to perceive it, the other person being, of course, in the wrong.
4. The consultant meets the senior registrar with the nursing staff to discuss how they can resolve their different attitudes and feelings; this proves not difficult to do, once the nature of the problem is clear.
5. In meetings with the children the staff discuss their disagreement and their ability to resolve their differences.
6. As the 'good' and 'bad' staff are seen by the boy to be now working consistently together, he becomes less agressive, less paranoid, and more

depressed, but now in a way that seems appropriately and more healthily sad. From then on he begins to make and maintain progress.

7. The issue of the team's vulnerability to misunderstanding, work overload, and splitting is kept alive in staff meetings from organizational, teaching, and staff relationships point of view. The consultant and the unit's nursing officer work together to ensure that the unit's organization in terms of nurse staffing can cope with the current extra work load.

Roles, responsibilities, and relationships in the clinical team

This example also illustrates the range of quite different professional roles and relationships involved in work in a clinical team, and which should be

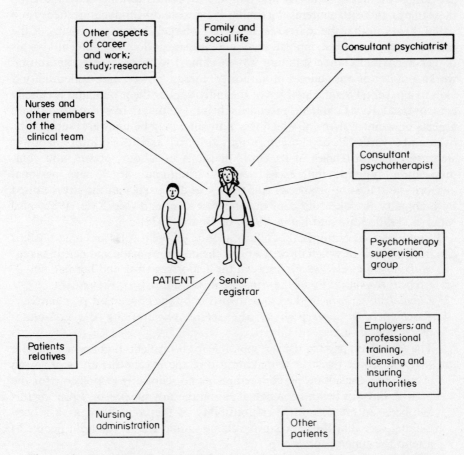

Figure 30   Examples of relationships network for one staff member: simplified

distinguished from each other. One way of looking at this is to begin with the position in this example of the senior registrar, though an equivalent network of roles and responsibilities could be drawn up for every member of staff. The diagram (Figure 30) is extended beyond the clinical team to include other aspects of the senior registrar's life that are inevitably influential in his or her work. It is also a much simplified representation of an organization; even a small psychiatric team is a focus of an immensely complex network of quite different professional hierarchies with their own characteristics and rules. A child guidance clinic, for example, will usually represent education and social services departments as well as the Area Health Authority, and within these broad groupings individuals, for example psychiatrist, psychologist, social worker, and psychotherapist have in addition considerable autonomy. Social organizations are immensely complex; in exploring what they do to and for the individuals who belong to them, providing resources, authority and support as well as lacking or withholding these things, there is an interesting similarity between psychodynamic theory and social theory in that the individual tends to be largely unaware of many of the competing expectations, opportunities, and pressures which are influential in his or her behaviour. Understanding how a clinical team or other organization works and its various sources of authority, energy, power, and vulnerability is akin to a psychodynamic analysis of the individual or the group, and is equally controversial. Ryle (1982) has provided a helpful summary in which she outlines aspects of social systems of which the individual may be unaware, such as the overt and covert goals of an organization; its formal and also its informal power structure; inconsistencies in its aims; divisions of labour, power, and communication systems; differences between traditional, legal, and personal authority; and the importance of role theory, and in particular the stress caused by ambiguity in role, role conflict, and role overload (see Ryle, 1982; also Menzies, 1970; Katz and Kahn, 1966; de Board, 1978).

To return to the example, the following quite different roles and relationships can be seen, each of which directly affects the decisions made and action taken:

1. A *therapeutic relationship* between the senior registrar and her patient.
2. *Clinical responsibility* of the consultant psychiatrist for the patient.
3. *Clinical supervision* of the senior registrar by the consultant psychiatrist.
4. *Psychotherapy supervision* of the senior registrar by the consultant psychotherapist.

   The consultant psychiatrist is responsible for his patients and for making sure that the senior registrar is making use of the psychotherapy supervision group. The consultant psychotherapist is not clinically responsible for the patient, only for being a competent psychotherapy supervisor. Ensuring this has been an *administrative* responsibility of the consultant, as has been making sure that the team's programme should enable the right people to attend the supervision group.

5. A *collaborative* relationship between psychiatrists, psychotherapist, and nursing staff. (The term is used here to describe the nature of the task, that is working together, although it is usually applied to collaboration *between* rather than *within* teams.)

6. The use of *clinical authority* when the psychiatrist made it clear that despite dissent and misgivings the treatment approach was the required one and would continue.

7. *Administration*, and *consultation* between consultant and senior nursing staff about how the team can adapt itself administratively to the requirements of the situation: the patient's need for nursing supervision around the clock, and the need for the nursing staff to be more fully informed about the treatment being undertaken and the misunderstandings that have arisen.

8. *Work with staff feelings and working relationships* on various formal and informal occasions but also in the staff groups, specifically for this purpose, and taken by a consultant from outside the unit's team.

9. *Teaching*, for example by consultant and by senior nursing staff among others. Clearly more explanation and discussion was needed about the treatment being used and why some members of staff knew of theoretical reasons why it seemed to be going according to plan, while others were aware only that the patient seemed to be getting worse as a result of psychotherapy and becoming harder to nurse.

10. *Training and staff development*. The process of resolving this problem depended on a number of shared attitudes among senior staff about multi-professional teamwork, and on machinery (for example staff meetings and how they operate) built into the unit's programme. It is important to appreciate, however, that such arrangements serve not only to cope with crisis, but also as the means by which such organizational and group dynamic processes are brought to the attention of staff and become part of their experience and therefore part of their training. This applies no less to senior staff, who may know of such group processes in theory, and indeed will have experienced them before, but none the less can always learn more from each incident, which always has its own unique qualities.

   Any organization which uses people's skills and relationships in therapy or in teaching, or to provide a setting in which these can proceed, requires attention to be given to such matters, which form the nuts and bolts of the group's structure. It is particularly important in the care of disturbed children and adolescents where reasonably coherent, consistent, skilled, adaptable, and rewarding working relationships need to be developed out of circumstances which have many inherent qualities that work against this aim, something which has been much discussed in this field of work (see Whitmore, 1974; Steinberg, 1981c; Child Guidance Trust, 1981; and Part One of this book) and remains full of controversy.

CONSULTATION AND RELATED WORK

Consultation is a term used in a variety of different ways; Caplan (1970) has pointed out that it is sometimes used to refer to practically any professional activity. The necessity for different professional workers to share experience, skills, and indeed time on overlapping problems has resulted in increasing interest in the methods by which this can be achieved, and they include a variety of professional skills and relationships of which consultation is one.

The example given above illustrates the range of quite different activities and relationships available to professional workers in addition to these that are primarily therapeutic. Administrative, teaching, supervisory, and collaborative functions are usually easy to distinguish from each other, but in circumstances when they are not considerable problems and misunderstandings can result. Thus the consultant psychotherapist in the example was supervising what was happening in the psychotherapeutic sessions, but the consultant psychiatrist remained clinically responsible for his patient and shared administrative responsibility for the team's activities with the senior nurse. Occasionally it may happen that a professional worker agrees to offer consultation to a children's home or school, and later discovers that the establishment's managers had expected supervision of the staff, which is a different task, and such misunderstandings can have quite serious consequences. Although such distinctions may sometimes seem rather fine, the realities of work with children and adolescents, with several different adults having substantially different relationships with them and with each other, and undertaking different responsibilities, makes it important at least to be able to differentiate between them (see also Steinberg, 1982b; Steinberg and Yule, 1983).

Consultation as the term is used here is based on the concept developed by G. Caplan (1964, 1970) of work in which one professional worker (the consultant) helps another (the consultee) clarify and resolve a problem or issue arising in his work. The consultant's task is to enable problems to be explored, and he may direct attention to issues to do with the consultee's work setting, his goals and objectives, and his relationship with his client, to help the consultee make the best use of his own experience and skills and the resources available to him in his work. Essential to this view of consultation is that it can be a peer exercise in a way which supervision or teaching is not; that responsibility for the problem and for what use is made of the consultative session remains with the consultee; and that the consultee should learn from the consultation and be in a better position to handle future problems, so that some degree of professional development is part of the work.

Consultation may be a 'one-off' matter, for example a particular way of responding to a problem or a referral or it may be planned as a series of sessions to meet a particular need, for example to help school or children's home staff cope with recurring problems and use them as a focus for staff development.

Techniques of consultation are discussed by G. Caplan (1970) and Dare (1982).

Supervision implies seniority on the part of the supervisor, in experience of the work being supervised though often in terms of the administrative hierarchy too. The supervisor has responsibility for the work being undertaken, and the person being supervised is responsible for using the advice or direction given.

Collaboration simply means working together. It includes teamwork, liaison (information exchanging and task distribution) between teams, and often has a training component, for example when a psychologist helps the staff of a children's home or special school develop and apply behaviour modification techniques.

It is always worth clarifying (through consultation) the nature of the anticipated work to avoid later misunderstanding. A psychiatrist, invited to help an acute medical unit with patients who have taken overdoses, may be expected to offer a truly consultative service to the medical team, to offer a diagnostic and therapeutic service to some of the patients, or simply to arrange their 'disposal' as swiftly as possible. It is as well to be clear about what is expected.

Psychotherapy, it may seem, should be easily distinguished from consultation, but it is not always easy to differentiate between ordinary feelings which in some way are impeding work, and those which derive from and are affecting wider aspects of the consultee's life. Consultant and consultee should deal with work-focused issues only; the consultant should not become therapist, counsellor or marital expert towards the consultee, and the consultee should not expect him to. What consultation may do is to clarify for the consultee that psychotherapy or counselling of some sort would be helpful, and the consultee should decide this and arrange it for himself. Staff groups should operate on the same basis; they are consultative, not therapeutic, providing a forum to clarify what needs to be done outside the group, whether in terms of administrative moves, therapy or training. But the line is not easily drawn.

Teaching and learning

Similar considerations apply in relation to teaching. A training course is not the same thing as a series of consultative meetings; but the latter should result in professional development and, as Dare (1982) points out, systematic teaching can be appropriately undertaken within the bounds of the consultation contract. The consultant will usually be experienced in a relevant field, and there is no reason why he should keep information to himself that may be useful for the consultees. However, if he turned his consultation seminars into a series of didactic lectures he would not be helping his consultees find things out for themselves in a way that gets the best from consultation. If the consultant found the consultees to be so very deficient in knowledge or skills that extra training was most important, then, as with the need for psychotherapy, an important task within the consultation sessions would be to clarify that need, and hope that it becomes something the consultees will want.

Earlier chapters showed how so many of the problems that arise in adolescent psychiatry are not due simply to the familiar difficulties of understanding individual psychiatric disorder and its treatment. Some of the most challenging issues are to do with making the best use of the skills of parents, teachers, and others in the community, and encouraging their development; enhancing the work of professionals dealing with troubled adolescents by improving training and supervision; and considering how the settings from which they work can be most helpfully organized and administered. Clarification of such personal, professional, and organizational matters helps to demonstrate the questions about individual development and disorder that remain to be asked, both in general and in the case of the individual adolescent. Consultation brought into focus, learned, and taught as a particular way for professional workers to explore such matters together can thereby function as a third main method of enquiry alongside clinical investigation and systematic research.

References

Aarkrog, T. (1981). The borderline concept in childhood, adolescence and adulthood: borderline adolescents in psychiatric treatment and 5 years later. *Acta Psychiatrica Scandinavica*, Suppl. **293**, 64.

Abraham, K. (1927). A short study of the development of the libido viewed in the light of mental disorders. In *Selected Papers of Karl Abraham*, 1927. Translated by D. Bryan and A. Strachey. London: Hogarth Press.

Abramowitz, C. V. (1976). The effectiveness of group psychotherapy with children. *Archives of General Psychiatry*, **33**, 320–326.

Acton, W. P. (1970). Analytic group therapy with adolescents. *Proceedings of the Fifth Conference of the Association for the Psychiatric Study of Adolescents*, 49–59.

Adams, J. F. (1965). The interpersonal relationship: the core of guidance. In *Counselling and Guidance – a summary view*. J. F. Adams (ed.) New York: Macmillan.

Adams, P. L. (1973). *Obsessive children: a sociopsychiatric study*. London: Butterworth.

Adamson, J. W. (1938). Education. In *The Legacy of the Middle Ages*, C. G. Crump and E. F. Jacob (eds). Oxford: Clarendon Press.

Adelson, J., and O'Neill, R. (1966). The development of political thought in adolescence. *Journal of Personality and Social Psychology*, **4**, 295–308.

Adelstein, A., and Mardon, C. (1975). Suicides 1961–1974. In *Population Trends*. No. 2. London: Her Majesty's Stationery office.

Aichorn, A. (1935). *Wayward Youth*. New York: Viking Press.

Ainsworth, M. D., Blehar, M. C., Waters, E., and Wall, S. (1978). *Patterns of Attachment: Assessed in the Strange Situation and at Home*. Hillsdale, New Jersey: Lawrence Elbaum.

Aitken, R. C. B., Buglass, D., and Kreitman, N. (1969). The changing pattern of attempted suicide in Edinburgh 1962–1967. *British Journal of Preventive and Social Medicine*, **23**, 111–115.

Alden, M. (1909). Child Life and labour. London: Headley Brothers.

Alexander, J., and Parsons, B. (1973). Short-term intervention with delinquent families. *Journal of Abnormal Psychology*, **81**, 219–225.

Al-Kaisi, A. H., and McGuire, R. J. (1974). The effect of sulthiame on disturbed behaviour in mentally subnormal patients. *British Journal of Psychiatry*, **124**, 45–49.

Allchin, W. H., Dell, D. E., and Wills, M. A. (1967). Leigh House Adolescent Psychiatric Unit: a report of the first five years (unpublished paper).

Allen, A., and Morton, A. (1961). *This is Your Child: the story of the National Society for the Prevention of Cruelty to Children*. London: Routledge and Kegan Paul.

Allen, M. R. (1967). *Male Cults and Secret Initiations in Melanesia*. Melbourne University Press.

American Psychiatric Association (1979). *Diagnostic and Statistical Manual (DSM III)*, 3rd edn.

Anderson, L. S. (1981). Notes on the linkage between the sexually abused child and the suicidal adolescent. *Journal of Adolescence*, **4**, 157–162.

Angst, J., Baastrup, P., Grof, P., Hippius, H., Poldinger, W., and Weis, P. (1973). The course of monopolar depression and bipolar psychoses. *Psychiatry, Neurology and Neurosurgery*, **76**, 489–500.

Annals of the American Society for Adolescent Psychiatry (1972 and subsequent volumes) see Feinstein, Giovacchini, and Miller, 1972.

Annell, A. L. (1969a). Lithium in the treatment of children and adolescents. *Acta Psychiatrica Scandinavica*, Suppl. **207**, 19–30.

Annell, A. L. (1969 b). Manic depressive illness in children and effect of treatment with lithium carbonate. *Acta Paedopsychiatrica*, **36**, 292–300.

Annesley, P. T. (1961). Psychiatric illness in adolescence: presentation and prognosis. *Journal of Mental Science*, **107**, 268–278.

Anthony, E. J. (1957). An experiemental approach to the psychopathology of childhood encopresis. *British Journal of Medical Pscyology*, **30**, 146–175.

Anthony, E. J., and Scott, P. (1960). Manic depressive psychosis in childhood. *Journal of Child Psychology and Psychiatry*, **1**, 53–72.

Argyle, M. (1969). *Social Interaction*. London: Methuen.

Argyris, C. (1960). *Understanding Organisational Behaviour*. London: Tavistock.

Aries, P. (1962). *Centuries of Childhood*. New York: Knopf.

Asperger, H. (1944). Die autistischen Psychopathen in Kindes alter. Archiv für Psychiatie und Nervenkrankheit, **177**, 76–137. Quoted in Wolff and Chick, 1980. Schizoid personality in childhood: a controlled follow-up study. Psychological Medicine, **10**, 85–100.

Association for the Psychiatric Study of Adolescence (1976). Register of Psychiatric Adolescent Units.

Association for the Psychiatric Study of Adolescence. Symposia for conferences held in 1970, 1971, 1972, 1973, 1974, 1975, and 1976.

August, G. J., and Stewart, M. A. (1982). Is there a syndrome of pure hyperactivity? *British Journal of Psychiatry*. **140**, 305–311.

Bancroft, J. H. J., Skrimshire, A. M., Reynolds, F., Simkin, S., and Smith, J. (1975). Self-poisoning and self-injury in the Oxford area. Epidemiological Aspects 1969–1973. *British Journal of Preventive and Social Medicine*, **29**, 170–177.

Bandura, A. (1964). The stormy decade: fact or fiction? In *Psychology in Schools*. New York: Clinical Psychology Publishing Company.

Barker, P. (1974a). The results of in-patient care. In *The Residential Psychiatric Treatment of Children*. P. Barker (ed.). London: Crosby Lockwood Staples.

Barker, P. (1974b). Aims and nature of inpatient psychiatric treatment of children. In *The Residential Psychiatric Treatment of Children*. P. Barker (ed.). London: Crosby Lockwood Staples.

Barker, P. (1947c). History. In *The Residential Psychiatric Treatment of Children*. P. Barker (ed.). London: Crosby Lockwood Staples.

Barker, P., and Frazer, I. A. (1968). A controlled trial of haloperidol in children. *British Journal of Psychiatry*, **114**, 855–857.

Barkley, R. A. (1976). Predicting the response of hyperkinetic children to stimulant drugs: a review. *Journal of Abnormal Child Psychology*, **4**, 327–348.

Barkley, R. A. (1977). A review of stimulant drug research with hyperactive children. *Journal of Child Psychology and Psychiatry*, **18**, 137–165.

Barraclough, B., Shepard, D., and Jennings, C. (1977). Do newspaper reports of coroners' inquests incite people to commit suicide? *British Journal of Psychiatry*, **131**, 528–532.

Barrett, A. M. (1931). Manic-depressive psychoses in childhood. *International Clinics*, **3** (41), 205–217.

Bass, M. (1970). Sudden sniffing death. *Journal of the American Medical Association*, **212** (12), 2075–2079.

Bateson, G. (1958). *Naven*. California: Stanford University Press.

Bateson, G. (1971). The cybernetics of self: a theory of alcoholism. *Psychiatry*, **34**, 1–18.

Bateson, G. (1973). *Steps to an Ecology of Mind*. St Albans: Paladin.

Bateson, G. (1979). *Mind and Nature: A Necessary Unity*. London: Wildwood House.

Bateson, G., Jackson, D. D., Haley, J., and Weakland, J. H. (1956). Towards a theory of Schizophrenia. *Behavioural Science*, **1**, 251–264.

Bateson, P. P. G. 1976, Rules and reciprocity in behavioural development. In *Growing Points in Ethology*. P. P. G. Bateson and P. H. Klopfer (eds). New York: Plenum.

Bean, A., and Roberts, M. (1981). The effect of time-out release contingencies on changes in child non-compliance. *Journal of Abnormal Child Psychology*, **9** (1), 95–105.

Bearn, A. G. (1972). Wilson's disease. In *The Metabolic Basis of Inherited Disease*, J. B. Stanbury, J. B. Wyngaarden, and D. S. Frederickson, (eds). New York: McGraw-Hill.

Beck, A. T. (1967). *Depression: Clinical, Experimental and Theoretical Aspects*. New York: Hoeber.

Bedford, A. P., and Tennent, T. G. (1981). Behaviour training with disturbed adolescents. *News of the Association for Child Psychology and Psychiatry*, **7**, 6–12.

Bellman, M. (1966). Studies on encopresis. *Acta Paediatrica Scandinavica*, Suppl. 170.

Belson, W. A. (1978). *Television Violence and the Adolescent Boy*. Farnborough: Saxon House.

Benaim, S., Horder, J., and Anderson, J. (1973). Hysterical epidemic in a classroom. *Psychological Medicine*, **3**, 366–373.

Bentovim, A. (1972a). Emotional disturbances of handicapped pre-school children and their families: attitudes to the child. *British Medical Journal*, **3**, 579–581.

Bentovim, A. (1972b). Handicapped pre-school children and their families: effects on child's early emotional development. *British Medical Journal*, **3**, 634–637.

Bentovim, A., and Gilmour, L. (1981). A family therapy interactional approach to decision making in child care, access and custody cases. *Journal of Family Therapy*, **3**, 65–77.

Bentovim, A., and Kinston, W. (1978). Brief focal therapy when the child is the referred patient. I: Clinical. *Journal of Child Psychology and Psychiatry*, **19** (1), 57–62.

Berg, I. (1980). School refusal in early adolescence. In *Out of School: modern perspectives in truancy and school refusal*. L. Hersov. and I. Berg. (eds). Chichester: John Wiley.

Berg, I., Butler, A., Hullin, R., Smith, R., and Tyrer, S. (1978). Features of children taken to juvenile court for failure to attend school. *Psychological Medicine*, **8**, 447–453.

Berg, I., and Griffiths, B. (1970). Two years' admissions to a Regional adolescent psychiatry unit. *Medical Officer*, January 1970.

Berg, I., Hullin, R., Allsopp, M., O'Brien, P., and Macdonald, R. (1974). Bipolar manic-depressive psychosis in early adolescence: a case report. *British Journal of Psychiatry*, **125**, 416–417.

Berg, I., and Jones, K. V. (1964). Functional faecal incontinence in children. *Archives of Diseases of Childhood*, **39**, 465–472.

Berger, P. L., and Luckmann, T. (1967). *The Social Construction of Reality*. London: Allen Lane The Penguin Press.

Berkowitz, D. A. (1979). The disturbed adolescent and his family: problems of individuation. *Journal of Adolescence*, **2**, 27–39.

Berkowitz, I. H. (ed.) (1972). *Adolescents Grow in Groups: experiences in adolescent group psychotherapy*. New York: Brunner-Mazel.

Berkowitz, I. H., and Sugar, M. (1975). Indications and contraindications for adolescent group psychotherapy. In *The Adolescent in Group and Family Therapy*. M. Sugar (ed.). New York: Brunner-Mazel.

Beskind, H. (1962). Psychiatric in-patient treatment of adolescents: a review of clinical experience. *Comprehensive Psychiatry*, **3**, 354–369.

Bettelheim, B. (1950). *Love is Not Enough*. Illinois: Free Press of Glencoe.

Bettelheim, B. (1960). *The Informed Heart*. New York: The Free Press.

Bettelheim, B. (1976). *The Uses of Enchantment: the meaning and importance of fairy tales*. London: Thames and Hudson.

Bettelheim, B., and Sylvester, E. (1952). A therapeutic milieu. *American Journal of Orthopsychiatry*, **22**, 314–334.

Bhanji, S. (1979). Affective disorder. In *Essentials of Postgraduate Psychiatry*. P. Hill, R. Murray, and A. Thorley (eds). London: Academic Press.

Bibring, E. (1953). The mechanism of depression. In *Affective Disorders*. P. Greenacre (ed.). New York: International Universities Press.

Bicknell, J. (1975). *Pica. A Childhood Symptom*. London: Butterworths.

Biller, H. B. and Borstelmann, L. J. (1965). Intellectual level and sex role development in mentally retarded children. *American Journal of Mental Deficiency*, **70**, 443–447.

Birch, N. J. (1979). Bone side-effects of lithium. In *A Handbook of Lithium Therapy*. F. N. Johnson (ed.). Lancaster: MTP.

Birley, J. L. T., and Brown, G. W. (1970). Crises and life changes preceding the onset or relapse of acute schizophrenia: clinical aspects. *British Journal of Psychiatry*, **116**, 327–333.

Blackwell, B., and Currah, J. (1973). The psychopharmacology of nocturnal enuresis. In *Bladder Control and Enuresis*. I. Kolvin, R. McKeith, and S. Meadow, (eds). Clinics in Developmental Medicine No. 48/49. London: Heinemann.

Blackwell, R. D., and Wilkins, M. P. J. (1981). Beyond the family system. *Journal of Family Therapy*, **3**, 79–90.

Bleuler, E. (1911). *Dementia Praecox or the Group of Schizophrenias*. (Trans. J. Zinkin, 1950) New York. International Universities Press.

Blitzer, J. A., Rollins, N., and Blackwell, A. (1961). Children who starve themselves. *Psychosomatic Medicine*, **23**, 369–381.

Blos, P. (1962). *On Adolescence: A Psychoanalytic Interpretation*. New York: Free Press.

Blos, P. (1967). The second Individuation process of adolescence. *Psychoanalytic Study of the Child*, **22**, 162–186.

Blos, P. (1970). *The Young Adolescent: clinical studies*. London: Collier-MacMillan.

Blos, P. (1979). *The Adolescent Passage: developmental issues*. New York: International Universities Press.

Blumberg, H. (1977). Drug taking. In *Child Psychiatry–Modern Approaches*. M. Rutter and L. Hersov (eds). Oxford: Blackwell.

Bolthauser, E., and Wilson, J. (1976). Value of brain biopsy in neurodegenerative disease in childhood. *Archives of Disease in Childhood*, **51**, 264–268.

Bolton, D., Collins, S., and Steinberg, D. (1983). The Treatment of Obsessive–Compulsive disorder in Adolescence: A report of 15 cases. *British Journal of Psychiatry*, **142**, 456–464.

Booker, C. (1969). *The Neophiliacs: a study of the revolution in English life in the fifties and sixties*. London: Collins.

Bowden, P. (1979). A short history of the management of the insane. In *Essentials of Postgraduate Psychiatry*. P. Hill, R. Murray, and A. Thorley (eds). London: Academic Press.

Bower, E. M. (1960). *Early Identification of Emotionally Handicapped Children in School.* Springfield. Illinois: Charles C. Thomas.

Bower, E. M., Shellhamer, T. A., and Daily, J. M. (1960). School characteristics of male adolescents who later become schizophrenic. *American Journal of Orthopsychiatry*, **30**, 712–729.

Bowlby, J. (1961). Processes of mourning. *International Journal of Psychoanalysis*, **62**, 317–340.

Bowlby, J. (1969). *Attachment and Loss.* Vol. 1: *Attachment.* London: Hogarth.

Bowlby, J. (1973). *Attachment and Loss.* Vol. 2: *Separation: Anxiety and Anger.* London: Hogarth Press.

Bowlby, J. (1977). The making and breaking of affectional bonds. *British Journal of Psychiatry*, **130**, 201–210 and 421–431.

Bowlby, J. (1979). *The Making and Breaking of Affectional Bonds.* London: Tavistock.

Bowlby, J. (1980). *Attachment and Loss.* Vol. 3: *Loss.* London, Hogarth Press.

Boyson, R. (1974). The need for realism. In *Truancy.* B. Turner (ed.). London: Ward Lock Educational.

Bray, G. A. (1976). *The Obese Patient.* Vol. IX: *Major Problems in Internal Medicine.* Philadelphia: W. R. Saunders.

Brett, E. M., and Lake, B. D. (1975). Reassessment of rectal approach to neuropathology in children. Review of 307 biopsies over 11 years. *Archives of Disease in Childhood*, **50**, 753–762.

Breunlin, C., and Breunlin, D. C. (1979). The family therapy approach to adolescent disturbances: a review of the literature. *Journal of Adolescence*, **2**, 153–169.

Brewer, C., and Lait, J. (1980). *Can Social Work Survive?* London: Temple Smith.

Bridgeland, M. (1971). *Pioneer Work with Maladjusted Children.* London: Staples Press.

British Medical Journal (1975). Nature and nurture in childhood obesity. *British Medical Journal* **2**, 706.

Brodie, H. K. H., and Leff, M. J. 1971. Bipolar depression – a comparative study of patient characteristics. *American Journal of Psychiatry*, **127**, 1086–1090.

Brook, C. G. D. 1980. The fat child. *British Journal of Hospital Medicine*, **24** (6), 517–522.

Brook, C. G. D. 1981. Delayed puberty. *British Journal of Hospital Medicine*, **26** (6) 573–580.

Brougham and Vaux, Henry Lord: Bell, Sir Charles (1845). In *Paley's Natural Theology*, **3**, p. 19. London: Charles Knight.

Brown, B. J., and Christie, M. (1981). *Social Learning Practice in Residential Child Care.* Oxford: Pergamon.

Brown, F. (1966). Childhood breavement and subsequent psychiatric disorder. *British Journal of Psychiatry*, **112**, 1035–1041.

Brown, G. W., Bhrolchain, M. V., and Harris, T. (1975). Social class and psychiatric disturbance among women in an urban population. *Sociology*, **9**, 225–254.

Brown, G. W. and Birley, J. L. T. (1968). Crisis and life changes and the onset of schizophrenia. *Journal of Health and Social Behaviour*, **9**, 203–214.

Brown, G. W., Birley, J. L. T., and Wing, J. K. (1972). Influence of family life on the course of schizophrenic disorders: a replication. *British Journal of Psychiatry*, **121**, 241–258.

Brown, G. W. and Harris, T. (1978). *Social Origins of Depression: a study of psychiatric disorder in women.* London: Tavistock.

Brown, G. W., Harris, T., and Copeland, J. R. (1977). Depression and loss. *British Journal of Psychiatry*, **130**, 1–8.

Brown, G. W., Monck, E. M., Carstairs, G. M., and Wing, J. K. (1962). Influence of family life on the course of schizophrenic illness. *British Journal of Preventive and Social Medicine*, **16**, 55–68.

Brown, J. A. C. (1961). *Freud and the Post-Freudians*. Harmondsworth: Penguin Books.

Bruce, T. (1975). Adolescent psychotherapy groups. *Therapeutic Education*, 3, 38–42.

Bruce, T. (1978). Group work with adolescents. *Journal of Adolescence*, 1, 47–54.

Bruch, H. (1971). Obesity in adolescence. In *Modern Perspectives in Adolescent Psychiatry*. I. G. Howells (ed.). Edinburgh: Oliver and Boyd.

Bruch, H. (1974). *Eating Disorders*. London: Routledge and Kegan Paul.

Bruch, H. (1978). *The Golden Cage: the enigma of anorexia nervosa*. London: Open Books.

Bruggen, P. (1979). Authority in work with young adolescents: a personal review. *Journal of Adolescence*, 2, 345–354.

Bruggen, P., Byng-Hall, J., and Pitt-Aikens, T. (1973). The reason for admission as a focus of work in an adolescent unit. *British Journal of Psychiatry*, 122, 319–329.

Bruggen, P., and Davies, G. (1977). Family therapy in adolescent psychiatry. *British Journal of Psychiatry*, 131, 433–447.

Bruggen, P., and Westland, P. (1979). Difficult to place adolescents: are more resources required? *Journal of Adolescence*, 2, 245–250.

Brumback, R. A., and Weinberg, W. A. (1977). Mania in childhood II: Therapeutic trial of lithium carbonate and further description of manic-depressive illness in children. *American Journal of Diseases of Children*, 131, 1122–1126.

Bryant, P. (1977). Piaget: causes and alternatives. In *Child Psychiatry: Modern Approaches*. M. Rutter and L. Hersov (eds). Oxford: Blackwell.

Bullough, V. L. (1981). Age at menarche: a misunderstanding. *Science*, 213, 365–366.

Burlingham, D. and Freud, A. (1943). *Infants without Families*. London: George Allen and Unwin.

Burn, M. (1964). *Mr Lyward's Answer: a successful experiment in education*. London: Hamish Hamilton.

Burnham, J. (1942). *The Managerial Revolution*. London: Putnam.

Burrell, S. (1982). Glue sniffing. Personal Communication.

Burton, R. (1927). *The Anatomy of Meloncholy: new impression*. London: Chatto and Windus.

Butcher, H. J. (1970). *Human Intelligence: Its Nature and Assessment*. London: Methuen.

Butler, A. M. and Ritchie, R. H. (1960). Simplification and improvement in estimating drug dosage and fluid and dietary allowances for patients of varying sizes. *New England Journal of Medicine*, 262, 903–908.

Byng-Hall, J. and Bruggen, P. (1974). Family admission decisions as a therapeutic tool. *Family Process*, 13, 443–459.

Cadbury, G. S. (1938). *Young Offenders Yesterday and Today*. London: George Allen and Unwin, quoting Judicia Civitatis Lundoniae Subrege Aethalstano edita (British Museum).

Camden and Islington Area Health Authority (Teaching) (1981). *Solvent Sniffing: notes designed for professionals*. London Borough of Islington Social Services Department.

Campbell, J. D. (1952). Manic depressive psychosis in children: report of 18 cases. *Journal of Nervous and Mental Diseases*, 116, 424–439.

Campbell, M. (1975). Pharmacotherapy in early infantile autism. *Biological Psychiatry*, 10, 399–423.

Campbell, M. (1976). Biological interventions in psychoses of childhood. In *Psychopathology and Child Development*. E. Schopler and R.J. Reichler (eds.). London: Plenum Press.

Campbell M., Fish, B., Korein, J., Shapiro T., Collins, P., and Koh, C. (1972). Lithium and chlorpramazine: A controlled crossover study in hyperactive severely disturbed young children. *Journal of Autism and Childhood Schizophrenia*, 2, 234–263.

Canning, H., and Mayer, J. (1966). Obesity: its possible effect on college acceptance. *New England Journal of Medicine*, **285**, 1402–1407.

Canning, H., and Mayer, J. (1967). Obesity: an influence on high school performance. *American Journal of Clinical Nutrition*, **20**, 352–354.

Cantril, H. (1950). *The 'Why' of Man's Experience*. New York: MacMillan.

Cantwell, D. (1975). A critical review of therapeutic modalities with hyperactive children. *The Hyperactive Child: Diagnosis, Management and Current Research*. D. Cantwell (ed.). New York: Spectrum Publications.

Cantwell, D. (1977). Hyperkinetic syndrome. In *Child Psychiatry: modern approaches*. M. Rutter and L. Hersov (eds). Oxford: Blackwell.

Cantwell, D. P., Sturzenberger, S., Burroughs, J., Salkin, B., and Green, J. K. (1977). Anorexia nervosa: an affective disorder? *Archives of General Psychiatry*, **34**, 1087–1093.

Capes, M., Gould, E., and Townsend, M. (1971). *Stress in Youth*. London: Oxford University Press.

Caplan, G. (1964). *Principles of Preventive Psychiatry*. London: Tavistock.

Caplan, G. (1970). *The Theory and Practice of Mental Health Consultation*. London: Tavistock.

Caplan, H. L. (1970). Hysterical 'Conversion' Symptoms in Childhood. University of London: M. Phil Dissertation.

Caplan, M. G., and Douglas, V. I. (1969). Incidence of parental loss in children with depressed mood. *Journal of Child Psychology and Psychiatry*, **10**, 225–232.

Carney, M. W. P., Roth, M. P., and Garside, R. F. (1965). The diagnosis of depressive syndromes and the prediction of ECT response. *British Journal of Psychiatry*, **111**, 659–674.

Carr, A. T. (1974). Compulsive neurosis: a review of the literature. *Psychological Bulletin*, **81** (5), 311–318.

Cartwright, G. E. (1978). Diagnosis of treatable Wilson's disease. *New England Journal of Medicine*, **298**, 24.

Cawson, P. (1979). *Children Referred to a Closed Unit*. London: Her Majesty's Stationery Office.

Centre for the Study of Adolescence, London. Monographs for 1968, 1969, 1970, 1972 and 1974.

Chess, S. (1960). Diagnosis and treatment of the hyperactive child. *New York State Journal of Medicine*, **60**, 2379–2385.

Chess, S. (1973). Marked anxiety in children. *American Journal of Psychotherapy*, **17**, 390–395.

Chess, S. (1980). Developmental theory revisited. In *Annual Progress in Child Psychiatry and Child Development*. S. Chess and A. Thomas (eds.). New York: Brunner Mazel.

Chess, S., and Hassibi, M. (1978). *Principles and Practice of Child Psychiatry*. New York and London: Plenum Press.

Child Guidance Trust (1981). Interdisciplinary Work in Child Guidance. Report of the Interdisciplinary Standing Committee.

Children's and Young Persons Act (1969). London: Her Majesty's Stationery Office.

Chisholm, D. D. (1978). Obesity in Adolescence. *Journal of Adolescence*, **1**, 177–194.

Clare, A. (1976). *Psychiatry in Dissent*. London: Tavistock.

Clare, A. (1979a). The disease concept in psychiatry. In *Essentials of Postgraduate Psychiatry*. P. Hill, R. Murray, and A. Thorley (eds). London: Academic Press.

Clare, A. (1979b). Psychosurgery and electroconvulsive therapy. In *Essentials of Postgraduate Psychiatry*. P. Hill, R. Murray, and A. Thorley (eds). London: Academic Press.

Clark, D. H. (1977). The therapeutic community. *British Journal of Psychiatry*, **13**, 553–564.

Clark, A. W., and Yeomans, N. T. (1969). *Fraser House: Theory, Practice and Evolution of a Therapeutic Community*. New York: Springer.

Clarke, D. F. (1966). Behaviour therapy of Gilles de la Tourette's syndrome. *British Journal of Psychiatry*, **112**, 771–778.

Clarke, R. V. G. (ed.) (1978). *Tackling Vandalism*. Home Office Research Study No. 47. London: Her Majesty's Stationery Office.

Clarke, R. V. G., and Cornish, D. B. (1978). The effectiveness of residential treatment for delinquents. *In Aggression and Antisocial Behaviour in Childhood and Adolescence*. L. Hersov, M. Berger and D. Shaffer (eds). Oxford: Pergamon.

Clarke, R. V. G., and Martin, D. N. (1971). *Absconding from Approved Schools*. London: Her Majesty's Stationery Office.

Clausen, J. A. (1975). The social meaning of Differential physical and sexual maturation. In *Adolescence in the Life Cycle: psychological change and social context*. S. E. Dragastin and G. H. Elder (eds). London: Halsted Press.

Cobb, E. (1977). *The Ecology of Imagination in Childhood*. New York: Columbia University Press.

Cohen, D. (1976). The diagnostic process of child psychiatry. *Psychiatric Annals*, **6**, 29–56.

Cohen, D. and Young, J. (1977). Neurochemistry of child psychiatry. *Journal of the American Academy of Child Psychiatry*, **16**, 353–411.

Cohen, S. (ed.) (1971). *Images of Deviance*. Harmondsworth: Penguin.

Cohen, W. J., and Cohen, N. H. (1974). Lithium carbonate, haloperidol and irreversible brain damage. *Journal of the American Medical Association*. **230**, 1283–1287.

Coleman, J. C. (1978). Current contradictions in adolescent theory. *Journal of Youth and Adolescence*, **7**, 1–12.

Coleman, J. C. (1979). Current views on the adolescent process. In *The School Years*. J. C. Coleman (ed.). London: Methuen.

Coleman, J. C. (1980). *The Nature of Adolescence*. London: Methuen.

Conger, J. J. (1977). *Adolescence and Youth*. New York: Harper and Row.

Connell, P. H. (1958). *Amphetamine Psychosis*. Institute of Psychiatry: Maudsley Monograph No. 5.

Connell, P. (1977). Clinical aspects of drug misuse. In *Child Psychiatry – modern approaches*. M. Rutter and L. Hersov (eds). Oxford: Blackwell.

Connell, P. H., Corbett, J. A., Horne, D. J., and Matthews, A. M. (1967). Drug treatment of adolescent ticqueurs: a double-bind study of diazepam and haloperidol. *British Journal of Psychiatry*, **113**, 375–381.

Conners, C., Kramer, R., Rothschild, G., Schwartz, L., and Stone, A. (1971). Treatment of young delinquent boys with diphenylhydantoin sodium and methylphenidate: a controlled comparison. *Archives of General Psychiatry*, **24**, 156–160.

Conners, C. K., and Werry, J. S. (1979). Pharmacotherapy. In *Psychopathological Disorders of Childhood*. H. C. Quay and J. S. Werry (eds). Chichester: John Wiley.

Cooper, D. (1967). *Psychiatry and Anti-Psychiatry*. London: Tavistock.

Corbett, J. A. (1975). Aversion for the treatment of self-injurious behaviour. *Journal of Mental Delinquency Research*, **19**, 79–95.

Corbett, J. A. (1977a). Mental retardation – psychiatric aspects. In *Child Psychiatry: modern approaches*. M. Rutter and L. Hersov (eds). Oxford: Blackwell.

Corbett, J. A. (1971). The nature of tics and Gilles de la Tourette's syndrome. *Journal of Psychosomatic Research*, **15**, 403–409.

Corbett, J. A. (1976). *Medical Management in Early Childhood Autism*. L. Wing (ed.). Oxford: Pergamon.

Corbett, J. A. (1977b). Tics and Tourette's Syndrome. In *Child Psychiatry: modern approaches*. M. Rutter and L. Hersov (eds). Oxford: Blackwell.

Corbett, J. A., and Campbell, H. J. (1981). Causes of severe self-injurious behaviour. In *New Frontiers in Mental Retardation*. Vol. II: *Biomedical Aspects*. P. Mittler and F. De Jong (eds). Baltimore: University Park Press.

Corbett, J. A., Harris, R., Taylor, E., and Trimble, M. (1977). Progressive disintegrative psychosis of childhood. *Journal of Child Psychology and Psychiatry*, **18**, 211–219.

Corbett, J. A., Matthews, A. M., Connell, P. H., and Shapiro, D. A. (1969). Tics and Gilles de la Tourette's syndrome: a follow-up study and critical review. *British Journal of Psychiatry*, **115**, 1229–1241.

Cornell, W. F., Stroobant, R. E., and Sinclair, K. E. (1975). *Twelve to Twenty: studies of city youth*. Sydney: Hicks and Sons.

Cornfield, R. B., and Feeling, S. D. (1980). Impact of the threatening patient on ward communications. *American Journal of Psychiatry*, **137** (5), 616–619.

Corte, H. E., Wolf, M. M., and Locke, B. J. (1971). A comparison of procedures for eliminating self-injurious behaviour in retarded adolescents. *Journal of Applied Behaviour Analysis*. Quoted in Corbett, 1975.

Cowen, E. L., Peterson, A., Babigian, H., Izzo, L. D. and Trost, M. A. (1973). Long-term follow-up of early detected vulnerable children. *Journal of Consulting and Clinical Psychology*, **41**, 438–446.

Cox, A., Holbrook, D., and Rutter, M. (1981a). Psychiatric interviewing techniques. VI: Experimental study: eliciting feelings. *British Journal of Psychiatry*, **139**, 144–152.

Cox, A., Hopkinson, K., and Rutter, M. (1981b). Psychiatric interviewing techniques. II: Naturalistic study: eliciting factual information. *British Journal of Psychiatry*, **138**, 283–291.

Cox, A., and Rutter, M. (1977). Diagnostic appraisal and interviewing. In *Child Psychiatry: modern approaches*. M. Rutter and L. Hersov (eds). Oxford: Blackwell.

Cox, A., Rutter, M., and Holbrook, D. (1981c). Psychiatric interviewing techniques. V: Experimental study: eliciting factual information. *British Journal of Psychiatry*, **139**, 29–37.

Coyne, J. C. (1976). Towards an interactional description of depression. *Psychiatry*, **39**, 28–40.

Crabtree, L. H., and Grossman, W. K. (1974). Administrative clarity and redefinition for an open adolescent unit. *Psychiatry*, **37**, 350–359.

Craft, A., and Craft, M. (1979). Personal relationships and partnerships for the mentally handicapped. in *Tredgold's Mental Retardation*. M. Craft (ed.). London: Bailliere Tindall.

Craft, A., and Craft, M. (1980). Sexuality and the mentally handicapped. In *The Modern Management of Mental Handicap*. G. B. Simon (ed.). Lancaster: MTP Press.

Craft, A., and Craft, M. (1981). Sexuality and mental handicap: a review. *British Journal of Psychiatry*, **139**, 494–505.

Craig, W. S. (1946). *Child and Adolescent Life in Health and Disease. A Study in Social Paediatrics*. Edinburgh: Livingstone.

Crammer, J. L. (1977). Lithium – effects and side effects. In *Advanced Medicine* vol. 13. G. M. Besser (ed.). Tunbridge Wells: Pitman Medical.

Crammer, J. L., Barraclough, B., and Heine, B. (1978). *The Use of Drugs in Psychiatry*. London: Gaskell Books and the Royal College of Psychiatrists.

Crammer, J. L., Rosser, R., and Crane, G. (1974). Blood levels and management of Lithium treatment. *British Medical Journal*, **3**, 650–654.

Creak, M., and Pampiglione, G. (1969). Clinical and EEG studies on a group of 35 psychotic children. *Developmental Medicine and Child Neurology*, **11**, 218–227.

Crichton Miller, H., (1925). *The New Psychology and the Parent*. London: Jarrolds.

Crisp, A. H. (1974). Primary anorexia nervosa or adolescent weight phobia. *Practitioner*, **212**, 525–535.

Crisp, A. H. (1978). Prevalence of anorexia nervosa. *British Medical Journal*, **2**, 500.

Crisp, A. H. (1980). *Anorexia Nervosa: let me be*. London: Academic press.

Crisp, A. H. (1982). Personal Communication.

Crisp, A.H., Palmer, R. L., and Kalucy, R. S. (1976). How common is anorexia nervosa? A prevalence study. *British Journal of Psychiatry*, **128**, 549–554.

Cutting, J. (1978). A re-appraisal of alcoholic psychoses. *Psychological Medicine*, **8**, 285–296.

Cytryn, L., and McKnew, D. H. (1975). Factors influencing the changing clinical expression of the depressive process in children. In *Annual Progress in Child Psychiatry and Child Development*. S. Chess and T. Thomas (eds). New York: Brunner Mazel.

Dalby, M. A. (1971). Antiepileptic and psychotropic effect of carbamazepine in the treatment of psychomotor epilepsy. *Epilepsia*, **12**, 325–334.

Dally, P. (1981). Treatment of anorexia nervosa. *British Journal of Hospital Medicine*, **25** (5), 434–440.

Dally, P. (1982). Community psychiatry. *Bulletin of the Royal College of Psychiatrists*, **6** (4), 66 (Correspondence).

Dally, P. Gomez, J., and Isaacs, A. J. (1979). *Anorexia Nervosa*. London: Heinemann.

Daniel, W. A. (1977). *Adolescents in Health and Disease*. St Louis: C. V. Mosby.

Dare, C. (1975). A classification of interventions in child and conjoint family therapy. *Psychotherapy and Psychosomatics*, **25**, 116–125.

Dare, C. (1977). Psychoanalytic theories. In *Child Psychiatry: modern approaches*, M. Rutter and L. Hersov, (eds). Oxford: Blackwell.

Dare, C. (1982). Techniques of consultation. In *Consultation from Child and Adolescent Psychiatric Settings*. C. Dare, R. Ryle, D. Steinberg, and W. Yule (eds). *News of the Association for Child Psychology and Psychiatry*. No. 11, July.

Davidson, W. S., and Seidman, E. (1974). Studies of behaviour modification and juvenile delinquency: a review, methodological critique and social perspective. *Psychological Bulletin*, **81**, 998–1011.

de Board, R. (1978). *The Psycho-Analysis of Organisations*. London: Tavistock.

De Mause, L. (ed.) (1974). *The History of Childhood*. London: Souvenir Press.

Demerath, N. J. (1943). Adolescent status demands and the student experiences of 20 schizophrenics. *Americal Sociological Review*, **8**, 513–518.

Department of Health and Social Security (1970). *Care and Treatment in a Planned Environment*. London: Her Majesty's Stationery Office.

Department of Health and Social Security (1977). Unpublished report of a conference on the problems of difficult to place adolescents.

Department of Health and Social Security/Department of Education and Science (1973). Circular on Child Guidance.

Department of Health and Social Security (DHSS) (1977). *Health and Personal Service Statistics*. London: Her Majesty's Stationery Office.

Despert, J. L. (1955). Differential diagnosis between obsessive–compulsive neurosis and schizophrenia in children. In *Psychopathology of Childhood*. P. Hoch and J. Zubin (eds). New York: Grune and Stratton.

Dicks, H. V. (1970). *Fifty Years of the Tavistock Clinic*. London: Routledge and Kegan Paul.

Dimascio, A. (1973). The effect of benzodiazepines on aggression: reduced or increased. In the Benzodiazepines. S. Garratini, E. Mussini, and L. O. Randall (eds). New York: Raven Press.

Dixon, J. (1981). The welfare of urban youth in China, 1949–1979. *Journal of Adolescence*, **4**, 1–12.

Dockar-Drysdale, B. (1968). Residential treatment of 'frozen' children. In *Therapy in Child Care*. London: Longman Green.

Donnan, S., and Haskey, J. (1977). Alcoholism and cirrhosis of the liver. *Population Trends*, **7**, 18–24.

Dostal, T., and Zvolsky, P. (1970). Antiaggressive effect of lithium salts in severely mentally retarded adolescents. *International Pharmacopsychiatry*, **5**, 203–207.

Douglas, J. W. B. (1964). *The Home and the School*. London: MackGibbon and Kee.

Dubowitz, V., and Hersov, L. (1976). Management of children with non-organic (hysterical) disorders of motor function. *Developmental Medicine and Child Neurology*, **18**, 358–368.

Dunham, J. (1980). Conflict and competence in inter-professional communication in the services for adolescents. In *Social Work with Adolescents*. R. Jones and C. Pritchard (eds). London: Routledge and Kegan Paul.

Dunn, J. (1980). Individual differences in temparament. In *Scientific Foundations of Developmental Psychiatry*. M. Rutter (ed.). London: Heinemann.

Dunn, J. F., and Kendrick, C. (1980). The arrival of a sibling: changes in patterns of interaction between mother and first-born child. *Journal of Child Psychology and Psychiatry*, **21**, 119–132.

Dusek, D., and Girdano, D. A. (1980). *Drugs*. California: Addison-Wesley.

Easson, W. M. (1968). Ego defects in nonpsychotic adolescents. *Psychiatric Quarterly*, **42**, 156–168.

Eisenberg, L. (1958). School phobia: a study in the communication of anxiety. *American Journal of Psychiatry*, **114**, 712–718.

Eisenberg, L. (1966). The management of the hyperkinetic child. *Developmental Medicine and Child Neurology*, **8**, 593–598.

Eisenberg, L. (1972). Principles of Drug Therapy in Child Psychiatry with Special Reference to Stimulant Drugs. *American Journal of Orthopsychiatry*, **41** (3), 371–379.

Eisenberg, L. (1973). The future of psychiatry. *Lancet*, **2**, 1371–1375.

Eisenberg, L. (1975). The ethics of intervention: acting amidst ambiguity. *Journal of Child Psychology and Psychiatry*, **16**, 93–104.

Eisenberg, L. (1977). Development as a unifying concept in psychiatry. *British Journal of Psychiatry*, **131**, 225–237.

Eisenberg, L., Ascher, E. A., and Kanner, L. (1959). A clinical study of Gilles de la Tourette's disease (maladie des tics) in children. *American Journal of Psychiatry*, **115**, 715–726.

Eisenberg, L., and Connors C. K. (1971). Psychopharmacology in childhood. In *Behavioral Science in pediatric Medicine*. S. Kagan and L. Eisenberg (eds). Philadelphia: W. B. Saunders.

Eissler, K. R. (1958). Notes on problems of technique in the psychoanalytic treatment of adolescents. *Psychoanalytic Study of the Child*, **13**, 223–254.

Elkind, D. (1966). Conceptual orientation shifts in children and adolescents. *Child Development*, **37**, 493–498.

Elkind, D. (1967). Egocentrism in adolescence. *Child Development*, **38**, 1025–1034.

Elkins, R. Rapoport, J. L., and Lipsky, A. (1980). Obsessive–compulsive disorder of childhood and adolescence. A neurobiological viewpoint. *Journal of the American Academy of Child Psychiatry*, **19**, 511–524.

Ellenberger, H. F. (1970). *The Discovery of the Unconscious: The History and Evolution of Dynamic Psychiatry*. London: Allen Lane, The Penguin Press.

Ellis, M. J. L. (1980). Conflict in an institutional setting: training and treatment considerations. *Journal of Adolescence*, **3**, 115–131.

Ellis, M. J. L. (1982). Psychotherapy in Borstal. *Journal of Adolescence*, **5**, 39–50.

Engel, G. L. (1977). The need for a new medical model. A challenge for biomedicine. *Science*, **196**, 129–136.

Erikson, E. (1964). *Insight and Responsibility*. New York: W. W. Norton and Company.

Erikson, E. (1965). *Childhood and Society*. London: Hogarth Press.

Erikson, E. (1968). *Identity, Youth and Crisis*. London: Faber.

Esterson. A. (1970). *The Leaves of Spring: schizophrenia, family and sacrifice*. London: Tavistock.

Evans, J. (1965). In-patient analytic group therapy of neurotic and delinquent adolescents. *Psychotherapy and Psychosomatics*, **13**, 265–270.

Evans, J. (1966). Analytic group therapy on delinquents. *Adolescence*, **1**, 180–196.

Evans, J. (1980). Ambivalence and how to turn it to your advantage: adolescence and paradoxical intervention. *Journal of Adolescence*, **3**, 273–284.

Evans, J., and Acton, W. P. (1972). A psychiatric service for disturbed adolescents. *British Journal of Psychiatry*, **120**, 429–432.

Evans, P. 1972. Henri Ey's concepts of the organisation of consciousness and its disorganisation: an extension of Jacksonian theory. *Brain*, **95** (2), 413–440.

Eveleth, P. and Tanner, J. (1977). *World Wide Variation in Human Growth*. Cambridge: Cambridge University Press.

Eysenck, H. J. (1953). *Uses and Abuses of Psychology*. Harmondsworth: Penguin Books.

Eysenck, H. J. (1957). *Sense and Nonsense in Psychology*. Harmondsworth: Penguin Books.

Eysenck, H. J. (ed.) (1960). *Behaviour Therapy and the Neuroses*. Oxford: Pergamon.

Eysenck, H. J. (1975). *The Future of Psychiatry*. London. Methuen.

Eysenck, H. J. and Rachman, S. J. (1965). The application of learning theory to child psychiatry. In *Modern Perspectives in Child Psychiatry*. J. G. Howells (ed.). Edinburgh: Oliver and Boyd.

Fairburn, C. G. (1980). Self-induced vomiting. *Journal of Psychosomatic Research*, **24**, 193–197.

Fairburn, C. G., and Cooper, P. J. (1982). Self-induced vomiting and bulimia nervosa: an undetected problem. *British Medical Journal*, **284**, 1153–1155.

Falstein, E. I., Feinstein, E. C., and Judas, I. (1956). Anorexia nervosa in the male child. *American Journal of Orthopsychiatry*, **26**, 751–772.

Family Therapy (1979). Editorial, **1**, 1–5.

Farrington, D. (1980). Truancy, delinquency, the home and the school. In *Out of School: modern perspectives in truancy and school refusal*. Chichester: Wiley.

Farrington, D. P. (1973). Self-reports of deviant behaviour: predictive and stable? *Journal of Criminal law and Criminology*, **64**, 99–110.

Feinstein, S. C., Giovacchini, P. L., and Miller, A. A. (1972). *Adolescent Psychiatry*. Vol. 1: *Developmental and Clinical Studies*. New York: Basic Books.

Festinger, L. (1957). *A Theory of Cognitive Dissonance*. Illinois: Row, Peterson and Co.

Field, J. R., Corbin, K. B., Goldstein, N. P., and Klass, D. W. (1966). Gilles de la Tourette's Syndrome. *Neurology*, **16**, 453–462.

Fine, R. (1973). Family therapy and a behavioural approach to childhood obsessive–compulsive neurosis. *Archives of General Psychiatry*, **28**, 695–697.

Fish, B. (1971). The 'one child, one drug' myth of stimulants in hyperkinesis: importance of diagnostic categories in evaluating treatment. *Archives of General Psychiatry*, **25**, 193–203.

Fleck, S. (1972). Some basic aspects of family pathology. In *Manual of Child Psychopathology*. B. Wolman (ed.). New York: McGraw Hill.

Fletcher, R. (1973). *The Family and Marriage in Britain: an analysis and moral assessment*. Harmondsworth: Penguin Books.

Flexner, A. (1915). Is social work a profession? *Proceedings of the National Conference of Charities and Correction*.

Flugel, J. C. (1933). *A Hundred Years of Psychology*. London: Duckworth.

Forrest, D. W. (1974). *Francis Galton: the life and work of a Victorian genius*. London: Paul Elek.

Foucault, M. (1967). *Madness and Civilization*. London: Tavistock.

Foucault, M. (1970). *The Order of Things: an archaeology of the human sciences*. New York: Random House.

Foulkes, S. H. and Anthony, E. J. (1965). *Group Psychotherapy: the psychoanalytic approach*. Harmondsworth: Penguin.

Fowler, D. R., and Longabaugh, E. D. (1975). The problem-oriented record. *Archives of General Psychiatry*, **32**, 831–834.

Framrose, R. (1975). The first seventy admissions to an adolescent unit in Edinburgh: general characteristics and treatment outcome. *British Journal of Psychiatry*, **126**, 380–389.

Frank, M. G. and Zilbach, J. (1968). Current trends in group therapy with children. *International Journal of Group Psychotherapy*, **18**, 447–460.

French, E. L. (1963). Residential treatment for emotionally disturbed young people. *Mental Hospitals*, **14**, 386–389.

Freud, A. (1936). *The Ego and the Mechanisms of Defence*. London: Hogarth Press.

Freud, A. (1958). Adolescence. *Psychoanalytic Study of the Child*, **13**, 255–278.

Freud, A. (1966). *Normality and Pathology in Childhood*. London: Hogarth Press.

Freud, S. (1905). Three essays on sexuality. In *Standard Edition of Freud's Works*. J. Strachey (ed.) 1922. London: Hogarth Press.

Freud, S. (1908). Creative writers and day-dreaming. In *Standard Edition of the Complete Works of Sigmund Freud*, vol. 9. J. Strachey (ed.) 1959. London: Hogarth Press.

Freud, S. (1917). Mourning and melancholia. In *Standard Edition of the Collected Works of Sigmund Freud*, vol. 14. J. Strachey (ed.) 1957; London: Hogarth Press.

Freud, S. (1922). *Introductory Lectures on Psychoanalysis*. George Allen and Unwin.

Freudenberger, H. J. (1975). The staff burnout syndrome in alternative institutions. *Psychotherapy*, spring 1975, 73–82.

Friedmann, C. T. H. and Silvers, F. M. (1977). A multimodality approach to inpatient treatment of obsessive compulsive disorder. *American Journal of Psychotherapy*, **31**, 456–465.

Frith, U. (1980). Reading and spelling skills. In *Scientific Foundations of Developmental Psychiatry*, M. Rutter (ed.). London: Heinemann.

Frommer, E. A. (1967). Treatment of childhood depression with antidepressant drugs. *British Medical Journal*, **1**, 729–732.

Frommer, E. A. (1968). Depressive illness in childhood. In *Recent Developments in Affective Disorders*. A. Coppen and A. Walk (eds). Ashford: Headley Brothers.

Fyvel, T. R. (1961). *The Insecure Offenders: rebellious youth in the welfare state*. London: Chatto and Windus.

Gallagher, J. R., and Harris, H. I. (1964). *Emotional Problems of Adolescents*. New York: Oxford University Press.

Garmezy, N. (1974a). Children at risk: the search for antecedents of schizophrenia. Part 1, conceptual models and research methods. *Schizophrenia Bulletin*, **8**, 14–90.

Garmezy, N. (1974b). Children at risk: the search for antecedents of schizophrenia. Part II, ongoing research programmes, issues and intervention. *Schizophrenia Bulletin*, **9**, 55–125.

Garralda H. M. E. (1980). Trainees' attitudes in child psychiatry. *The Bulletin of the Royal College of Psychiatrists,* Feb. 1980, 26–27.

Gath, A. (1972). The effects of mental Subnormality on the family. *British Journal of Hospital medicine*, **8**(2), 147–150.

Gath, D. (1968). Child guidance and the general practitioner: a study of factors influencing referrals made by general practitioners to a child psychiatric department. *Journal of Child Psychology and Psychiatry*, **9**, 213–227.

Gath, D., Cooper, B., and Gattoni, F. E. G. (1972). Child guidance and delinquency in a London Borough. *Psychological Medicine*, **2**, 185–191.

Geleerd, E. R. (1961). Some aspects of ego vicissitudes in adolescence. *Journal of the American Psychoanalytic Association*, **9**, 394–405.

Gibbens, T. (1977). Treatment of delinquents. In *Child Psychiatry: modern approaches*. Oxford: Blackwell.

Gibbens, J. S., Elliott, J., Urwin, P., and Gibbons, J. L. (1978). The urban environment and deliberate self-poisoning trends in Southampton. 1972–1977. *Social Psychiatry*, **13**, 159–166.

Gittelman-Klein, R., and Klein, D. F. (1971). Controlled imipramine treatment of school phobia. *Archives of General Psychiatry*, **25**, 204–207.

Gittelman-Klein, R., and Klein, D. G. (1973). School phobia: diagnostic considerations in the light of imipramine effects. *Journal of Nervous and Mental Disease*, **156**, 199–215.

Gittelman-Klein, R., and Klein, D. (1980). Separation anxiety in school refusal and its treatment with drugs. In *Out of School*, L. Hersov, and I. Berg. (eds). Chichester: Wiley.

Glaser, K. (1967). Masked depression in children and adolescents. *American Journal of Psychotherapy*, **21**, 265–574.

Goffman, E. (1961). *Asylums: essays on the social situation of mental patients and other inmates.* New York: Doubleday.

Goffman, E. (1963). *Stigma: notes on the management of spoiled identity.* New Jersey: Prentice Hall.

Goffman, E. (1968). *Asylums.* Harmondsworth: Penguin Books.

Goldberg, D., and Huxley, P. (1980). *Mental Illness in the Community: the pathway to psychiatric care.* London: Tavistock.

Goodman, N. Richardson, S. A., Dornbusch, S. M., and Hastorf, A. H. (1963). Variant reactions to physical disabilities. *American Sociological Review*, **38**, 429–435.

Goodwin, D., Guze, S., and Robins, E. (1969). Follow up studies in obsessional neurosis. *Archives of General Psychiatry*, **20**, 182–187.

Gostin, L. (1981). *Patients' Rights Handbook.* London: National Association for Mental Health.

Gould, M. S., Wunsch-Hitzig, R., and Dohrenwend, B. (1981). Estimating the prevalence of childhood psychopathology: a critical review. *Journal American Academy of Child Psychiatry*, **20**, 462–476.

Graham, P. (1974a). Depression in prepubertal children. *Developmental Medicine and Child Neurology*, **16**, 340–349.

Graham, P. (1974b). Child psychiatry and psychotherapy. *Journal of Child Psychology and Psychiatry*, **15**, 59–66.

Graham, P. (1980). Moral development. In *Scientific Foundations of Developmental Psychiatry.* M. Rutter (ed.). London: Heinemann.

Graham, P., and Rutter, M. (1968). Organic brain dysfunction and child psychiatric disorder, *British Medical Journal*, **3**, 695–700.

Graham, P., and Rutter, M. (1973). Psychiatric disorder in the young adolescent. *Proceedings of the Royal Society of Medicine*, **66**, 1226–1229.

Graham, P., and Rutter, M. (1977). Adolescent disorders. In *Child Psychiatry: modern approaches*. M. Rutter and L. Hersov, (eds). Oxford: Blackwell.

Graham, P., Rutter, M., and George, S. (1973). Temperamental characteristics as predictors of behavior disorders in children. *American Journal of Orthopsychiatry*, **43**, 328–339.

Gray, G., Smith, A., and Rutter, M. (1980). School attendance and the first year of employment. In *Out of School*, L. Hersov and I. Berg (eds.). Chichester: Wiley.

Green, D., (1980). A behavioural approach to the treatment of obsessional rituals: an adolescent case study. *Journal of Adolescence*, **3**, 297–306.

Green, R. (1975). Sexual identity: research strategies. *Archives of Sexual Behaviour*, **4** (4), 337–352.

Green, R. (1977). Atypical psychosexual development. In *Child Psychiatry: modern approaches*. M. Rutter and L. Hersov. (eds). Oxford: Blackwell.

Greenacre, P. (1937). Review of practical examination of personality and behaviour disorders. *Psychoanalytic Quarterly*, **6**, 134.

Greenwood, J. (1982a). Community psychiatry. *Bulletin of the Royal College of Psychiatrists*, **6**, (1), 6–8.

Greenwood, J. (1982b). Community psychiatry. *Bulletin of the Royal College of Psychiatrists*, **6**(4), 67 (Correspondence).

Grinker, R., Werble, B., and Drye, R. (1968). *The Borderline Syndrome*. New York: Basic Books.

Group for the Advancement of Psychiatry: Committee on Adolescence (1974). *Normal Adolescence: its dynamics and impact*. London: Crosby Lockwood Staples.

Gruber, T. (1980). The preadmission screening process. In *A Psychodynamic Approach to Adolescent Psychiatry*. D. R. Heacock (ed.). New York: Marcel Dekker.

Gull, W. W. (1874). Anorexia nervosa. In *Abnormal Psychology: collected readings*. M. Hamilton (ed.) Harmondsworth: Penguin.

Gunderson, J. and Singer, M. (1975). Defining borderline patients. An overview. *American Journal of Psychiatry*, **132**, 1–10.

Haley, J. (1975). Family therapy. In *Comprehensive Textbook of Psychiatry*. Vol. 2, 2nd edn. A. M. Freedman, H. I. Kaplan, and B. J. Sadock, (eds). Baltimore: Williams and Wilkins.

Haley, J. (1980). *Leaving Home: the therapy of disturbed young people*. New York: McGraw-Hill.

Hall, G. S. (1904). *Adolescence: its psychology and its relations to physiology, anthropology, sociology, sex, crime, religion and education*. Vols. I and II. New York: Appleton.

Hall, M. B. (1952). Our present knowledge about manic-depressive states in childhood. *Nervous Child*, **9**, 319–325.

Hallam, R. S. (1974). Extinction of ruminations: a case study. *Behaviour Therapy*, **5**, 565–568.

Hamilton, M. (1976). *Fish's Schizophrenia*. Bristol: Wright.

Harris, H. (1970). Development of moral attitudes in white and Negro boys. *Developmental Psychology*, **2**, 376–383.

Harris, R. (1977). The EEG. In *Child Psychiatry: modern approaches*. M. Rutter and L. Hersov (eds.) Oxford: Blackwell.

Hatfield, J. S., Ferguson, J. R., and Alpere, R. (1967). Mother–child interaction and the socialisation process. *Child Development*, **38**, 365–414.

Hatrick, J. A., and Dewhurst, K. (1970). Delayed psychosis due to LSD. *Lancet*, **2**, 742–744.

Hauser, S. L., Delong, G. R., and Rosman, N. P. (1975). Pneumographic findings in the infantile autism syndrome: a correlation with temporal lobe disease. *Brain*, **98**, 667–688.

Hawton, K., Cole, D., O'Grady, J., and Osborn, M. (1982a). Motivational aspects of deliberate self-poisoning in adolescents. *British Journal of Psychiatry*. **141**, 286–291.

Hawton, K., O'Grady, J., Osborn, M., and Cole, D. (1982b). Adolescents who take overdoses: their characteristics, problems and contacts with helping agencies. *British Journal of Psychiatry*, **140**, 118–123.

Hawton, K., Osborn, M., O'Grady, J., and Cole, D. (1982c). Classification of adolescents who take overdoses. *British Journal of Psychiatry*, **140**, 124–131.

Hay, G. G., and Leonard, J. C. (1979). Anorexia nervosa in males. *Lancet*, **2**, 574–576.

Hazel, N. (1978). Family placement-a hopeful alternative. *Journal of Adolescence*, **1**, 363–369.

Hazel, N. (1981). *A Bridge to Independence*. Oxford: Blackwell.

Heacock, D. R. (ed.) (1980a). *A Psychodynamic Approach to Adolescent Psychiatry: the Mount Sinai experience*. New York: Marcel Dekker.

Heacock, D. R. (1980b). The diagnostic home visit. In *A Psychodynamic Approach to Adolescent Psychiatry*. D. R. Heacock (ed.). New York: Marcel Dekker.

Heacock, D. R. (1980c). Therapeutic groups with hospitalised adolescents. In *A Psychodynamic Approach to Adolescent Psychiatry*. D. R. Heacock, (eds). New York: Marcel Dekker.

Heal, K. and Cawson, P. (1975). Organisation and change in children's institutions. In *Varieties of Residential Experience*. J. Tizard, I. Sinclair, and R. V. G. Clarke (eds). London: Routledge and Kegan Paul.

Heard, D. H. (1974). Crisis intervention guided by attachment concepts – a case study. *Journal of Child Psychology and Psychiatry*, **15**, 111–122.

Heard, D. H. (1978). From object relations to attachment theory: a basis for family therapy. *British Journal of Medical Psychology*, **51**, 67–76.

Heard, D. H. (1981). The relevance of attachment theory to child psychiatric practice. *Journal of Child Psychology and Psychiatry*, **22**, 89–96.

Helliwell, M., and Murphy, M.˙ (1979). Drug induced neurological disease. *British Medical Journal*, **1**, 1283–1284 (Correspondence).

Henderson, S. (1974). Care-eliciting behaviour in man. *Journal of Nervous and Mental Disease*, **159** (3), 172–181.

Hersov, L. (1960a). Persistent non-attendance at school. *Journal of Child Psychology and Psychiatry*, **1**, 130–136.

Hersov, L. (1960b). Refusal to go to school. *Journal of Child Psychology and Psychiatry*, **1**, 137–145.

Hersov, L. (1977a). School refusal. In *Child Psychiatry: modern approaches*. M. Rutter and L. Hersov (eds). Oxford: Blackwell.

Hersov, L. (1977b). Faecal soiling. In *Child Psychiatry: modern approaches*. M. Rutter and L. Hersov (eds). Oxford: Blackwell.

Hersov, L. (1977c). Emotional disorders. In *Child Psychiatry: modern approaches*. M. Rutter and L. Hersov (eds). Oxford: Blackwell.

Hersov, L. and Bentovim, A. (1977). In-patient units and day hospitals. In *Child Psychiatry: modern approaches*. M. Rutter and L. Hersov (eds). Oxford: Blackwell.

Hersov, L., and Berg, I. (1980). *Out of School: modern perspectives in truancy and school refusal*. L. Hersov and I. Berg (eds). Chichester: Wiley.

Hertzig, M. A., and Birch, H. G. (1966). Neurologic organisation in psychiatrically disturbed adolescent girls. *Archives of General Psychiatry*, **15**, 590–599.

Hertzig, M. A., and Birch, H. G. (1968). Neurologic organisation in psychiatrically disturbed adolescents. *Archives of General Psychiatry*, **19**, 528–537.

Heston, L. L., and Denny, D. (1968). Interactions between early life experience and biological factors in schizophrenia. In *The Transmission of Schizophrenia*. D. Rosenthal and S. S. Kety (eds). Oxford: Pergamon.

Heymann, K. 1965. Some thoughts on the fundamental nature of depression. *The Practitioner*, **194**, 668–672.

Hibbert, C. (1963). *The Roots of Evil: a social history of crime and punishment*. London: Weidenfeld and Nicolson.

Hildebrand, J., Jenkins, J., Carter, D., and Lask, B. (1981). The introduction of a full family orientation in a child psychiatric in-patient unit. *Journal of Family Therapy*, **3**, 139–152.

Hilgard, E. K., and Atkinson, R. C. (1967). *Introduction to Psychology*. New York: Harcourt, Brace, and World.

Hinde, R. A. (1976). On describing relationships. *Journal of Child Psychology and Psychiatry*, **17**, 1–19.

Hinde, R. A. (1979). *Towards Understanding Relationships*. London: Academic Press.

Hinde, R. A. (1980). Family influences. In *Scientific Foundation of Developmental Psychiatry*. Ed. M. Rutter (ed.). London: Heinemann.

Hindley, C. B., and Owen, C. F. (1978). The extent of individual changes in I.Q. for ages between 6 months and 17 years in a British Longitudinal sample. *Journal of Child Psychology and Psychiatry*, **19**, 329–350.

Hirsch, S. R., and Leff, J. P. (1975). *Abnormalities in Parents of Schizophrenics*. Institute of Psychiatry, Maudsley Monograph No. 22. London: Oxford University Press.

Hobson, R. F. (1953). Prognostic factors in electric convulsive therapy. *Journal of Neurology, Neurosurgery and Psychiatry*, **16**, 275–281.

Hodgman, C. H., and Braiman, A. (1965). College phobia: school refusal in university students. *American Journal of Psychiatry*, **12**, 801–805.

Hodgson, R. and Rachman, J. (1972). The effect of contamination and masking in obsessional patients. *Behaviour Research and Therapy*, **10**, 111–117.

Hoghughi, (1978). *Troubled and Troublesome: coping with severely disordered children*. London: André Deutsch.

Holding, T. A., Buglass, D., Duff, J. C., and Krettman, N. (1977). Parasuicide in Edinburgh: a seven year review 1968–1974, *British Journal of Psychiatry*, **130**, 534–543.

Hollingsworth, C. E., Tanguay, P. E., Grossman, L., and Pabst, P. (1980). Long-term outcome of obsessive–compulsive disorder in childhood. *Journal of the American Academy of Child Psychiatry*, **19**, 134–144.

Hood, R., and sparks, R. (1970). *Key Issues in Criminology*. London: Weidenfeld and Nicolson.

Hopkinson, K., Cox, A., and Rutter, M. (1981). Psychiatric intervening techniques. III Naturalistic study: eliciting feelings. *British Journal of Psychiatry*, **138**, 406–415.

Horowitz, H. A. (1977). Lithium and the treatment of adolescent manic-depressive illness. *Diseases of The Nervous System*, **38**, 480–483.

House, W. C., Miller, S. I., and Schlachter, R. H. (1978). Role definitions among mental health professionals. *Comprehensive Psychiatry*, **19** (5), 469–476.

Howard, A. N., Dub, I., and MacMahon, M. (1971). The incidence, cause and treatment of obesity in Leicester school children. *Practitioner*, **207**, 662–668.

Howlin, P. (1980). Language. In *Scientific Foundations of Developmental Psychiatry*. M. Rutter (ed.). London: Heinemann.

Howlin, P., Hersov, L., Holbrook, D., Rutter, M., and Yule, W. (1978). Treating autistic children in a family context. In *Autism: a reappraisal of concepts and treatment*. M. Rutter and E. Schopler (eds). New York: Plenum.

Howlin, P., Marchant, R., Rutter, M., Berger, M., Hersov, L., and Yule, W. (1973). A home-based approach to the treatment of autistic children. *Journal of Autism and Childhood Schizophrenia*, **3**, 308–336.

Hudson, L. (1966). The question of creativity. In *Contrary Imaginations*. London: Methuen.

Humphrey, G. (1932). *the Wild Boy of Aveyron*. New York: The Century Company.

Hunter, R., and MaCalpine, I. (1963). *Three Hundred Years of Psychiatry, 1535–1860*. London: Oxford University Press.

Hutt, S. J., Jackson, P. M., Belsham, A., and Higgins, G. (1968). Perceptual motor behaviour in relation to blood phenobarbitone levels. *Developmental Medicine and Child Neurology*, **10**, 626–632.

Hyslop, T. B. (1925). *The Great Abnormals*. London: Philip Allan and Co.

Idestrom, G. M., Schalling, D., Carlquist, V., and Shoquist, F. (1972). Acute effects of diphenylhydantoin in relation to plasma levels. Behaviour and psychophysiological studies. *Psychological Medicine*, **2**, 111–120.

Ingram, T. T. S. (1956). A characteristic form of overactive behaviour in brain damaged children. *Journal of Mental Science*, **102**, 550–558.

Inhelder, B., and Piaget, J. (1958). *The Growth of Logical Thinking*. London: Routledge and Kegan Paul.

Illich, I. (1977). *Limits to Medicine*. Harmondsworth. Penguin Books.

Irwin, E. M. (1977). *Growing Pains: a study of teenage distress*. Plymouth: Macdonald and Evans.

Jackson, J. Hughlings (1884). Remarks on evolution and dissolution of the nervous system. In *Selected Writings II, 1932*. London: Hodder and Stoughton.

Jacobi, J. (1968). *The Psychology of C. G. Jung*. London: Routledge and Kegan Paul.

Jansson, B. (1968). The prognostic significance of various types of hallucinations in young people. *Acta Psychiatrica Scandinavica*, **44**, 401–409.

Johnson, F. N. (1979). *A handbook of Lithium Therapy*. Lancaster: MTP.

Johnson, S. M., and Brown, R. A. (1969). Producing behaviour change in parents of disturbed children. *Journal of Child Psychology and Psychiatry*, **10**, 107–121.

Joint Committee on Higher Psychiatric Training (1976). Requirements for approval of training programme in Child and Adolescent Psychiatry. (CAPS AS/1) Royal College of Psychiatrists.

Jones, G. P. (1981). Using early assessment of prehomosexual boys as a counselling tool: an exploratory study. *Journal of Adolescence*, **4**, 231–238.

Jones, M. (1946). Rehabilitation of forces neurosis patients to civilian life. *British Medical Journal*, **1**, 533–535.

Jones, M. (1968). *Social Psychiatry in Practice: the idea of the therapeutic community*. Harmondsworth: Penguin.

Jones, R. M., Allen, D. J., Wells, P. G., and Morris, A. (1978). An adolescent unit assessed: attitudes to a treatment experience for adolescents and their families. *Journal of Adolescence*, **1**, 371–383.

Journal of Adolescence (1978). Editorial, **1**, 1–2.

Journal of Family Therapy (1979). Editorial, **1**, 1–5.

Judd, L. (1965). Obsessive–compulsive neurosis in children. *Archives of General Psychiatry*, **12**, 136–143.

Jung, C. G. (1936). The archetypes and the collective unconscious. In *Collected Works*, vol. 9. London: Routledge and Kegan Paul.

Jung, C. G. (1963). *Memories, Dreams, Reflections.* London: Routledge and Kegan Paul.

Kagan, J. (1965). Reflection–impulsivity and reading ability in primary grade children. *Child Development,* **36,** 609–628.

Kalucy, R. S. (1978). An approach to the therapy of anorexia nervosa. *Journal of Adolescence,* **1,** 197–228.

Kanner, L. (1943). Autistic disturbances of affective contact. *Nervous Child,* **2,** 217–250.

Kanner, L. (1949). Problems of nosology and psychodynamics of early childhood autism. *American Journal of Orthopsychiatry.* **19,** 416–426.

Kashani, J. H., Venzke, R., and Miller, E. A. (1981). Depression in children admitted to hospital for orthopaedic procedures. *British Journal of Psychiatry,* **138,** 21–25.

Katchadourian, H. (1977). *The Biology of Adolescence.* San Francisco: Freeman.

Katz, D., and Kahn, R. L. (1966). *Social Psychology or Organisations.* Chichester and New York: John Wiley.

Kaufman, I., Heims, L. W., and Reiser, D. E. (1961). A re-evaluation of the psychodynamics of firesetting. *American Journal of Orthopsychiatry,* **22,** 63–72.

Keesing, R. M., and Keesing, F. M. (1971). *New Perspectives in Cultural Anthropology.* New York: Holt, Rinehart and Winston.

Kellam, S. A., Branch, J. D., Hendrickes Brown, C., and Russell, G. (1981). Why teenagers came for treatment. A ten year prospective study in Woodlawn. *Journal of the American Academy of Child Psychiatry,* **20,** 477–495.

Kempton, W. (1972). *Guidelines for Planning a Training Course on Human Sexuality and the Retarded.* Philadelphia: Planned Parenthood Association.

Kendell, R. E. (1976). The classification of depressions: a review of contemporary confusion. *British Journal of Psychiatry,* **129,** 15–28.

Kendell, R. E. (1979). Alcoholism: a medical or political problem? *British Medical Journal,* **1,** 367–371.

Kennedy, I. (1981). *The Unmasking of Medicine: the 1980 Reith Lectures.* London: George Allen and Unwin.

Kernberg, O. (1975). *Borderline Conditions and Pathological Narcissism.* New York. Aronson.

Kernberg, O. (1976). *Object–Relations Theory in Clinical Psychoanalysis.* New York: Aronson.

Kessler, E. S. (1979). Individual psychotherapy with adolescents. In *The Short Course in Adolescent Psychiatry.* J. R. Novello (ed.). New York: Brunner Mazel.

Kety, S. S. (1974). From rationalisation to reason. *American Journal of Psychiatry,* **131,** 957–963.

Kety, S. S., Rosenthal, D., Wender, P. H. and Schulsinger, F. (1968). The types and prevalence of mental illness in the biological and adoptive families of adopted schizophrenics. In *The Transmission of Schizophrenia.* D. Rosenthal and S. S. Kety (eds). Oxford: Pergamon.

King, L. J., and Pittmann, G. D. (1971). A follow-up of 65 adolescent schizophrenic patients. *Diseases of the Nervous System,* **32,** 328–334.

King, M., Day, R., Oliver, J., Lush, M., and Watson, J. (1981). Solvent encephalopathy. *British Medical Journal,* **2,** 663–665.

Kinston, W., and Bentovim, A. (1978). Brief focal therapy when the child is the referred patient. II Methodology and results. *Journal of Child Psychology and Psychiatry,* **19** (2), 119–143.

Kipling, Rudyard, (1973). *Something of Myself.* London: MacMillan.

Kirman, B. (1977). Mental retardation – medical aspects. In *Child Psychiatry: modern approaches.* M. Rutter and L. Hersov (eds). Oxford: Blackwell.

Klein, M. (1950). *Contributions to Psychoanalysis*. London: Hogarth Press.

Klopp, H. I. (1932). The children's institute of the Allentown State Hospital. *American Journal of Psychiatry*, **88**, 1108–1118.

Knight, R. R. (1954). Borderline states. In *Psychoanalytic Psychiatry and Psychology*. New York: International Universities Press.

Knobloch, H., and Pasamanick, B. (1962). Medical progress: mental subnormality. *New England Journal of Medicine*, **266**, 1045–1051. 1092–1097, 1155–1161.

Koestler, A. (1969). *The Act of Creation*. London: Hutchinson.

Kohlberg, L., and Kramer, R. (1969). Continuities and discontinuities in child and adult moral development. *Human Development*, **12**, 93–118.

Kohn, M. L., and Clausen, J. A. (1955). Social isolation and schizophrenia. *American Sociological Review*, **20**, 265–273.

Kolansky, N., and Moore, W. T. (1971). Effects of marijuana on adolescents and young adults. *Journal of the American Medical Association*, **216**, 486–492.

Kolvin, I. (1971a). Psychoses in childhood – a comparative study. In *Infantile Autism: concepts, characteristics and treatment*. M. Rutter (ed.). London: Churchill-Livingstone.

Kolvin, I. (1971b). Studies in the childhood psychoses: I. Diagnostic criteria and classification. *British Journal of Psychiatry*. **118**, 381–384.

Kolvin, I., MacKeith, R. C., and Meadow, S. R. (1973). *Bladder Control and Enuresis*. Clinics in Developmental Medicine Nos 48/49. London: Heinemann.

Kolvin, I., Ounsted, C., Humphrey, M., and Mcnay, A. (1971). Studies in the childhood psychoses: II. The phenomenology of childhood psychoses. *British Journal of Psychiatry*, **118**, 385–395.

Kolvin, I., Taunch, J., Currah, J., Garside, R. F., Nolan, J., and Shaw, W. B. (1972). Enuresis: a descriptive analysis and a controlled trial. *Developmental Medicine and Child Neurology*, **14**, 715–726.

Kraepelin, E. (1899). *Clinical Psychiatry*. Translated by A. R. Diefendorf. 1902. New York: MacMillan.

Kraft, I. A. (1968). An overview of group therapy with adolescents. *International Journal of Group Psychotherapy*, **18**, 461–480.

Kramer, E. (1978). *Art Therapy with Children*. New York: Shocken.

Kramer, A. D., and Feiguine, B. A. (1981). Clinical effect of amitriptyline in adolescent depression. A pilot study. *Journal of the American Acadamy of Child Psychiatry*, **20**, 636–644.

Kreitman, N., and Schreiber, M. (1979). Parasuicide in young Edinburgh women 1968–75. *Psychological Medicine*, **9**, 469–479.

Kringley, E. (1965). Obsessional neurosis: long-term follow-up. *British Journal of Psychiatry*, **111**, 709–722.

Krohn, A., Miller, D., and Looney, J. (1974). Flight from autonomy: problems of social change in an adolescent inpatient unit. *Psychiatry*, **37**, 360–371.

Kumar, K., and Wilkinson, J. C. M. (1971). Thought stopping: a useful treatment for phobias of internal stimuli. *British Journal of Psychiatry*, **119**, 305–307.

Kymissis, P., Padrusch, B., and Schulman, D. (1979). The use of lithium in cyclical behavior disorders of adolescence: a case report. *The Mount Sinai Journal of Medicine*, **46**, 141–142.

Lader, M. (1977). *Psychiatry on Trial*. Harmondsworth: Penguin.

Laing, R. D. (1960). *The Divided Self*. London: Tavistock.

Laing, R. D. (1967). *The Politics of Experience and the Bird of Paradise*. Harmondsworth: Penguin.

Laing, R. D., and Esterson, A. (1964). *Sanity, Madness and the Family*. London: Tavistock.

Lampen, J. (1978). Drest in a little brief authority: controls in residential work with adolescents. *Journal of Adolescence*, **1**, 163–175.

Lampen, J. (1981). Different perspectives. *Journal of Adolescence*, **4**, 199–209.

Lange, J. (1928). The endogeneous and reactive affective disorders and the manic-depressive constitution. In *Handbook of Mental Diseases*. O. Bumke (ed.). Berlin: Springer. Quoted in J. S. Price, 1968.

Langsley, D., Pittman, F., Machotka, P., and Flomenhaft, K. (1968). Family crisis therapy – results and implications. *Family Process*, **7**, 145–158.

Langsley, D., Flomenhaft, K., and Machotka, P. (1969). Follow-up evaluation of family crisis therapy. *American Journal of Orthopsychiatry*, **39** 753–759.

Lask, B. (1979). Family therapy outcome research 1972–8. *Journal of Family Therapy*, **1**, 87–91.

Lask, B., and Kirk, M. (1979). Childhood asthma: family therapy as an adjunct to routine management. *Journal of Family Therapy*, **1**, 33–49.

Laufer, M. A. (1964). Ego ideal and pseudo ego-ideal in adolescence. *Psychoanalytic Study of the Child*, **19**, 196–221.

Laufer, M. A. (1968). *The Work of the Brent Consultation Centre and the Centre for the Study of Adolescence*. Monograph No. 1 of the Centre for the Study of Adolescence. 3–7.

Laufer, M. A. (1980). Which adolescents must be helped and by whom ?*Journal of Adolescence*, **3**, 265–272.

Lazarus, A. (1960). The elimination of children's phobias by deconditioning. In *Behaviour Therapy and the Neuroses*. H. J. Eysenck (ed.). Oxford: Pergamon.

Lazarus, R. S. (1966). *Psychological Stress and the Coping Process*. New York: McGraw-Hill.

Lazarus, R. S. (1969). *Patterns of Adjustment and Human Effectiveness*. New York: McGraw-Hill.

Leach, E. (1976). *Culture and Communication: the logic by which symbols are connected*. Cambridge: Cambridge University Press.

Leese, S. M. (1969). Suicide behaviour in 20 adolescents. *British Journal of Psychiatry*, **115**, 479–480.

Leff, J. P., and Wing, J. K. (1971). Trial of Maintenance Therapy in Schizophrenia. *British Medical Journal*, **3**, 599–604.

Lefkowitz, M. M., Eron, L. D., Walder, L. O., and Huesmann, L. R. (1977). *Growing up to be Violent: a longitudinal study of aggression*. Oxford: Pergamon.

LeHorne, D. J. (1981). A case of severe obsessive–compulsive behaviour treated by nurse therapists in an in-patient unit. *Behavioural Psychotherapy*, **9**, 46–54.

Lena, B., Surtees, S. J., and Maggs, R. (1977). The efficacy of lithium in the treatment of emotional disturbance in children and adolescents. In *Lithium in Medical Practice*. F. N. Johnson and S. Johnson (eds). Lancaster: MTP.

Lenhoff, F. G., and Lampen, J. C. (1968). *Learning to Live*. Shrewsbury: Shotton Hall.

Lenhoff, F. G., and Lampen, J. C. (1975). *Towards Self-Discipline*. Shrewsbury: Shotton Hall.

Leslie, S. A. (1974). Psychiatric disorder in the young adolescents of an industrial town. *British Journal of Psychiatry*, **125**, 113–124.

Lesser, L. I., Ashenden, R. J., Debuskey, M., and Eisenberg, L. (1960). Anorexia nervosa in children. *American Journal of Orthopsychiatry*, **30**, 572–580.

Levine, R. J. (1977). Epidemic faintness and syncope in a school marching band. *Journal of the American Medical Association*, **238**, 2373–2376.

Levine, R. J., Sexton, D. J., Romm, F. J., Wood, B. T., and Kaiser, J. (1974). Outbreak of psychosomatic illness at a rural elementary school. *Lancet*, **2**, 1500–1503.

Levi-Strauss, C. (1966). *The Savage Mind*. Chicago: University of Chicago Press.

Levinson, D. F., and Crabtree, L. H. (1979). Ward tension and staff leadership in a therapeutic community for hospitalized adolescents. *Psychiatry*, **42**, 220–240.

Lewin, K. (1935). *A Dynamic Theory of Personality*. New York: McGraw.

Lewis, A. J. (1934). Melancholia: a clinical survey of depressive states. *Journal of Mental Science*, **80**, 277.

Lewis, A. J. (1936). Problems of obsessional illness. *Proceedings of the Royal Society of Medicine*, **29**, 325–336.

Lewis, A. J. (1936). Melancholia: prognostic study and case material. *Journal of Mental Science*, **82**, 488–588.

Lewis, A. J. (1951). Social aspects of psychiatry. *Edinburgh Medical Journal*, **58**, 214–247.

Lewis, A. J. (1955). Health as a social concept. *British Journal of Sociology*, **4**, 109–124.

Lewis, A. J. (1963). Medicine and the affections of the mind. *British Medical Journal*, **2**, 1549–1557.

Lewis, M., and Lewis, D. O. (1973). Paediatric management of psychologic crises. *Current Problems in Paediatrics*, **3** (12), 1–48.

Lewis, M. L., and Sarrel, P. M. (1969). Some psychological aspects of seduction, incest and rape in childhood. *Journal of the American Academy of Child Psychiatry*, **8**, 606–619.

Lewis, N. D. C., and Yarnell, H. (1951). *Pathological Firesetting*. Nervous and Mental Disease Monographs. No. 82. New York: The Coolidge Foundation.

Liberman, R. P., and Raskin, D. E. (1971). Depression: a behavioural formulation. *Archives of General Psychiatry*, **24**, 515–523.

Lidz, T. (1958). Schizophrenia and the family. *Psychiatry*, **21**, 21–27.

Lidz, T. (1968). The family, language and the transmission of schizophrenia. In *The Transmission of Schizophrenia*, D. Rosenthal and S. Kety (eds.) Oxford: Pergamon.

Liebman, R., Honig, P., and Berger, H. (1976). An integrated treatment program for psychogenic pain. *Family Process.*, **15**, 397–406.

Lindemann, E. (1964). Adolescent behavior as a community concern. *American Journal of Psychotherapy*, **18**, 405–417.

Lipowski, Z. J. (1977). Psychiatric consultation: concepts and controversies. *American Journal of Psychiatry*, **134** (5), 523–528.

Lishman, W. A. (1968). Brain damage in relation to psychiatric disability after head injury. *British Journal of Psychiatry*, **114**, 373–410.

Lishman, W. A. (1978). *Organic Psychiatry: the psychological consequences of cerebral disorder*. Oxford: Blackwell.

Liston, E. H. (1976). Use of problem-oriented medical record in psychiatry a survey of university based residency training programmes. *American Journal of Psychiatry*, **133**, 700–703.

Litt, I. F., Cohen, M. I., and Schonberg, S. K. (1972). Liver disease in the drug-using adolescent. *Journal of Paediatrics*, **81** (2), 238–242.

London, I. D. and London, M. B. (1970). Attitudes of mainland youth towards traditional Chinese customs and beliefs. *Chinese Culture*, **11**, 51–53.

Loney, J., Langhorne, J. E., and Paternite, C. E. (1978). An empirical basis for subgrouping the hyperkinetic minimal brain Dysfunction syndrome. *Journal of Abnormal Psychology*, **87**, 431–441.

Looker, A., and Conners, C. (1970). Diphenylhydantoin in children with severe temper tantrums. *Archives of General Psychiatry*, **23**, 80–89.

Lorand, S. (1961). Treatment of adolescents. In *Adolescents: psychoanalytic approach to problems and therapy*. S. Lorand and H. I. Schneer (eds). New York: Hoeber.

Loranger, A. W., and Levine, P. M. (1978). Age of onset of bipolar affective illness. *Archives of General Psychiatry*, **35**, 1345–1348.

Lotter, V. (1966). Epidemiology of autistic conditions in young children. I: Prevalence. *Social Psychiatry*, **1**, 124–137.

Lotter, V. (1967). Epidemiology of autistic conditions in young children. II: Some characteristics of the parents and children. *Social Psychiatry*, **1**, 163–173.

Loudon, J. B., and Waring, H. (1976). Toxic reactions to lithium and haloperidol. *Lancet*, **2**, 1088.

Lubove, R. (1971). *The Professional Altruist: the emergence of social work as a career, 1880–1930*. Cambridge, Massachusetts: Harvard University Press.

Lucas, A. Kauffman, P., and Morris, E. (1967). Gilles de la Tourette's disease: a clinical study of fifteen cases. *Journal of the American Academy of Child Psychiatry*, **6**, 700–722.

Lucas, A. R., and Weiss, M. (1971). Methylphenidate hallucinosis. *Journal of the American Medical Association*, **217**, 1079–1081.

Lum, L. C. (1982). Total allergy. *British Medical Journal*, **284**, 1044–1045. Correspondence.

Lumsden Walker, W. (1980). Intentional self-injury in school age children. A study of 50 cases. *Journal of Adolescence*, **3**, 217–228.

Lynd, S. (1942). *English Children*. London: Collins.

Macaskill, N. D., and Macaskill, A. (1981). The use of term 'borderline patient' by Scottish psychiatrists: a preliminary survey. *British Journal of Psychiatry*, **139**, 397–399.

Maccoby, E. E., and Jacklin, C. N. (1980). Psychological sex differences. In *Scientific Foundations of Developmental Psychiatry*. M. Rutter (ed.) London: Heinemann.

MacFarlane, J. W., Allen, L., and Honzik, M. P. (1954). *A Developmental Study of the Behaviour Problems of Normal Children between 21 Months and 14 Years*. Berkeley: University of California Press.

Mackay, D. (1982). Cognitive Behaviour therapy. *British Journal of Hospital Medicine*, **27**,(3), 242–247.

MacKeith, R. (1976). The Association for Child Psychology and Psychiatry 1956–1976. *Journal of Child Psychology and Psychiatry*, **17**, 249–250.

Macklin, R. (1973). The medical model in psychoanalysis and psychotherapy. *Comprehensive Psychiatry*, **14**(1), 49–69.

Maddox, G. L. Buck, K. W. and Liederman, V. R. (1968). Overweight versus social deviance and disability. *Journal of Health and Social Behaviour*, **9**, 287–298.

Madge, N., and Tizard, J. (1980). Intelligence. In *Scientific Foundations of Developmental Psychiatry*. M. Rutter (ed.). London: Heinemann.

Mahler, M. (1971). The study of the separation–individuation process and its possible application to borderline phenomenon in the psychoanalytic situation. *Psychoanalytic study of the Child*, **26**, 403–425.

Main, T. F. (1946). The hospital as a therapeutic institution. *Bulletin of the Menninger Clinic*, **10**, 66–70.

Malmquist, C. P. (1971). Depressions in childhood and adolescence. *New England Journal of Medicine*, **284**, 887–893 and 955–961.

Malmquist, E. (1958). *Factors Leading to Reading Disabilities in the First Grade of Elementary School*. Stockholm: Almquist.

Manning, N. P. (1975). What Happened to the Therapeutic Community? *In Yearbook of Social Policy 1975*, M. Jones (ed.). London: Routledge and Kegan Paul.

Manning, N. P. (1976). Innovation in social policy: the case of the therapeutic community. *Journal of Social Policy*, **5**(3), 265–279.

Marks, I. M. (1969). *Fears and Phobias*. London: Heinemann.

Marks, I. M., Stern, R. S., Mawson, D., Cobb, J., and McDonald, R. (1980). Clomipramine and exposure for obsessive–compulsive rituals. I. *British Journal of Psychiatry*, **136**, 1–25.

Martin, A. J. Landau, L. F., and Phelan, P.D. (1982). Asthma from childhood at age 21: the patient and his disease. *British Medical Journal*, **284**, 380–382.

Martin, D. V. (1962). *Adventure in Psychiatry: social change in a mental hospital.* Oxford: Bruno Cassirer.

Martindale, B., and Bottomley, V. (1980). The management of families with Huntington's chorea: a case study to illustrate some recommendations. *Journal of Child Psychology and Psychiatry*, **21**, 343–351.

Maslach, C. (1976). Burned-out. *Human Behaviour*, **5**, 16–22.

Masterson, J. F. (1967). *The Psychiatric Dilemma of Adolescence.* London: Churchill.

Masterson, J. F. (1972). *Treatment of the Borderline Adolescent: a developmental approach.* New York: Wiley-Interscience.

Masterson, J. F. (1973). The borderline adolescent. In *Adolescent Psychiatry,* Vol. II. S. C. Feinstein and P. Giovacchini, (eds). New York: Basic Books.

Masterson, J. F. and Costello, J. L. (1980). *From Borderline Adolescent to Functioning Adult: the test of time.* New York: Brunner Mazel.

Masterton, G. (1979). The management of solvent abuse. *Journal of Adolescence*, **2**, 65–75.

Matson, J. L. (1981) Use of independence training to teach shopping skills to mildly mentally retarded adults *American Journal of Mental Deficiency*, **86**(2), 178–183.

Matsumura, M., Ingue, N., and Ohnishi, A. (1972). Toxic polyneuropathy due to glue sniffing. *Clinical Neurology* (Tokio), **12**(6), 290–296.

Mattinson, J. (1975). *Marriage and Mental Handicap.* London: Institute of Marital Studies, the Tavistock Institute of Human Relations.

Mattsson, A. (1972). Long-term physical illness in childhood: a challenge to psychosocial adaptation. *Paediatrics*, **50**, 801–811.

Maudsley, H. (1981). Insanity of early life. Chapter 2 (259–268). In *Physiology and Pathology of the Mind.* London: MacMillan.

Maxwell, C., and Seldrup, J. (1971). Imipramine in the treatment of childhood enuresis. *Practitioner*, **207**, 809–814.

McAndrew, J. B., Case, Q., and Treffert, D. A. (1972). Effects of prolonged phenothiazine intake on psychotic and other hospitalised children. *Journal of Autism and Childhood Schizophrenia*, **2**, 75–91.

McCabe, M. S. Fowler, R. C., Cadoret, R. J., and Winokur, G. (1971). Familial differences in schizophrenia with good and poor prognosis. *Psychological Medicine*, **1**, 326–332.

McDonald, M. (1965). Psychiatric evaluation in children. *Journal of the American Academy of Child Psychiatry*, **5**, 569–612.

McEvedy, C. P. Griffith, A., and Hall, T. (1966). Two school epidemics. *British Medical Journal,* **2**, 1300–1302.

McIntyre, N., Day, R. C., and Pearson, A. J. G. (1972). Can we write better medical notes? Introduction to problem orientated medical records: the Weed approach. *British Journal of Hospital Medicine*, **7**(5), 603–61.

McLachlan, P. (1981). Teenage experience in a violent society, *Journal of Adolescence*, **4**, 285–294.

Mead, M. (1928). *Coming of Age in Samoa.* New York: William Morrow & Company.

Mead, M. (1930). *Growing Up In New Guinea.* Harmondsworth: Penguin Books.

Mead, M. (1953). National Character. In *Anthropology Today.* A. L. Kroeber (ed.). Chicago: University of Chicago Press.

Mednick, S. A., Schulsinger, F., Higgins, J., and Bell, B. (1974). *Genetics, Environment and Psychopathology.* New York: American Elsever.

Mednick, S. A., Schulsinger, F., Teasdale, T. W., Schulsinger, H., Venables, P. H., and Rock, D. R. (1978). Schizophrenia in high-risk children: sex differences in predisposing factors. In *Cognitive Development of Mental Illness*, New York: Brunner Mazel.

Meeks, J. E. (1971). *The Fragile Alliance*. Baltimore: Williams and Wilkins.

Meeks, J. E. (1974). Adolescent development and group cohesion. In *Adolescent Psychiatry*, vol. III. S. C. Feinstein and P. Giovacchmi (eds). New York: Basic Books.

Meichenbaum, D. H. (1977). *Cognitive Behaviour Modification*. New York: Plenum Press.

Menzies, I. E. P. (1970). *The Functioning of Social Systems as a Defence against Anxiety*. London: Tavistock.

Meyer, V., and Chesser, E. S. (1970). *Behaviour Therapy in Clinical Psychiatry*. Harmondsworth: Penguin.

Meyersburg, H. A., and Post, R. M. (1979). A holistic development view of neural and psychological processes: a Neurobiologic–psychoanalytic integration. *British Journal of Psychiatry*, **135**, 139–155.

Micklem, N. (1948). *Religion*. London: Home University Library.

Midwinter, E. (1977). The professional–lay relationship: a Victorian legacy. *Journal of Child Psychology and Psychiatry*, **18**(2), 101–113.

Miller, D. (1969). *The Age Between: adolescents in a disturbed society*. London: Cornmarket/Hutchinson.

Miller, D. (1974). *Adolescence: psychology, psychopathology and psychotherapy*. New York: Jason Aronson.

Miller, E. (ed.) (1940). *The Neuroses in War*. London: MacMillan.

Miller, G. A. (1964). *Psychology: the science of mental life*. London: Hutchinson.

Miller, L. C. (1959). Short-term therapy with adolescents. *American Journal of Orthopsychiatry*, **29**, 772–779.

Millham, S. (1981). The therapeutic implications of locking up children. *Journal of Adolescence*, **4**(1), 13–26.

Millham, S., Bullock, R., and Hosie, K. (1978a). *Locking Up Children: secure provision within the child care system*. Farnborough: Saxon House.

Millham, S., Bullock, R., and Hosie, K. (1978b). Juvenile unemployment: a concept due for recycling? *Journal of Adolescence*, **1**, 11–24.

Minde, K. (1978). Coping styles of 34 adolescents with cerebral palsy. *American Journal of Psychiatry*, **135**, 1349–1355.

Minuchin, S. (1974). *Families and Family Therapy*. London: Tavistock.

Minuchin, S., Baker, L., Rosman, B., Liebman, R., Milman, L., and Todd, T. (1975). A conceptual model of psychosomatic illness in children. *Archives of General Psychiatry*, **32**, 1031–1038.

Minuchin, S., Montalvo, B., Guerney, B. G., Rosman, B. L., and Schumer, F. (1967). *Families of the Slums*. New York: Basic Books.

Minuchin, S., Rosman, B. L., and Baker, L. (1980). *Psychosomatic Families: anorexia nervosa in context*. Cambridge Massachusetts: Harvard University Press.

Mitchell, K. M., Bozarth, J. S., and Krauft, C. C. (1977). A reappraisal of the therapeutic effectiveness of accurate empathy, non-possessive warmth and genuineness. In *Effective Psychotherapy: a handbook of research*. A. S. Gurman and A. M. Razin (eds). Oxford: Pergamon.

Mitchell, S., and Shepherd, M. (1967). The child who dislikes going to school. *British Journal of Educational Psychology*, **37**, 32–40.

Mohr, G. S., and Despres, M. A. (1958). *The Stormy Decade: Adolescence*. New York: Random House.

Mohr, P. D., and Bond, M. J. (1982). A chronic epidemic of hysterical blackouts in a comprehensive school. *British Medical Journal*, **284**, 961–962.

Monello, L. F., and Mayer, J. (1963). Obese adolescent girls: an unrecognized 'minority' group. *American Journal of Clinical Nutrition*, **13**, 35–39.

Money, J. (1970). Hormonal and genetic extremes at puberty. In *The Psychopathology of Adolescence*. J. Zubin and A. Freedman (eds). New York: Grune and Stratton.

Money, J., and Erhardt, A. A. (1972). *Man and Woman: Boy and Girl*. Baltimore: Johns Hopkins Press.

Morgan, H. G., Burns-Cox, J., Pocock, H., and Pottle, S. (1975). Deliberate self-harm: clinical and socioeconomic characteristics of 368 patients. *British Journal of Psychiatry*, **127**, 564–574.

Morris, D. P., Soroker, E., and Burruss, C. (1954). Follow up studies of shy withdrawn children. I: Evaluation of later adjustment. *American Journal of Orthopsychiatry*, **24**, 743–754.

Morse, M. (1965). *The Unattached*. A Report of the Three Year Project Carried Out By the National Association of Youth Clubs. Harmondsworth: Penguin Books.

Morton, R. (1689). Phthisiologia; or, a Treatise of Consumption. Quoted in *Three Hundred Years of Psychiatry*, R. Hunter and I. Macalpine. 1963. London: Oxford University Press.

Moss, P. (1975). Residential care of children: a general view. In *Varieties of Residential Experience*, J. Tizard, I. Sinclair and R. V. G. Clarke (eds). London: Routledge and Kegan Paul.

Moss, P. D., and McEvedy, C. (1966). An epidemic of overbreathing among schoolgirls. *British Medical Journal*, **2**, 1295–1300.

Mrazek, P. B. (1980). Sexual abuse of children. *Journal of Child Psychology and Psychiatry*, **21**, 91–95.

Mulcock, D. (1955). Juvenile suicide. *Medical Officer*, **94**, 155–160.

Mullen, P. (1979). Phenomenology of disordered mental function. In *Essentials of Postgraduate Psychiatry*. P. Hill, R. Murray, and A. Thorley (eds). London: Academic Press.

Mungham, G., and Pearson, G. (eds) (1976). *Working Class Youth Culture*. London: Routledge and Kegan Paul.

Murphy, G. E., Woodruff, R. A., Herjanic, M., and Super, G. (1974). Variability of the clinical course of primary affective disorder. *Archives of General Psychiatry*, **30**, 757–761.

Murray, R. (1979). Schizophrenia. In *Essentials of Postgraduate Psychiatry*. P. Hill, R. Murray, and A. Thorley (eds). London: Academic Press.

Muss, R. E. (1980). Peter Blos' modern psychoanalytic interpretation of adolescence. *Journal of Adolescence*, **3**, 229–252.

Mwanalushi, M. (1979). Discontinuity and adolescent stress in Zambia. *Journal of Adolescence*, **3**, 91–100.

Nannarello, J. J. (1953). Schizoid *Journal of Nervous and Mental Disease*, **118**, 237–249.

National Association for Mental Health (1965). *Child Guidance and Child Psychiatry as an Integral Part of Community Service*. London: NAMH.

Newman, O. (1975). Reactions to the 'defensible space' study and some further findings. *International Journal of Mental Health*, **4**, 48–70.

Newsome, A. (1980). Doctors and counsellors: collaboration or conflict? *Bulletin of the Royal College of Psychiatrists*, July 1980, 102–104.

Newsome, A., Thorne, B. J., and Wyld, K. L. (1975). *Student Counselling in Practice*. London: University of London Press.

Nunn, C. M H. (1981). What should psychiatrists do? A personal view. *The Bulletin of the Royal College of Psychiatrists*, **5**(6), 102–103.

O'Connor, D. J. (1979). A profile of solvent abuse in school children. *Journal of Child Psychology and Psychiatry*, **20**, 365–368.

O'Donughue, E. G. (1929). *Bridewell Hospital: place, prisons, schools*. Volume 2. 1603–1929. London: John Lane, Bodley Head.

Office of Population Censuses and Surveys (1978). *Mortality Statistics*. London: Her Majesty's Stationery Office.

Offord, D. K., and Cross, L. A. (1969). Behavioural antecedents of adult schizophrenia. *Archives of General Psychiatry*, **21**, 267–283.

Oliver, J. E. (1970). Huntington's chorea in Northamptonshire. *British Journal of Psychiatry*, **116**, 241–253.

Olshansky, S., (1963). Chronic sorrow. *Social Casework*, **43**(4), 2–43.

O'Malley, J. E., Kocher, G., Foster, D., and Slavin, L. (1979). Psychiatric sequelae of surviving childhood cancer. *American Journal of Orthopsychiatry*, **49**(4), 608–616.

O'Neal, P., and Robins, L. N. (1958). Childhood patterns predictive of adult schizophrenia: a 30 year follow up study. *American Journal of Psychiatry*, **115**, 385–391.

Opie, I., and Opie, P. (1959). *The Lore and Language of schoolchildren*. London: Oxford University Press.

Orwell, G. (1946). James Burnham and the Managerial Revolution. *Polemic* No. 3, May 1946. In *The Collected Essays, Journalism and Letters of George Orwell 1968*. S. Orwell and I. Angus (eds). London: Secker and Warburg.

Ounsted, C. (1955). The hyperkinetic syndrome in epileptic children. *Lancet*, **2**, 303–311.

Ounsted, C. (1972). Biographical science: an essay on developmental medicine. In *Psychiatric Aspects of Medical Practice*, B. M. Mandelbrote and M. G. Gelder (eds). London: Staples Press.

Ounsted, C., Lindsay, J., and Norman, R. (1966). *Biological Factors in Temporal Lobe Epilepsy*. Clinics in Developmental Medicine No. 22. London: Heinemann.

Palkes, H., and Stewart, M. (1972). Intellectual ability and performance of hyperactive children. *American Journal of Orthopsychiatry*, **42**, 35–39.

Parkes, C. M. (1969). Separation anxiety: an aspect of the search for a lost object. In *Studies of Anxiety*. M. H. Lader (ed.). London: Royal Medico-Psychological Association and Ashford: Headley Brothers.

Parkes, C. M. (1971). Psycho-social transitions: a field for study. *Social Science and Medicine*, **5**, 101–115.

Parkin, J. M., and Fraser, M. S. (1972). Poisoning as a complication of enuresis. *Developmental Medicine and Child Neurology*, **14**, 727–730.

Patterson, G. R. (1969). Behavioral techniques based upon social learning: an additional base for developing behavior modification technologies. In *Behavior Therapy: appraisal and status*. C. M. Franks (ed.) New York: McGraw-Hill.

Patterson, G. R. (1971). *Families: applications of social learning theory to family life*. Champaign, Illinois: Research Press.

Patterson, G. R. (1973). Multiple evaluations of a parent training programme. In *Proceedings of the International Symposium on Behaviour Modification*. T. Thompson and W. S. Dockens (eds). New York: Appleton-Century-Crofts.

Patterson, G. R. (1974). Interventions for boys with conduct problems: multiple settings, treatments and and criteria. *Journal of Consulting and Clinical Psychology*, **42**, 471–481.

Paykel, E. S., Myers, J. K., Dienelt, M. N., Klerman, G. L., Lindenthal, J. J., and Pepper, M. P. (1969). Life events and depression. *Archives of General Psychiatry*, **21**, 753–760.

Payne, G. H. (1916). *The Child in Human Progress*. New York: Putnam.

Pearce, J. B. (1978). The recognition of depressive disorder in children. *Journal of the Royal Society of Mecicine*, **71**, 494–500.

Pease, J. J. (1979). A social skills training group for early adolescents. *Journal of Adolescence*, **2**, 229–238.

Perinpanayagam, K. S. (1978). Dynamic approach to adolescence: treatment. *British Medical Journal*, **1**, 563–566.

Perris, C. (1968). The course of depressive psychoses. *Acta Psychiatrica Scandinavica*, **44**, 238–248.

Peterson, E. B. (1980). *Disturbed Adolescents: the case for integration of young people's services*. London: Origen Communication.

Philips, I. (1967). Psychopathology and mental retardation. *American Journal of Psychiatry*, **124**, 29–35.

Philips, I., and Williams, N. (1975). Psychopathology and mental retardation: a study of 100 mentally retarded children. I: Psychopathology. *American Journal of Psychiatry*, **132**, 12.

Phillips, E. L., (1968). Achievement place: token reinforcement procedures in a home-style rehabilitation setting for predelinquent boys. *Journal of Applied Behaviour Analysis*, **1**, 213–223.

Piaget, J. (1955). *The Child's Construction of Reality*. London: Routledge and Kegan Paul.

Piaget, J. (1972). Intellectual evolution from adolescence to adulthood. *Human Development*, **5**, 1–12.

Piaget, J., and Inhelder, B. (1958). *The Growth of Logical Thinking from Childhood to Adolescence*. London: Routledge and Kegan paul.

Pichel, J. I. (1975). A long-term follow up study of sixty adolescent psychiatric outpatients. In *Annual Progress in Child Psychiatry and Child Development*. S. Chess and T. Thomas (eds). New York: Brunner Mazel.

Pless, I. B., and Roghmann, K. J. (1971). Chronic illness and its consequences. Observations based on three epidemologic surveys. *Journal of Paediatrics*, **79**, (3) 351–359.

Pollack, M. (1960). Comparison of childhood, adolescent and adult schizophrenics. *Archives of General Psychiatry*, **2**, 652–660.

Pollit, J. (1957). Natural history of obsessional states. *British Medical Journal*, **1**, 194–198.

Pomeroy, J. C., Behar, D., and Stewart, M. A. (1981). Abnormal sexual behaviour in pre-pubescent children. *British Journal of Psychiatry*, **138**, 119–125.

Post, F. (1966). *Persistent Persecutory States of the Elderly*. Oxford: Pergamon.

Post, R. M. (1975). Cocaine psychosis: a continuum model. *American Journal of Psychiatry*, **132** (3), 225–231.

Poster, M. (1978). *Critical Theory of the Family*. London: Pluto Press.

Potter, H. W. (1934). The treatment of problem children in a psychiatric hospital. *American Journal of Psychiatry*, **91**, 869–880.

Power, M. J., Benn, R. T., and Morris, J. N. (1972). Neighbourhood, school and juveniles before the courts. *British Journal of Criminology*, **12**, 111–132.

Poznanski, E. O. (1973). Children with excessive fears. *American Journal of Orthopsychiatry*, **43** (3), 428–438.

Press, E., and Done, A. K. (1967). Physiologic effects and community control measures for intoxication from the inhalation of organic solvents. *Paediatrics*, **39**, 451–461 and 611–622.

Price, J. S. (1968). The genetics of depressive behaviour. In *Recent Developments in Affective Disorders*. A. Coppen and A. Walk (eds). Royal Medico-Psychological Association and Ashford: Headley Brothers.

Pringle, M. L. K., Butler, N. R., and Davie, R. (1967). *11,000 7-year-olds. National Bureau for cooperation in child care*. London: Longman.

Proceedings of the Fifth Conference of the Association for the Psychiatric Study of Adolescence (1970). APSA.

Pyle, R. L., Mitchell, J. E., and Eckert, E. D. (1981). Bulimia: a report of 34 cases. *Journal of Clinical Psychiatry*, **42**, 60–64.

Quinton, D. (1980). Cultural and community influences. In *Scientific Foundations of Developmental Psychiatry*. M. Rutter (ed.). London: Heinemann.

Quitkin, F., Rifkin, A., and Klein, D. F. (1976). Neurological soft signs in schizophrenia and character disorder. *Archives of General Psychiatry*, **33**, 834–853.

Rachman, S. (1971). Obsessional ruminations. *Behaviour Research and Therapy*, **9**, 229–235.

Rachman, S. (1972). Clinical applications of observational learning, imitation and modeling. *Behaviour therapy*, **3**, 379–397.

Rachman, S. (1974). *The Meanings of Fear*. Harmondsworth: Penguin.

Raddock, D. M. (1977). *Political Behaviour of Adolescents in China: the Cultural Revolution in Kwangchow*. Tuscon: University of Arizona Press.

Rae, M., Hewitt, P., and Hugill, B. (1981). *First Rights: a guide to legal rights for young people*. London: National Council for Civil Liberties.

Ragg, N. M. (1977). *People Not Cases: a philosophical approach to social work*. London: Routledge and Kegan Paul.

Rahe, R. H., Fleistad, I., Bergan, R., Ringdale, R., Gerhardt, R., Gunderson E. K., and Arthur, R. J. (1974). A model for life changes and illness research. *Archives of General Psychiatry*, **31**, 172–177

Rapoport, R. N. (1960). *Community as Doctor: new perspectives an a therapeutic community*. London: Tavistock.

Rapoport, J., Elkins, R., Langer, D. H., Sceery, W., Buchsbaum, M. S., Gillin, J. C., Murphy, D. L., Zahn, T.P., Lake, R., Ludlow, C., and Mendelson, W. (1981). Childhood obsessive–compulsive disorder. *American Journal of Psychiatry*, **138**(12), 1545–1554.

Rapoport, J. L., and Gittelman, R. (1979). The diagnostic spectrum in adolescent psychiatry: DSM II and DSM III. In *The Short Course in Adolescent Psychiatry*. J. R. Novello (ed.). New York: Brunner Mazel.

Rapoport, J., Quinn, P. O., Bradbard, G., Riddle, K. D., and Brooks, E. (1974). Imipramine and methylphenidate treatment of hyperactive boys. *Archives of General Psychiatry*, **30**, 789–793.

Rathod, N. H. (1975). Cannabis psychosis. In *Cannabis and Man*. P. H. Connell and N. Dorn (eds). Edinburgh: Churchill Livingstone.

Redl, F., and Wineman, D. (1951). *Children who Hate*. Glencoe: The Free Press.

Redl, F., and Wineman, D. (1952). *Controls from Within*. Glencoe: The Free Press.

Registrar General (1979). *1977–2017 Population Projection*. Series PP2, 9. London: Her Majesty's Stationery Office; Office of Population Censuses and Surveys.

Reid, J.B., Hawkins, N., Keutzer, C. McNeal, S. A., Phelps, R. E., Reid, K. M., and Mees, H. L. (1967). A marathon behaviour modification of a selectively mute child. *Journal of Child Psychology and Psychiatry*, **8**, 27–30.

Renton, G. (1978). The East London Child Guidance Clinic. *Journal of Child Psychology and Psychiatry*, **19**, 309–312.

Rinsley, D. M. (1963). Psychiatric hospital treatment with special reference to children. *Archives of General Psychiatry*, **9**, 489–496.

Rioch, D. M., and Stanton, A. H. (1953). Milieu therapy. *Psychiatry*, **16**, 65–72.

Ritson, B. (1981). Alcohol and young people. *Journal of Adolescence*, **4**, 93–100.

Rivinus, T. M., Jamison, D. L., and Graham, P. J. (1975). Childhood Organic Neurological Disease Presenting as Psychiatric Disorder. *Archives of Diseases of Childhood*, **50**, 115–119.

Roberts, J. M. (1976). *The Hutchinson History of the World*. London: Hutchinson.

Robins, L. N. (1966). *Deviant Children Grown Up*. Baltimore: Williams and Wilkins.

Robins, L. N. (1979). Follow-up studies. In H. Quay and J. S. Werry (eds). *Psycholpathological Disorders in Childhood*. New York: Wiley.

Robins, L. N., and Ratcliff, K. S. (1980). The long-term outcome of truancy. Modern perspectives in truancy and school refusal. In *Out of School*. L. Hersov and I. Berg (eds) Chichester: Wiley.

Robins, E., and Guze, S. B. (1972). Classification of affective disorders: the primary–secondary, the endogenous–reactive and the neurotic–psychotic concepts. In T. A. Williams, M. M. Katz, and J. A. Shield (eds). *Recent Advances in Psychobiology of Depressive Illness*. Washington: DHEW Publication No. (HSM) 70–9053.

Robinson J. F. (ed.) (1957). *Psychiatric In-patient Treatment of Children*. Washington: American Psychiatric Association.

Rodriguez, A., Rodriguez, M., and Eisenberg, L. (1959). The outcome of school phobia: a follow-up study based on 41 cases. *American Journal of Psychiatry*, **116**, 540–544.

Roff, M., Sells, S. B., and Golden, M. M. (1972). *Social Adjustment and Personality Development in Children*. Minneapolis: University of Minnesota Press.

Rogers, C R. (1942). Mental health findings in 3 elementary schools *Educational Research Bulletin*, **21** (66) 69–79.

Rogers, C. R. (1951). *Client-Centered Therapy*. Boston, Massachusetts: Houghton, Mifflin Co.

Roghmann, K. J., and Haggerty, R. J. (1970). Rochester child health surveys. 1. Objectives, organisation and methods. *Medical Care*, **8**, 47.

Rose, M. (1977). *Residential Treatment: a Total Therapy*. David Wills lecture, London, November 1977.

Rosen, B. M., Bahn, A. K., Shellow, R., and Bower, E. M. (1965). Adolescent patients served in outpatient psychiatric clinics. *American Journal of Public Health*, **55**, 1563–1577.

Rosen, G. (1968). Madness in society. Chapters in *The Historical Sociology of Mental Illness*. London: Routledge and Kegan Paul.

Rosen, G. (1970). The revolt of youth: some historical comparisons. In *The Psychopathology of Adolescence*. J. Zubin and A. M. Freedman (eds). New York: Grune and Stratton.

Rosen, M. (1972). Psychosexual adjustment of the mentally handicapped. In *Sexual Rights and Responsibilities of the Mentally Retarded*. M. S. Bass (ed.). Proceedings of the Conference of the American association of Mental Deficiency, Newark, Delaware.

Rosenblatt, D. B. (1980). Play. In *Scientific Foundations of Developmental Psychiatry*. M. Rutter (ed.). London: Heinemann.

Rosenthal, D. (1975). The genetics of schizophrenia. In *Genetic Research in Psychiatry*. R. R. Fieve, D. Rosenthal, and H. Brill (eds). Baltimore: Johns Hopkins Press.

Rosenthal, D., Wender, P. H., Kety, S. S., Welner, J., and Schulsinger, F. (1971). The adopted-away offspring of schizophrenics. *American Journal of Psychiatry*, **128**, 307–311.

Ross, J. (1964). A *Follow-up Study of Obsessional Illness Presenting in Childhood and Adolescence*. University of London: DPM Dissertation.

Ross, M., and Moldofsky, H. (1978). A Comparison of pimozide and haloperidol in the treatment of Gilles de la Tourette's syndrome. *American Journal of Psychiatry*, **135**, 585–587.

Royal College of Psychiatrists (1978). Memorandum on the role, responsibilities and work of the child and adolescent psychiatrist. *Bulletin of the Royal College of Psychiatrists*, July 1978, 127–131.

Royal College of Psychiatrists (1979). *Guidelines for the Training of General Psychiatrists in Child and Adolescent Psychiatry*.

Russell, G. F. M. (1977a). The present status of anorexia nervosa. *Psychological Medicine*, **7**, 363–367.

Russell, G. F. M. (1977b). General management of anorexia nervosa and difficulty in assessing the efficacy of treatment. In *Anorexia Nervosa*. R. Vigersky (ed.). New York: Raven Press.

Russell, G. F. M. (1979). Bulimia nervosa: an ominous variant of anorexia nervosa. *Psychological Medicine*, **9**, 429–448.

Russell, G. F. M. (1981). The current treatment of anorexia nervosa. *British Journal of Psychiatry*, **138**, 164–166.

Rutter, M. (1965). Classification and categorisation in child psychiatry. *Journal of Child Psychology and Psychiatry*, **6**, 71–83.

Rutter, M. (1966). *Children of Sick Parents: an environmental and psychiatric study*. Oxford University Press and Institute of Psychiatry: Maudsley Monographs.

Rutter, M. (1968). Concepts of autism: a review of research. *Journal of Child Psychology and Psychiatry*, **9**, 1–25.

Rutter, M. (1970). Autistic children: infancy to adulthood. *Seminars in Psychiatry*, **2**, 435–450.

Rutter, M. (1971a). Psychiatry. In *Mental Retardation*, Vol. III. An Annual Review. J. Wortis (ed.). New York: Grune and Stratton.

Rutter, M. (1971b). Parent–child separation: psychological effects on the children. *Journal of Child Psychology and Psychiatry*, **12**, 233–260.

Rutter, M. (1977c). Normal psychosexual development. *Journal of Child Psychology and Psychiatry*, **11**, 259–283.

Rutter, M. (1972a). Childhood schizophrenia reconsidered. *Journal of Autism and Childhood Schizophrenia*, **2**, 315–337.

Rutter, M. (1972b). *Maternal Deprivation Reassessed*. Harmondsworth: Penguin.

Rutter, M. (1972c). Relationships between child and adult psychiatric disorders: some research considerations. *Acta Psychiatrica Scandinavica*, **48**, 3–21.

Rutter, M. (1974). Emotional disorder and educational underachievement. *Archives of Diseases of Childhood*, **49**, 249–256.

Rutter, M. (1975). *Helping Troubled Children*. Harmondsworth: Penguin.

Rutter, M. (1976). Prospective studies to investigate behavioral change. In *Methods of Longitudinal Research in Psychopathology*. J. S. Strauss, H. M. Barbigian, and M. Roff (eds). New York: Plenum Press. Quoted in A. Cox and M. Rutter, 1977.

Rutter, M. (1977a). Other family influences. In *Child Psychiatry: modern approaches*. M. Rutter and L. Hersov (eds). Oxford: Blackwell.

Rutter, M. (1977b). Infantile autism and other child psychoses. In *Child Psychiatry: modern approaches*. M. Rutter and L. Hersov (eds). Oxford: Blackwell.

Rutter, M. (1971c). Speech delay. In *Child Psychiatry: modern approaches*. M. Rutter and L. Hersov (eds). Oxford: Blackwell.

Rutter, M. (1977d). Classification. In *Child Psychiatry: modern approaches*. M. Rutter and L. Hersov (eds). Oxford: Blackwell.

Rutter, M. (1977e). Individual differences. In *Child Psychiatry: modern approaches*. M. Rutter and L. Hersov (eds). Oxford: Blackwell.

Rutter, M. (1979a). *Changing Youth in a Changing Society. Patterns of Adolescent Development and Disorder*. London: Nuffield Provincial Hospitals Trust.

Rutter, M. (1979b). Maternal separation 1972–1978: New findings, new concepts, new approaches. *Child Development*, **50**, 283–305.

Rutter, M. (1979c). Separation, loss and family relationships. In *Child Psychiatry: modern approaches*. M. Rutter and L. Hersov (eds). Oxford: Blackwell.

Rutter, M. (1980a). Introduction. In *Scientific Foundations of Developmental Psychiatry*. M. Rutter (ed.). London: Heinemann.

Rutter, M. (1980b). Psychosexual development. In *Scientific Foundations of Developmental Psychiatry*. M. Rutter (ed.). London: Heinemann.

Rutter, M. (1980c). Emotional development. In *Scientific Foundations of Developmental Psychiatry* M. Rutter (ed.). London: Heinemann.

Rutter, M., and Cox, A. (1977). Diagnostic appraisal and interviewing. In *Child Psychiatry: modern approaches*. M. Rutter and L. Hersov (eds). Oxford: Blackwell.

Rutter, M., and Cox, A. (1981). Psychiatric interviewing techniques: I. Methods and measures. *British Journal of Psychiatry*, **138**, 273–282.

Rutter, M., Graham, P., and Birch, H. G. (1966). Inter-relations between choreiform syndrome, reading disability and psychiatric disorder in children of 8–11 years. *Developmental Medicine and Child Neurology*, **8**, 149–159.

Rutter, M., Graham, P., Chadwick, O., and Yule, W. (1976). Adolescent turmoil: fact or fiction? *Journal of Child Psychology and Psychiatry*, **17**, 35–56.

Rutter, M., and Lockyer, L. (1967). A five to fifteen year follow-up of infantile psychosis. I. Description of sample. *British Journal of Psychiatry*, **113**, 1169–1182.

Rutter, M., and Madge, N. (1977). *Cycles of Disadvantage: a review of research*. London: Heinemann.

Rutter, M., Maughan, B., Mortimore, P., and Ouston, J. (1979). *Fifteen Thousand Hours: secondary schools and their effects on children*. London: Open Books.

Rutter, M. and Quinton, D. (1977). Psychiatric disorder – ecological factors and concepts of causation. In *Ecological Factors in Human Development*. H. McGurk (ed.). Amsterdam: North-Holland. Quoted in M. Rutter, 1979 *Changing Youth in a Changing Society*. London: Nuffield Provincial Hospitals Trust.

Rutter, M., and Shaffer, D. (1980). DSM III: a step forward or back in terms of the classification of child psychiatric disorders? *Journal of the American Academy of Child Psychiatry*, **19**, 371–394.

Rutter, M., Shaffer, D., and Shepherd, M. (1975a). *A Multi-Axial Classification of Child Psychiatric Disorders*. Geneva: WHO.

Rutter, M., Shaffer, D., and Stureg, C. (1975b). *Guide to a Multi-Axial Classification Scheme for Psychiatric Disorders in Childhood and Adolescence*. London: Institute of Psychiatry.

Rutter, M., Tizard, J., and Whitmore, K. (1970). *Education, Health and Behaviour*. London: Longman.

Rutter, M., and Yule, W. (1973). Specific reading retardation. In *The First Review of Special Education*. L. Mann and D. Sabatino (eds). Philadelphia: J. S. E. Press.

Rutter, M., and Yule, W. (1977). Reading difficulties. In *Child Psychiatry: modern approaches* M. Rutter and L. Hersov (eds). Oxford: Blackwell.

Rutter, M., Yule, W., and Graham, P. (1973). Enuresis and behavioural deviance: some epidemiological considerations. In *Bladder Control and Enuresis*. I. Kolvin, R. C. Mackeith and S. R. Meadow (eds). Clinics in Developmental Medicine, Nos. 48/49 London: Heinemann.

Ryle, A. (1973). *Student Casualties*. Harmondsworth: Penguin.

Ryle, R. (1982). Understanding organisations. In *Consultation from Child and Adolescent Psychiatric Settings*. C. Dare, R. Ryle, D. Steinberg, and W. Yule (eds). *News of the Association for Child Psychology and Psychiatry*, No. 11, July.

Safer, D. J., and Allen, R. P. (1973). Factors influencing the suppressant effect of two stimulant drugs on the growth of hyperactive children. *Paediatrics*, **51**, 660–667.

Safer, D. J., Allen, R. P., and Barr, E. (1975). Growth rebound after termination of stimulant drugs. *Journal of Paediatrics*, **86**, 113–116.

Salzman, C., Kochansky, G. E., Shader, R. I., Porrino, L. J., Harmatz, J. S., and Swett, C. P. (1974). Chlordiazepoxide-induced hostility in a small group setting. *Archives of General Psychiatry*, **31**, 401–405.

Sandberg. S. T., Rutter, M., and Taylor, E. (1978). Hyperkinetic disorder in psychiatric clinic attenders. *Developmental Medicine and Child Neurology*, **20**, 279–299.

Sandler, J., and Joffe, W. (1965). Notes on childhood depression. *International Journal of Psychoanalysis.* **46**, 88–96.

Sands, D. E. (1953). A special mental hospital unit for the treatment of psychosis and neurosis in juveniles. *Journal of Mental Science*, **99**, 123–129.

Sands, D. E. (1956). The psychoses of adolescence. *Journal of Mental Science*, **102**, 308–316.

Sarason, I. G. (1968). Verbal learning, modeling and juvenile delinquency. *American Psychologist*, **23**, 254–266.

Sargant, W. (1951). *Battle for the Mind.* London: Heinemann.

Sargant, W. (1957). *The Unquiet Mind.* London: Heinemann.

Satterfield, J. H. (1973). EEG issues in children with minimal brain dysfunction. *Seminars in Psychiatry*, **5**, 35–47.

Scally, B. G. (1973). Marriage and mental retardation: some observations in Northern Ireland. In *Human Sexuality and the Mentally Retarded.* F. F. de la Cruz and G. D. La Veck (eds). New York: Brunner Mazel.

Scheffler, H. W. (1965). *Choiseul Island Social Structure.* Berkeley: University of California Press.

Scheinberg, I. A. Sternlieb, I., and Richman, J. (1968). Psychiatric manifestations in patients with Wilson's disease. In *Wilson's Disease*, D. Bergsma (ed.). New York: The National Foundation.

Schneider, K. (1959). *Clinical Psychopathology.* Translation of 5th ed. by M. R. Hamilton. New York; Grune and Stratton.

Schofield, M. (1965). *The Sexual Behaviour of Young People.* London: Longman.

Schopler, E., Andrews, C. E., and Strupp, K. (1979). Do autistic children come from upper middle class parents? *Journal of Autism and Developmental Disorders*, **9**(2), 139–152.

Schowlater, J. E. (1977). Psychological reactions to physical illness and hospitalization in adolescence. *Journal of the American Academy of Child Psychiatry*, **16**, 500–516.

Schulsinger, F., and Mednick, S. A., (1975). Nautre–nurture aspects of Schizophrenia. In *Studies of Schizophrenia*. M. H. Lader (ed.). Ashford: Headley Brothers.

Schwartzberg, A. Z. (1979). Diagnostic evaluation of adolescents. In *The Short Course in Adolescent Psychiatry*. J. R. Novello (ed.). New York: Brunner Mazel.

Sedman, G., and Kenna, J. C. (1965). The use of LSD 25 as a diagnostic aid in doubtful cases of schizophrenia. *British Journal of Psychiatry*, **111**, 96–100.

Seligman, R., Gleser, G., Rauh, J., and Harris, L. (1974). The effect of earlier parental loss in adolescence. *Archives of General Psychiatry*, **31**, 475–479.

Selvini-Palazzoli, M. (1974). *Self-Starvation: from the intrapsychic to the transpersonal approach to anorexia nervosa.* Trans. A. Pomerans. London: Chaucer.

Shaffer, D. (1974). Suicide in childhood and early adolescence. *Journal of Child Psychology and Psychiatry*, **15**, 275–291.

Shaffer, D. (1977a). Enuresis. In *Child Psychiatry: modern approaches.* M. Rutter and L. Hersov (eds). Oxford: Blackwell.

Shaffer, D. (1977b). Brain injury. In *Child Psychiatry: modern approaches.* M. Rutter and L. Hersov (eds). Oxford: Blackwell.

Shaffer, D. (1977c). Drug treatment. In *Child Psychiatry: modern approaches* M. Rutter and L. Hersov (eds). Oxford: Blackwell.

Shaffer, D. (1978). 'Soft' neurological signs and later psychiatric disorder – a review. *Journal of Child Psychology and Psychiatry*, **19**, 63–65.

Shaffer, D., Costello, A. J., and Hill, I. D. (1968). Control of enuresis with imipramine. *Archives of Diseases of Childhood*, **43**, 665–671.

Shaffer, D., McNamara, N., and Pincus, U. H. (1974). Controlled observations on patterns of activity, attention and impulsivity in brain damaged and psychiatrically disturbed boys. *Psychological Medicine*, **4**, 4–18.

Shapiro, A. K., Shapiro, E. S., Bruun, R. D., and Sweet, R. D. (1978). *Gilles de la Tourette syndrome*. Raven Press: New York.

Shapiro, R. (1978). The adolescent, the therapist and the family: the management of external resistances to the psycho-analytic therapy of adolescents. *Journal of Adolescence*, **1**, 1–8.

Shapiro, R. J., and Budman, S. H. (1973). Defection, termination and continuation in family and individual therapy. *Family Process*, **12**, 55–67.

Shaw, C. H., and Wright, C. H. (1960). The married mental defective. *Lancet*, **1**, 273–274.

Shayer, M., Kuchemann, D. E., and Wylam, H. (1976). The distribution of Piagetian stages of thinking in British middle and secondary school children. *British Journal of Educational Psychology*, **46**, 164–173.

Sheard, M. (1975). Lithium in the treatment of aggression. *Journal of Nervous and Mental Disease*, **160**, 108–118.

Shearin, R. B., and Jones, R. L. (1979). Puberty and associated medical disorders of adolescence. In *The Short Course in Adolescent Psychiatry*. J. R. Novello (ed.). New York: Brunner Mazel.

Shepherd, M. N., Oppenheim, A. N., and Mitchell, S. (1966). Childhood behaviour disorders and the child guidance clinic – an epidemiological study. *Journal of Child Psychology and Psychiatry*, **7**, 39–52.

Shepherd, M., Oppenheim, B., and Mitchell, S. (1971). *Childhood Behaviour and Mental Health*. London: University of London Press.

Sherman, L., Kim, S., Benjamin, F., and Kolodny, H. (1971). Effects of chlorpromazine on serum growth hormone concentration in man. *New England Journal of Medicine*, **284**, 72–74.

Sherrington, C. S. (1906). *Integrative Action of the Nervous System* (1961 reprint). New Haven: Yale University Press.

Shields, J., and Gottesman, I. I. (1973). *Genetic Studies of Schizophrenia as Signposts to Biochemistry*. Biochemical Society Special Publication **1**, 165–174.

Shirley, H. (1963). The physically handicapped child. In *Paediatric Psychiatry*. Boston: Harvard University Press.

Sigal, J., Barrs, C., and Doubilet, A. (1976). Problems in measuring the success of family therapy in a common clinical setting; impasse and solutions. *Family Process*, **7**, 225–234.

Silverstone, J. T., and Russell, G. F. M. (1967). Gastric 'hunger' contractions in anorexia nervosa. *British Journal of Psychiatry*, **113**, 257–263.

Sinclair, I. A. C. (1971). *Hostels for Probationers*. London: Her Majesty's Stationery Office.

Skuse, D., and Burrell, S. (1982). A review of solvent abusers and their management by a child psychiatric outpatient service. *Human Toxicology*, **1**, 321–329.

Skynner, A. C. R. (1969). Indications and contraindications for conjoint family therapy. *International Journal of Social Psychiatry*, **15**, 245–249.

Skynner, A. C. R. (1971). The minimum sufficient network. *Social Work Today*, **2**, 3–7.

Skynner, A. C. R. (1974). School phobia: a reappraisal. *British Journal of Medical Psychology*, **47**, 1–16.

Skynner, A. C. R. (1975). The large group in training. In *The Large Group*. L. Kreeger (ed.). London: Constable.

Skynner, A. C. R. (1976a). *One Flesh – Separate Persons*. London: Constable.

Skynner, A. C. R. (1976b). *Systems of Family and Marital Psychotherapy*. New York: Brunner Mazel.

Slade, P. D., and Russell, G. F. M. (1973). Awareness of body dimensions in anorexia nervosa: cross-sectional and longitudinal studies. *Psychological Medicine*, **3**, 188–199.

Slaff, B. (1980). The evaluative process in adolescent hospital psychiatry. In *A Psychodynamic Approach to Adolescent Psychiatry*. D. R. Heacock (ed.). New York: Marcel Dekker.

Slater, E. (1965). Diagnosis of hysteria. *British Medical Journal*, **1**, 1395–1399.

Slater, E., and Roth, M. (1969). *Clinical Psychiatry*. London: Baillière Tindall and Cassell.

Slipp, S., Ellis, S., and Kressel, K. (1974). Factors associated with engagement in family therapy. *Family Process*, **18**, 413–428.

Slivkin, S. E., and Bernstein, N. R. (1970). Group approaches to treating retarded adolescents. In *Psychiatric Approaches to Mental Retardation*. F. J. Menolascino (ed.). New York: Basic Books.

Smayling, L. M. (1959). Analysis of six cases of voluntary mutism. *Journal of Speech and Hearing Disorders*, **24**, 55–58. Quoted by M. Rutter, 1977c.

Smythe, T. (1981). The role of MIND (The National Association for Mental Health) in relation to psychiatry. Talk given at the winter quarterly meeting of the Royal College of psychiatrists; and *Bulletin of the Royal College of Psychiatrists*, August 1981, 140–143.

Smythies, J. R. (1966). *The Neurological Foundations of Psychiatry: an outline of the mechanisms of emotion, memory, learning and the organisation of behaviour, with particular regard to the limbic system*. Oxford: Blackwell.

Snaith, R. P. (1981). Correspondence. *The Bulletin of the Royal College of Psychiatrists*, **5** (9), 170.

Speck, R. V., and Attneave, C. L. (1971). Social Network intervention. In *Changing Families*. J. Haley (ed.) New York: Grune and Stratton.

Speck, R. V., and Attneave, C. L. (1973). *Family Networks*. New York: Pantheon Press.

Speck, R. V., and Rueventi, V. (1969). Network therapy – a developing concept. *Family Process*, **13**, 182–191.

Spencer, D. J. (1971). Cannabis-induced psychosis. *International Journal of Addictions*, **6**, 323–362.

Spitzer, R. L. and Cantwell, D. P. (1980). The DSM. III Classification of the psychiatric disorders of infancy, childhood and adolescence. *Journal of the American Academy of Child Psychiatry*, **19**, 356–370.

Spivack, G., and Spotts, J. (1967). Adolescent symptomatology. *American Journal of Mental Deficiency*, **72**, 74–95.

Stafford-Clark, D. (1967). *What Freud Really Said*. Harmondsworth: Penguin.

Stanley, L. (1980). Treatment of ritualistic behaviour in an 8-years-old girl by response prevention: a case report. *Journal of Child Psychology and Psychiatry*, **21**, 85–90.

Stearns, S. (1959). Self-destructive behaviour in young patients with diabetes mellitus. *Diabetes*, **8**, 379–382.

Stein, G. S., Hartshorn, S., Jones, J., and Steinberg, D. (1982). Lithium in a case of severe anorexia nervosa. *British Journal of Psychiatry*, **140**, 526–528.

Stein, Z., and Susser, M. (1967). Social factors in the development of sphincter control. *Developmental Medicine and Child Neurology*, **9**, 692–706.

Steinberg, D. (1972). Illness, Improvement and Coping Behaviour in 20 Patients with Phobic Disorders. University of London. M. Phil. Thesis.

Steinberg, D. (1979). Some common psychiatric problems in adolescence. *Journal of the Irish Medical Association*, **72** (9), 366–370.

Steinberg, D. (1980). The use of lithium carbonate in adolescence. *Journal of Child Psychology and Psychiatry*, **21**, 263–271.

Steinberg, D. (1981a). Adolescence: normal development. *Midwife, Health Visitor and Community Nurse*, **17** (11), 454–455.

Steinberg, D. (1981b). Adolescence: problems. *Midwife, Health Visitor and Community Nurse*, **17** (12), 508–514.

Steinberg, D. (1981c). *Using Child Psychiatry: the functions and operations of a specialty*. London: Hodder and Stoughton.

Steinberg, D. (1982a). Treatment, training, care or control? The functions of adolescent units. *British Journal of Psychiatry*, **141**, 306–309.

Steinberg, D. (1982b). In *Consultation from Child and Adolescent Psychiatric Settings*. C. Dare, R. Ryle, D. Steinberg, and W. Yule (eds). *News of the anexiation for Child Psychology and Psychiatry*: No. 11, July.

Steinberg, D. (1983). Psychotic disorders in adolescence. In *Child Psychiatry: modern approaches*. 2nd edn. M. Rutter and L. Hersov (eds). Oxford: Blackwell.

Steinberg, D., Galhenage, D. P. C., and Robinson, S. C. (1981). Two years' referrals to a regional adolescent unit: some implications for psychiatric services. *Social Science and Medicine*, **15**, 113–122.

Steinberg, D., and Heard, D. H. (1976). Attachment theory and its application to the role of an adolescent unit. Paper presented at the Conference of the Child Psychiatry Specialist Section of the Royal College of Psychiatrists, Oxford, September 1976. Unpublished.

Steinberg, D., Hirsch, S. R., Marston, S. D., Reynolds, K., and Sutton, R. N. P. (1972). Influenza infection causing manic psychosis. *British Journal of Psychiatry*, **120**, 531–535.

Steinberg, D., Merry, J., and Collins, S. (1978). The introduction of small group work to an adolescent unit. *Journal of Adolescence*, **1**, 331–344.

Steinberg, D. and Yule, W. (1983). Consultative work. In *Child Psychiatry: modern approaches*. 2nd edn. Oxford: Blackwell.

Stengel, E. (1959). Classification of mental disorders. *Bulletin of the World Health Organisation*, **21**, 601–663.

Stephens, J. H., Astrup, C., and Mangrum, J. C. (1967). Prognostic factors in recovered and deteriorated schizophrenics. *American Journal of Psychiatry*, **122**, 1116–1121.

Stern, R. S. (1970). Treatment of a case of obsessional neurosis using thought-stopping technique. *British Journal of Psychiatry*, **117**, 441–442.

Stern, R. S. (1978). Obsessive thoughts: the problem of therapy. *British Journal of Psychiatry*, **132**, 200–205.

Stern, R. S., and Cobb, J. P. (1978). Phenomenology of obsessive-compulsive neurosis. *British Journal of Psychiatry*, **132**, 233–239.

Stewart, M. A. De Blois, C. S., and Cummings, C. (1980). Psychiatric disorder in the parents of hyperactive boys and those with conduct disorder. *Journal of Child Psychology and Psychiatry*, **21**, 283–292.

Stewart, M. A., and Culver, K. W. (1982). Children who set fires: the clinical picture and a follow up. *British Journal of Psychiatry*, **140**, 357–363.

Stewart, M. A., Cummings, C., Singer, S., and De Blois, C. S. (1981). The overlap between hyperactive and unsocialised aggressive children. *Journal of Child Psychology and Psychiatry*, **22**, 35–45.

Stoller, R. J. (1968). *Sex and Gender*. New York: Jason Aronson.

Stoller, R. J. (1975). *Sex and Gender*. Vol. II: *The Transsexual Experiment*. New York: Jason Aronson.

Stores, G. (1975). Behavioural effects of anti-epileptic drugs. *Developmental Medicine and Child Neurology*, **17**, 647–658.

Stores, G. (1978). Anticonvulsants. In *Paediatric Psychopharmacology: the use of behaviour modifying drugs in children*. J. Werry (ed.). New York: Brunner Mazel.

Storr, A. (1972). *The Dynamics of Creation*. London: Secker and Warburg.

Storr, A. (1973). *Jung*. London: Collins/Fontana.

Strachan, J. G. (1981). Conspicuous firesetting in children. *British Journal of Psychiatry*, **138**, 26–29.

Stranahan, K., Schwartzmann, C., and Atkin, E. (1957). Group therapy for emotionally disturbed and potentially delinquent boys and girls. *American Journal of Orthopsychiatry*, **27**, 518–527.

Straughan, J. H., Potter, W. K., and Hamilton, S. H. (1965). The behavioural treatment of an elective mute. *Journal of Child Psychology and Psychiatry*, **6**, 125–130.

Strauss, J. S., and Carpenter, W. T. (1972). The prediction of outcome in schizophrenia. 1: Characteristics of outcome. *Archives of General Psychiatry*, **27**, 739–746.

Stuart, D. M. (1926). *The Boy through the Ages*. London: George C. Harrap.

Stuart, D. M. (1933). *The Girl through the Ages*. London: George G. Harrap.

Stunkard, A., d'Aquilie, E., Fox, S., and Filion, R. D. L. (1972). Influence of social class on obesity and thinness in children. *Journal of the American Medical Association*, **221**, 579–584.

Surgeon-General. (1972). *Television and Growing Up: the impact of televised violence*. Washington DC Superintendent of Documents, US Government Printing Office. Quoted in Rutter, 1979a.

Symonds, A., and Herman, M. (1957). The problems of schizophrenia in adolescence. *Psychiatric Quarterly*, **31**, 521–530.

Szasz. T. (1961). *The Myth of Mental Illness*. New York: Hoeber Harper.

Szasz T. (1971). *The Manufacture of Madness. A comparative study of the inquisition and the mental health movement*. London: Routledge and Kegan Paul.

Szasz. T. (1973). *Ideology and Insanity*. London: Calder and Boyars.

Szasz, T. (1974). *The Second Sin*. London: Routledge and Kegan Paul.

Talbot, M. (1957). Panic in school phobia. *American Journal of Orthopsychiatry*, **27**, 286–295.

Tanner, J. M. (1962). *Growth at Adolescence*. Oxford: Blackwell Scientific Publications.

Tanner, J. M., Whitehouse, R. H., and Takaishi, M. (1966). Standards from birth to maturity for height, weight, height velocity and weight velocity in British children. *Archives of Diseases in Childhood*, **41**, 455–471.

Tattersall, R. B. and Lowe, J. (1981). Diabetes and adolescence. *Diabetologia*, **20**, 517–523.

Taylor, D. C. (1969). Some psychiatric aspects of epilepsy. In *Current Problems in Neuropsychiatry*. R. N. Hetherington (ed.). Ashford: Headley Brothers and Royal Medico-Psychological Association.

Taylor, D. C. (1972). Psychiatry and sociology in the understanding of epilepsy. In *Psychiatric Aspects of Medical Practice*. B. M. Mandelbroke and M. G. Gelder (eds). London: Staples.

Taylor, D. C. (1979). The components of sickness: diseases, illnesses and predicaments. *Lancet*, **ii**, 1008–1010.

Taylor, D. C. and Falconer, M. A. (1968). Clinical, socio-economic and psychological changes after temporal lobectomy for epilepsy. *British Journal of Psychiatry*, **114**, 1247–1261.

Taylor, E. (1979a). Mental retardation. In *Essentials of Postgraduate Psychiatry*. P. Hill, R. Murray, and A. Thorley (eds). London: Academic Press.

Taylor, E. (1979b). Food additives, allergy and hyperkinesis. *Journal of Child Psychology and Psychiatry*, **20**, 357–363.

Taylor, F. Kraupl, (1979). *Psychopathology*. Sunbury on Thames: Quatermaine House.

Taylor, I., Walton, P., and Young, J. (1973). *The New Criminology: a social theory of deviance*. London: Routledge and Kegan Paul.

Terman, L. M. (1919). *The Intelligence of Schoolchildren*. Boston: Houghton Mifflin.

Thomas, A., and Chess. S. (1976). Evolution of behaviour disorders into adolescence. *American Journal of Psychiatry*, **133**, 539–542.

Thomas, A., Chess, S., and Birch, H. G. (1968). *Temperament and Behaviour Disorders in Children*. New York: University Press.

Thomas, C. J. (1979). Brain damage with lithium and haloperidol. *British Journal of Psychiatry*, **134**, 552.

Thomas, S. (1982). Ethics of a predictive test for Huntington's chorea. *British Medical Journal*, **284**, 1383–1385.

Thompson, J. W. (1980). 'Burnout' in group home houseparents. *American Journal of Psychiatry*, **137** (6), 710–714.

Thorley, A., and Stern, R. (1979). Neurosis and personality disorder. In *Essentials of Postgraduate Psychiatry*. P. Hill, R. Murray, and A. Thorley (eds). London: Academic Press.

Tibbets, R. S. (1981). Neuropsychiatric aspects of tics and spasms. *British Journal of Hospital Medicine*, **25** (5), 454–464.

Timbury, G. C. (1981). Social workers and compulsory admission. Note in the *Bulletin of the Royal College of Psychiatrists*, **6**, (1), 15–16.

Tizard, J. (1974). The upbringing of other people's children: implications of research and for research. *Journal of Child Psychology and Psychiatry*, **15**, 161–173.

Tizard, J., Sinclair, I., and Clarke, R. V. G. (1975). *Varieties of Residential Experience*. London: Routledge and Kegan Paul.

Toffler, A. (1970). *Future Shock*. London: The Bodley Head.

Tolan, E. J., and Lingl, F. A. (1964). 'Model psychosis' produced by inhalation of gasoline fumes. *American Journal of Psychiatry*, **120**, 757–761.

Toolan, J. M. (1962). Depression in children and adolescents. *American Journal of Orthopsychiatry*, **32**, 404–415.

Torup, E. (1962). A follow up study of children with tics. *Acta Paediatrica*, **51**, 261–268.

Truax, C. B., and Carkhuff, R. R. (1967). *Towards Effective Counselling and Psychotherapy: training and practice*. Chicago: Aldine.

Turiel, C. (1974). Conflict and transition in adolescent moral development.*Child Development*, **45**, 14–29.

Turle, G. C. (1966). On opening an adolescent unit. *Journal of Mental Science*, **106**, 1320–1326.

Turner, T. H., and Bates, R. (1983). The early outcome of adolescent admission – a report on 100 cases. In preparation.

Tyerman, M. (1974). Who are the truants? In *Truancy*. B. Turner (ed.). London: Ward Lock Educational.

Tyrer, P. (1976). Towards a rational therapy with mono-amine oxidase inhibitors. *British Journal of Psychiatry*, **128**, 354–360.

Tyrer, P., and Steinberg, D. (1975). Symptomatic treatment of agoraphobia and social phobias: a follow up study. *British Journal of Psychiatry*, **127**, 163–168.

Tyrer, P., and Steinberg, D. *Models for Mental Disorder*. In preparation.

Ugurel-Semin, R. (1952). Moral behaviour and moral judgement of children. *Journal of Abnormal and Social Psychology*, **47**, 463–474.

Ullman, L. P., and Krasner, L. (1975). *A Psychological Approach to Abnormal Behaviour.* Englewood Cliffs: Prentice Hall.

Vaillant, G. E. (1962). The prediction of recovery in schizophrenia. *Journal of Nervous and Mental Diseases*, **135**, 534–543.

Vaillant, G. E. (1964). Prospective prediction of schizophrenic remission. *Archives of General Psychiatry*, **11**, 509–518.

Vale, J. A., and Meredith, T. J. (1981). *Poisoning: diagnosis and treatment.* Lancaster: MTP Press.

Vale, J. A., Meredith, T., and Goulding, K. (1981). *A Concise Guide to the Management of Poisoning.* 2nd edn. London: Poisons Unit, Guys Hospital and Dista Products.

Valman, H. B. (1982). Poisoning in young children. *British Medical Journal*, **284**, 1178–1182.

Vaughn, C., and Leff, J. P. (1976). The influence of family and social factors on the course of psychiatric illness. *British Journal of Psychiatry*, **129**, 125–137.

Venables, P. H. (1968). Experimental psychological studies of chronic schizophrenia. In *Studies in Psychiatry*, M. Shepherd and D. L. Davies (eds). London: Oxford University Press.

Venables, P. H. (1978). Psychophysiology and psychometrics. *Psychophysiology*, **15**, 302–315.

Venables, P. H. (1980). Autonomic reactivity. In *Scientific Foundations of Developmental Psychiatry*. M. Rutter (ed.). London: Heinemann.

Vere, D. W. (1965). Errors of complex prescribing. *Lancet*, **1**, 370–373.

Vernon, P. E. (1960). *Intelligence and Attainment Tests.* London: University of London Press.

Vernon, P. E. (ed.) (1970). *Creativity: selected readings.* Harmondsworth: Penguin.

Viorst, J. (1980). Creative writing and ego development. *Journal of Adolescence*, **3**, 285–296.

Von Bertalanffy, L. (1968). *General System Theory.* New York: George Brazillier.

Wakeling, A., De Souza, V. F. A., and Beardwood, C. J. (1977). Assessment of negative and positive feedback effects of administred oestrogen on gonadotrophin release in patients with anorexia nervosa. *Psychological Medicine*, **7**, 397–405.

Walker, S. (1969). The psychiatric presentation of Wilson's disease (hepatolenticular degeneration) with an etiologic explanation. *Behavioral Neuropsychiatry*, **1**, 38–48.

Waller, D. (ed.) (1978). *As We See It: approaches to art as therapy.* By students of the Department of Art Therapy. University of London: Goldsmiths College.

Walrond-Skinner, S. (1976). *Family Therapy – the treatment of natural systems.* London: Routledge and Kegan Paul.

Walrond-Skinner, S. (1978). Indications and contra-indications for the use of family therapy (Annotation).*Journal of Child Psychology and Psychiatry*, **19**, 57–62.

Walter, H. I., and Gilmore, S. K. (1973). Placebo versus social learning effects in parent training procedures designed to alter the behaviour of aggressive boys. *Behaviour Therapy*, **4**, 361–377.

Wardle, C. J. (1974). Residential care of children with conduct disorders. In *The Residential Psychiatric Treatment of Children*. P. Barker (ed.). London: Crosby Lockwood Staples.

Warren, W. (1949). Abnormal behaviour and mental breakdown in adolescence. *Journal of Mental Science*, **95**, 589–624.

Warren, W. (1952). Inpatient treatment of adolescents with psychological illness. *Lancet*, **1**, 147–150.

Warren, W. (1960). Some relationships between the psychiatry of children and of adults. *Journal Mental Science*, **106**, 815–826.

Warren, W. (1965a). A study of adolescent psychiatric inpatients and the outcome six or more years later. I: Clinical histories and hospital findings. *Journal of Child Psychology and Psychiatry*, **6**, 1–17.

Warren, W. (1965b). A study of psychiatric inpatients and the outcome six or more years later. II: The follow up study. *Journal of Child Psychology and Psychiatry*, **6**, 141–160.

Warren, W. (1968). A study of anorexia nervosa in young girls. *Journal of Child Psychology and Psychiatry*, **9**, 27–40.

Warren, W. (1971). You can never plan the future by the past. The development of child and adolescent psychiatry in England and Wales. *Journal of Child Psychology and Psychiatry*, **11**, 241–257.

Warren, W. (1975). Child psychiatry and the Maudsley Hospital: an historical survey. In *Institute of Psychiatry, 1924–1974*. London: Institute of Psychiatry.

Watson, J. M. (1977). Glue sniffing in profile. *Practitioner*, **218**, 255–259.

Watson, J. M. (1980). Solvent abuse by children and young adults: a review. *British Journal of Addiction*, **75**, 27–36.

Weaver, A. (1981). Psychotherapy through art. *The New Era*, **62** (1), 22–24.

Weed, L. L. (1968a). Medical records that guide and teach. *New England Journal of Medicine*, **278**, 593–599.

Weed, L. L. (1968b). Medical records that guide and teach (concluded). *New England Journal of Medicine*, **278**, 652–657.

Weed, L. L. (1969). *Medical Records, Medical Education and Patient Care*. Cleveland: The Press of Case Western Reserve University.

Weinberg, W. A., Rutman, J., Sullivan, L., Penick, E. C., and Dietz, S. G. (1973). Depression in children referred to an educational diagnostic centre: diagnosis and treatment. *Journal of Paediatrics*, **83**, 1065–1072.

Weiner, H. (1958). Diagnosis and symptomatology. In *Schizophrenia: a review of the syndrome*, L. Bellak (ed.). New York: Logos.

Weiner, I. B. (1970a). *Psychological Disturbance in Adolescence*. New York: Wiley Interscience.

Weiner, I. B. (1970b). Depression and suicide. In *Psychological Disturbance in Adolescence*. New York: Wiley Interscience.

Weisberg, P. S. (1979). Group therapy with adolescents. In *The Short Course in Adolescent Psychiatry*. J. R. Novello (ed.). New York: Brunner Mazel.

Wells, R. A., Dilkes, T. C., and Trivelli, N. (1972). The results of family therapy: a critical review of the literature. *Family Process*, **11**, 189–207.

Wells, P. G., Morris, A., Jones, R. M., and Allen, D. J. (1978). An adolescent unit assessed: a consumer survey. *British Journal of Psychiatry*, **132**, 300–308.

Wellner, A., Wellner, Z., and Fishman, R. (1979). Psychiatric adolescent in-patients: eight to ten year follow-up. *Archives of General Psychiatry*, **36**, 698–700.

Werry, J. S. (1970). Some clinical and laboratory studies of psychotropic drugs in children: an overview. In *Drugs and Cerebral Function*. W. L. Smith (ed.). Springfield. Illinois: Charles C. Thomas.

Werry, J. S. (1976). Discussion of Conners' paper 'Classification and treatment of childfhood depression and depressive equivalents'. In *Depression: behavioral, biochemical, diagnostic and treament concepts*. D. Gallant and C. Simpson (eds). New York: Spectrum.

Werry, J. S. (ed.) (1978). *Paediatric Psychopharmacology: the use of behaviour modifying drugs in children*. New York: Brunner Mazel.

Werry, J. S. (1979a). Organic factors. In *Psychopathological Disorders of Childhood*. H. C. Quay and J. S. Werry (eds). New York: Wiley.

Werry, J. S. (1979b). Psychosomatic disorders, psychogenic symptoms and hospitalisation. In *Psychopathological disorders of childhood*. H. C. Quay and J. S. Werry (eds). Chichester: Wiley.

Werry, J. S., Aman, M. G., and Diamond, E. (1980). Imipramine and methylphenidate in hyperactive children. *Journal of Child Psychology and Psychiatry*, **21**, 27–35.

Werry, J. S. and Cohrssen, J. (1965). Enuresis: an aetiologic and therapeutic study. *Journal of Paediatrics*, **67**, 423–431.

Werry, J. S., Dowrick, P., Lampen, E., and Vamos, M. (1975). Imipramine in enuresis–psychological and physiological effects. *Journal of Child Psychology and Psychiatry*, **16**, 289–300.

Werry, J. S., and Sprague, R. L. (1974). Methylphenidate in children: effects of dosage. *Australia and New Zealand Journal of Psychiatry*, **8**, 9–19.

Wertham, F. L. (1929). A group of benign chronic psychoses: prolonged manic excitements. *American Journal of Psychiatry*, **86**, 17–78.

West, C. (1848). *Lectures on the Diseases of Infancy and Childhood*. London: Longman.

West, D. (1977). Delinquency. In *Child Psychiatry: modern approaches*. M. Rutter, and L. Hersov, (eds). Oxford: Blackwell.

Wexler, L., Weissman, M. M., and Kasl, S. V. (1978). Suicide attempts 1970–1975: updating on US study and comparisons with international trends. *British Journal of Psychiatry*, **132**, 180–185.

Whitaker, C. (1975). The symptomatic adolescent: an A. W. O. L. family member. In *The adolescent in Group and Family Therapy*. M. Sugar (ed.). New York: Brunner Mazel.

White, J. H. (1981). The hyperactive child in adolescence: some pharmacologic approaches. *Journal of Adolescence*, **4**, 79–86.

White, R. W. (1959). Motivation reconsidered: the concept of competence. *Psychological Reviews*, **66**, (5), 297–333.

White, R. W. (1960). Competence and the Psychosexual Stages of Development. *Nebraska Symposium on Motivation*. Jones M. R. (ed.). Nebraska: Nebraska University Press.

Whiteley, J. S. (1970). The response of psychopaths to a therapeutic community. *British Journal of Psychiatry*, **116**, 517–529.

Whiteley, J. S. (1975). The large group as a medium for sociotherapy. In *The Large Group: dynamics and therapy*. L. Kreeger. (ed.). London; Constable.

Whiteley, J. S. and Zlatic, M. (1972). A reappraisal of staff attitudes to the therapeutic community. *British Journal of Social Psychiatry*, **3**, 2.

Whitmore, K. (1974). The Contribution of Child Guidance to the Community. Paper given at the 30th Child Guidance Inter-Clinic Conference, March 1974.

Wilder, J. and Silberman, J. (1972). *Beitrage Zum Ticproblem*. Berlin: Kalger. Quoted in J. A. Corbett, 1977: Tics and Tourette's syndrome. In *Child Psychiatry: modern approaches*. M. Rutter and L. Hersov (eds). Oxford: Blackwell.

Willcox, D. R. C., Gillan, R., and Hare, E. H. (1965). Do psychiatric out-patients take their drugs? *British Medical Journal*, **2**, 790–792.

Wilson, J. (1972). Investigation of degenerative disease of the central nervous system. *Archives of Disease in Childhood*, **74**, 163–170.

Wing, J. K., and Wing, L. (1976). Provision of Services. In *Early Childhood Autism*. L. Wing (ed.) Oxford: Pergamon.

Wing, L. (1971). Severely retarded children in a London area: prevalence and provision of services. *Psychological Medicine*, **1** (5), 405–415.

Wing, L. (1980). Childhood autism and social class: a question of selection? *British Journal of Psychiatry*, **137**, 410–417.

Winnicott, D. W. (1971). *Playing and Reality*, London: Tavistock.

Winnicott, D. W. (1972). *The Maturational Process and the Facilitating Environment*. London: Hogarth Press.

Winokur, G., Clayton, P., and Reich, T. (1969). *Manic Depressive Illness*. St Louis: C. V. Mosby.

Winsberg, B., Bialer, I., Kupietz, S., and Tobias, J. (1972). Effects of imipramine and dextroamphetamine on behavior of neuropsychiatrically impaired children. *American Journal of Psychiatry*, **128**, 1425–1431.

Wolf, M. M., Phillips. E. L., and Fixsen, D. L., (1975a). Achievement Place, Phase II: Final Report. University of Kansas: Department of Human Development.

Wolf, M. M., Phillips, E. L., and Fixen, D. L. (1975b). Achievement Place, Phase III: Final Report. University of Kansas: Department of Human Development.

Wolff, S., and Chick, J. (1980). Schizoid personality in childhood: a controlled follow up study. *Psychological Medicine*, **10**, 85–100.

Wolkind, S., (1977). Women who have been 'in care'–psychological and social status during pregnancy. *Journal of Child Psychology and Psychiatry*, **18**, 179–182.

Wolkind, S., and Renton. G. (1979). Psychiatric disorders in children in long-term residential care: a follow up study. *British Journal of Psychiatry*, **135**, 129–135.

Wolkind, S., and Rutter, M. (1973). Children who have been 'in care'–an epidemiological study. *Journal of Child Psychology and Psychiatry*, **14**, 97–105.

Wolpe, J. (1958). *Psychotherapy of Reciprocal Inhibition.* Stanford: Stanford University Press.

Wood, D. J. (1980). Cognitive development. In *Scientific Foundations of Developmental Psychiatry*. M. Rutter. (ed.). London: Heinemann.

Woodcock, J. (1976). Teaching about a volatile situation: suggested health education strategies for minimising casualties associated with solvent abuse. *Druglink*, vol. 2. Issues 1–2. Institute of the Study of Drug Dependence.

World Health Organisation (1973). *The International Pilot Study of Schizophrenia.* Vol. 1. Geneva.

Wright, H. L. (1968). A clinical study of children who refuse to talk in school. *Journal of the American Academy of Child Psychiatry*, **7**, 603–617.

Wynne, L. C. (1968). Methodological and conceptual issues in the study of schizophrenics and the families. In *The Transmission of Schizophrenia*. D. Rosenthal and S. S. Kety (eds). Oxford: Pergamon.

Wynne, L. C., Ryckoff, I., Day, J., and Hirsch, S. (1958). Pseudo-mutuality in the family relations of schizophrenics. *Psychiatry*, **21**, 205–220.

Wynne, L. C., and Singer, M. T. (1963). Thought disorder and family relations of schizophrenics. *Archives of General Psychiatry*, **9**, 191–206.

Wyss, D. (1966). *Depth Psychology: a critical history.* London; George Allen Unwin.

Yates, A. J. (1958). The application of learning theory to the treatment of tics. *Journal of Abnormal and Social Psychology*, **56**, 175–182.

Young, J. Z. (1964). *A Model of the Brain.* Oxford: Clarendon Press.

Young, M., and Willmott, P., (1957). *Family and Kinship in East London.* London: Routledge and Kegan Paul.

Youngerman, J., and Canino, I. A. (1978). Lithium carbonate use in children and adolescents. *Archives of General Psychiatry*, **35**, 216–224.

Yule, W. (1975). Teaching psychological principles to non-psychologists. II: Training parents in child management. *Journal of the Association of Educational Psychologists*, **10**, (3), 5–16.

Yule, W. (1976). Behavioural treatment of children and adolescents with conduct disorders. In *Aggression and Antisocial Behaviour in Childhood and Adolescence*. L. A. Hersov, M. Berger, and D. Shaffer (eds). Oxford: Pergamon.

Yule, W. (1977). Behavioural approaches. In *Child Psychiatry: modern approaches*. M. Rutter and L. Hersov (eds). Oxford: Blackwell.

Yule, W. (1978). Behavioural treatment of children and adolescents with conduct disorders. In *Aggression and Antisocial Behaviour in Childhood and Adolescence*. L. Hersov, M. Berger, and D. Shaffer, (eds). Oxford: Pergamon.

Yule, W., Hersov, L., and Treseder, J. (1980). Behavioural treatments of school refusal. In *Out of School: modern perspectives in truancy and school refusal*. L. Hersov and I. Berg (eds). Chichester: Wiley.

Yule, W., Rutter, M., Berger, M., and Thompson, J. (1974). Over- and under-achievement in reading: distribution in the general population. *British Journal of Educational Psychology*, **44**, 1–12.

Zausmer, D. (1954). Treatment of tics in childhood. *Archives of Disease in Childhood*, **29**, 537–542.

Zax, M. M, Cowen, E. L., Rapoport, J., Beach, D. R., and Laird, J. D., (1968). Follow up study of children identified early as emotionally disturbed. *Journal of Consulting and Clinical Psychology*, **32**, 369–374.

Zinner, J. and Shapiro, E. (1975). Splitting in families of borderline adolescents. In *Borderline States in Psychiatry*. J. Mack (ed.). New York: Grune and Stratton.

Index